FIGHTING RADIATION & CHEMICAL POLLUTANTS
WITH FOODS, HERBS, & VITAMINS

FIGHTING RADIATION & CHEMICAL POLLUTANTS

WITH FOODS, HERBS, & VITAMINS

Documented Natural Remedies that
Boost Your Immunity
& Detoxify

BY STEVEN R. SCHECHTER, N.D.

Introduction by C. Norman Shealy, M.D., Ph.D.
Contributions by Geoff Oelsner

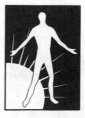

Vitality, Ink

1991

VITALITY, INK
P.O. Box 294
Encinitas, California 92024

ISBN 1-878412-04-3

Published in the United States of America

First Printing 1988
Second Edition 1990, revised
Third Printing 1991
Fourth Printing 1994

987654

Distributed to the natural food trade and to the book trade by
Vitality, Ink, P.O. Box 294, Encinitas, CA 92024, (619) 943-VITL(8485)

Cover and Illustrations by Richard Downs

This book is dedicated to our entire family of humankind. Every day, all of us absorb numerous different forms of radiation and chemical toxins. In addition, many people regularly ingest pharmaceuticals, alcohol, drugs, and other toxins, and inhale tobacco smoke and other airborne pollutants. The cumulative effects of these toxins continually stress our health, vitality, and immunity. May we learn to work together to heal ourselves and our planet, and to live long and healthy lives.

Author's Notes

I will donate 50 percent of the royalties from the sale of this book, above research expenses, to groups that are seeking to improve the quality of life on earth by working to create a non-nuclear, ecologically safe world. For information on these and other organizations, refer to Resource Groups in Appendix Six.

American Friends Service Committee
Committee for Nuclear Responsibility
Friends of the Earth
Physicians for Social Responsibility
Nuclear Information and Resource Service
Union of Concerned Scientists

To know is to care...
To care is to *act*.

For those who wish to receive regular updates on self-help information for boosting the immune system and dealing with radiation- and chemical pollutant-related problems, see Appendix Seven about subscribing to the *Optimal Health for the Nuclear Age* newsletter and joining the Optimal Health for the Nuclear Age Network, which is facilitated by Steve Schechter. Your membership contribution will sponsor further research.

This book contains instructions on the use of nutritional supplements, herbs, and other substances within the context of an overall health program. It is not intended to be a medical manual or to substitute for professional medical care. Not all of the substances mentioned should be used by all individuals. Every effort has been made to note when potentially adverse effects may be experienced from the ingestion of certain foods, supplements, or herbs, but neither the author nor the publisher can take responsibility for individuals' use of substances recommended herein.

Contents

PART III
DEVELOPING THE OPTIMAL LIFESTYLE FOR OUR
NUCLEAR/CHEMICAL AGE

Acknowledgements

I owe special thanks to my friend Geoff Oelsner, who became involved with this book soon after its inception in 1980. He served as a researcher, as my first editor, and as a contributor to some of the appendices. Geoff is a true renaissance man, and his assistance was of great help to me.

Dodie Horne, Leslie Oelsner, David Druding, Nancy and Gary Kahanak, Carrie Trinka, and Bill Browner also gave early help and important commentary.

Leonard Jacobs and Eliot Wadsworth II, publishers of East West Health Books, rendered valuable assistance. The first edition of this book was published by East West Health Books in 1988.

Mark Mayell, editor of East West Health Books, was always there for me at the other end of the phone. His sensitivity, quick understanding, and fine editing are especially appreciated.

Tom Monte was consistently professional and delightful to work with in every way. I quickly felt a kindred spirit with Tom and Mark and their families. Tom's contribution to Chapter 1 on the nature of radiation and his editorial suggestions throughout the book were quite valuable.

Though last to be mentioned, the following people will always be first in my heart. A special note of appreciation goes to Sonia, Jack, Ed, Carol, and Maurice Schechter, Phyllis and Steve Smilack, and Penelope Young Andrade. To Heather Chronert, a true Jill Friday Administrator with a wonderful heart and brain. Very special thanks also to Jacob Schechter, who was with me throughout this project and whose courage, emotional strength, enthusiasm, and goodness were the source of my inspiration.

To all of the above people, and to anyone I left out only because of space, I offer my sincerest thanks.

Certainly the time has come to present medically documented information on safe, effective, self-help remedies that vitalize and detoxify your life. This project does not end with the publication of this book; it continues on with you, the reader, the object of our deepest affection and most confident hopes.

Steven R. Schechter, N.D.
Encinitas, California
February 1990

Preface

In 1978 I was directing a health center in Austin, Texas. Numerous clients came to me because of exposure to environmental pollutants. One family from a small farm became quite sick every time the neighbors crop-dusted. Three workers at a city sanitation dump regularly suffered from allergic reactions. One of the workers developed severe liver and lymph problems. A thirty-seven-year-old woman was referred to me by her physician, who suspected that her chronic kidney problems had been induced by environmental pollutants. Others came for a wide variety of reasons related to environmental health and clinical ecology. Blood analyses of these clients often showed significant evidence of chemical toxicity.

My first client with radiation problems was a twenty-two-year-old man who had undergone extensive radiotherapy, including of the pelvic area, for several years, and was now suffering from leukemia. Surprisingly, his primary concern was not for himself but for the developing baby inside his wife's womb. They were worried that the child would be born with a birth defect or some other congenital problem.

Fortunately, I was able to help a majority of these and other clients. Some of the benefits reported by clients were higher energy levels, increased mental clarity, fewer allergies and infections, more balanced emotional lives, and improved sleeping patterns. Medical tests performed by a licensed physician indicated improved liver, kidney, and immune functions; lowered blood pressure, cholesterol, and triglycerides; and better results of other blood analyses.

As my research and experience with radiation and toxic chemicals expanded, I started helping more people create their own optimal health programs. At the time, my primary goals were both to help people heal themselves of a wide range of health problems due to radioactive or chemical toxins, and to prevent future degenerative diseases, such as cancers, immunological disorders, and birth defects caused by the cumulative effects of known toxins stored in the body.

By the beginning of 1979, word had spread from friend to friend that I might be able to help people help themselves with toxicity problems. I began regularly to receive long distance phone calls from individuals who felt they were suffering from problems related to exposure to "excessive" radioactive or chemical toxins. By then I was beginning to suspect that any exposure to unnecessary radiation or chemical pollutants could prove to be excessive.

Then, in the spring of 1979, the powerful movie "The China Syndrome" was released, and soon afterward Unit #2 at the Three Mile Island Nuclear Power Plant experienced a near meltdown. After that, I received more requests from people all over the country to provide them with information to help prevent or treat problems related to radiation and environmental pollutants. Unfortunately, many of these people were unable to come and see me, and often I knew of no practitioner in their area working with effective and safe therapies for these problems.

I felt caught in a terrible dilemma. Having felt the call of medicine since childhood, I wanted to help these people find someone in their area who could help them. Yet I did not know of anyone who had collected in-depth information on the subject of how foods, herbs, vitamins, and other substances could offer protection from the effects of radiation and industrial pollutants. I did not know if such information even existed, let alone in an organized, understandable, and useable format.

I felt that there was a national and international need for reliable, documented information on optimal dietary guidelines for the nuclear age. It seemed obvious that the community of humankind would quite literally have to begin facing and solving these problems together. But until we could evolve social solutions, I knew that more and more people would need effective, safe, self-help therapies to counteract radiation and common environmental pollutants.

By 1980, I had begun intensive research for this book. In 1981, a major national health magazine published a long, extensively documented self-help article I wrote entitled "Radiation: What You Can Do." In 1982 I had another article published entitled "Counteracting Radiation and Environmental Pollutants." At the end of these articles, I stated that I was working on a book about the same subject matter. As a result, more inquiries and even pleas for help came to me from across North America, Central America, and Europe. Because the pleas for self-help expressed such urgency, I subsequently had two more articles published—one immediately after the Chernobyl accident in 1986.

Today many people accept the fact that they need to make dietary and lifestyle changes in order to deal with health problems such as heart attacks, high blood pressure, diabetes, cancer, allergies, and so forth. There is growing concern about chemical dumping, the diminishing ozone layer, acid rain, and radioactivity in the environment. And there is a growing awareness that these environmental conditions can lead to cumulative health effects.

As our bodies have become increasingly stressed by the effects of radioactive isotopes and thousands of chemicals and pollutants, we have suffered a rapid increase in tumors, leukemia, congenital birth defects, and immunological problems such as AIDS, lowered resistance to bacteria and viruses, and a general decline in health and vitality. Unfortunately, radiation and chemical pollutants are so pervasive that trying to avoid them is physically impossible.

Thus, many people feel powerless to do anything about the invisible, yet pervasive, toxins in our air, water, food, homes, workplaces, and recreational environments. The problems seem so ubiquitous and so deeply ingrained in our nuclear age lifestyles, institutional technologies, and economy, that people make the choice either to ignore these problems or to work for political and social solutions on a local, state, or national level. Such work is of great importance for the long-term health of our society, and in Appendix Six I list ways to find numerous resource groups that promote effective programs for social change. On a strictly personal level, however, some people think that it is worthwhile solely to make dietary or lifestyle changes to address certain health problems obviously under individual control, such as heart disease (cut back on cholesterol and fat intake), hypertension (cut back on salt intake), hypoglycemia (cut back on sugar), and allergies (limit exposure to allergens).

The goal of this book is not to dwell on the extent or immediacy of the problems, nor to use scare tactics to excite, depress, or overwhelm you. The facts are compelling enough to motivate almost anyone. Rather, my goal is to share with you my research and clinical experience, and to thereby empower you to try some of the positive, self-help, documented remedies contained herein.

My opinion of current nuclear and pollutant-producing technologies is that some, certainly a minority, are useful. Regardless, for our personal and societal health, we need to learn how to use these technologies wisely, not excessively, and give people information on how to counteract their side effects. For example, I do not advocate that health professionals cease using x-rays. Certainly x-rays have proven beneficial and sometimes even life-saving. However, x-rays often are overused and unnecessary. Moreover, since the effects of radiation and chemical toxins may be cumulative, there are no "safe" or "nontoxic" exposures. Therefore, even if we learn how to use and control these technologies wisely, it is equally important that we learn how to counteract their already known side effects.

I have personally enjoyed working in the same clinics with medical doctors, a neurologist, an osteopath, chiropractors, nurses, and other naturopaths. I have worked with clients who subsequently healed themselves from a wide range of health concerns – including cancers, Epstein-Barr Virus, Candida, diminished energy/low blood sugar, and allergies. I have worked with environmentally injured (E. I.) clients who were previously reactive to everything from carpeting, felt pens, and photocopying chemicals to formaldehyde, benzene, lead, and other common indoor and outdoor pollutants.

From my clinical experience, I observed that clients can regain their independence and overcome the feelings of "helplessness" that frequently plague the chronically ill or toxically harmed. The optimal health program for the nuclear/chemical age that I developed has helped clients become fully functioning members of society through improved health.

My goal is to inspire hope and confidence. There are safe and effective personal solutions to the most pervasive problems facing all of humanity. If you are willing to make slow, gentle changes in your diet and lifestyle, you can control your vitality, health, and well-being despite the increasing industrial contaminants all of us are being subjected to. Our health is indeed our most important wealth.

Yes, there is hope. There are alternatives. *Fighting Radiation & Chemical Pollutants with Foods, Herbs, & Vitamins* documents effective natural therapies that boost your vitality, strengthen your immune system, and safely and reliably counteract environmental pollutants and radiation. Equally important, this book presents practical advice for both the prevention and treatment of common health problems resulting from routine exposure to toxins. It shows how to create an optimal health program for our nuclear and industrial age and thereby

- detoxify from chemical pollutants, radiation, x-rays, and drugs
- boost your immune system
- prevent degenerative diseases such as cancers and heart problems, and
- generate maximum vitality, health, and longevity.

The information, ability, and power is now yours if you wish to help yourself and those you care about.

Introduction

BY C. NORMAN SHEALY, M.D., PH.D.

In the 1990s, it is a toss-up as to whether chemical or radiation pollution will kill the most people before the AIDS epidemic kills an equal number of people. During the past forty-five years, America has contributed more pollution, either chemically or in the nuclear arena, than has been contributed in the entire history of the world by all other nations combined.

One of the decidedly most irresponsible misrepresentations ever perpetrated on the human race is the use of nuclear energy and other nuclear technologies. Someday there might be the possibility of using nuclear energy in a safe way. Now, however, over forty years after nuclear technology has been unleashed upon the world, the insufferable bureaucrats and greedy technocrats have not the foggiest notion of how to contain the waste products of the nuclear epidemic. I use the word epidemic advisedly. I believe that sooner or later we must come to grips with the fact that we are likely to wind up having huge epidemics of radiation sickness or radiation-induced illnesses. The best immediate answer would be to put a total stop to all use of nuclear energy until reasonable ways of storing the byproducts are found. Each year, we run tremendous risks of being wiped out or badly damaged by what already has been produced.

Each day our vitality and health are stressed by radiation in our air, water, soil, and food. Thousands of common devices that are used daily also emit radiation. Unfortunately, the myth that there is a safe level of exposure is more than just a myth—it is a fraud. There are no safe levels of exposure to any form of radiation, including x-rays, or to many chemical pollutants. All of these toxins produce cumulative side-effects which can become progressively more serious and complex.

In the chemical field we have even greater problems. There certainly are much more than just a few dangerous chemical pollutants being released in huge quantities each year. There are literally over fifty thousand toxic chemicals being produced and disposed of in reckless ways. A modest effort has been made in this country to restrict the use of some chemicals—a paltry number of pesticides and herbicides. Greedy companies export even these chemicals to Third World countries where these highly toxic substances are widely used on foods that are then imported back into this country. All of us, no matter where we live, are exposed to increasing concentrations of toxic chemicals and to greater amounts of unmonitored radiation, both of which have serious worldwide potential for ruining our air, water, and other vital resources.

I am impressed with the research that has been done in relation to the substances recommended in this book. Although there is considerable scientific documentation for many of the remedies for generating optimal vitality and health, strengthening the immune system, and detoxifying from radiation and chemical pollutants, some of my peers might argue that the usual FDA studies have not been done. All the materials in this extensive book however are well-documented. As far as I can tell, the recommendations being made to protect you are both safe and effective. I am well aware of the excellent work related to echinacea and astragalus, some work with Panax ginseng, and that with ligustrum. I have personally researched these herbs and believe there is enough scientific evidence to justify their use.

Ultimately each individual must make a decision personally as to how he or she will protect against both radiation and chemical poisoning. I believe that this book offers a rational approach for an intelligent person to begin making those decisions.

C. Normal Shealy, M.D., Ph.D.
Founder and Director, Shealy Institute for Comprehensive
Pain & Health Care
Founding President, American Holistic Medical Association
Research and Clinical Professor of Psychology, Forest Institute of
Professional Psychology
Author

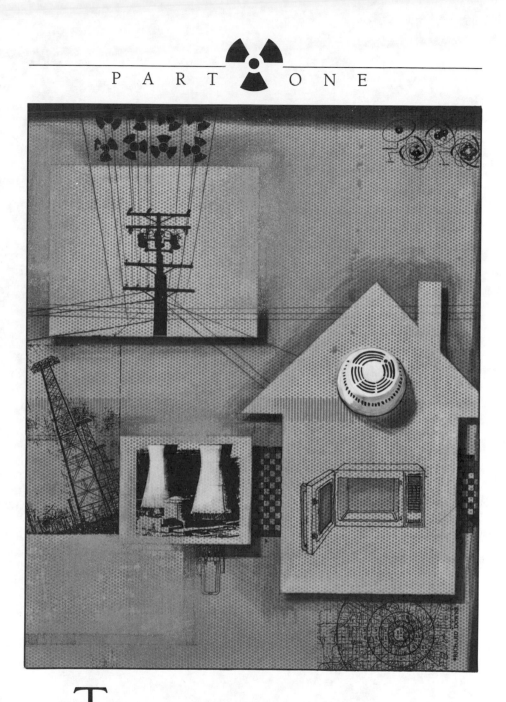
THE NUCLEAR & CHEMICAL THREATS TO HEALTH

CHAPTER 1

The Radiation Hazard

This book is about the effects of radiation and chemical pollutants on humans and the things we can do to protect ourselves against those effects. It is also about natural remedies that have been shown by scientific research to stimulate and strengthen the body's immune system.

Most discussions about radiation are arcane and abstract. Indeed, radiation itself is difficult to understand because most forms of it are invisible to the naked eye; we aren't even aware of it when it interacts with the tissues of our body. In fact, most low-level radiation—especially the kind we're most concerned with in this book, called ionizing radiation—is inaccessible to the other senses as well: you usually cannot feel it, hear it, taste it, or smell it. These characteristics make it ominous. It is the stuff horror movies are made of—a monster that strikes without apparent notice to cause sickness, deformity, and death.

Because radiation itself is difficult to perceive directly, it is beneficial to focus on the sources and the effects of radiation, both of which we can more easily perceive. As an example let's begin with the experience of people living in and around Utah in the early 1950s when the United States first began testing nuclear weapons at the Nevada Test Site (NTS) in southern Nevada.

WEAPONS FALLOUT COMES BACK TO HAUNT US

The first explosions of nuclear devices at the NTS in 1951 were greeted by the people of Nevada and Utah with patriotism and pride. Due to prevailing wind patterns, the people of southwest Utah, who were a mere 200 miles from the NTS, were among those potentially most affected by the tests. Yet they believed, as did most other Americans, that the nuclear explosions that shook the ground and caused radioactive dust and debris to rain down on their lands were essential to America's national defense system, a system that kept everyone safe from the threat of war. They even felt a swell of pride when Atomic Energy Commission (A.E.C.) officials told them that they were "participants in the nation's atomic test program." These were patriotic Americans, many of them Mormons with large families and spiritual roots in the red soil of Utah. Few questioned the public statements by the A.E.C. that the radioactive fallout released during the tests was well within safety levels. It represented a mere fraction of the radiation used in a chest x-ray, the A.E.C. officials said. Such statements, however, did not remain reassuring for very long.

The citizens of Cedar City and St. George, Utah realized that something was terribly wrong when, soon after the first series of tests, their livestock started dying. At first a few head became ill, then a few dozen. Soon hundreds and even thousands lay dead on the rough scrub of southwest Utah. By 1953, just two years after the tests had begun, the patina of patriotism had worn off and real fear took its place. And with good reason. Local health officials, using their own equipment to monitor the fallout from the explosions, saw their Geiger counter readings "going off the scale" whenever a test was conducted.

Radioactive fallout and debris had rained down upon the people of southwest Utah like pink snow. Children wrote their names in the radioactive dust. Other children actually ate the fallout as it fell from the skies, thinking that it was a strange snow shower.

Between 1951 and 1962, when the above-ground tests stopped, nearly 100 nuclear explosions took place at the Nevada Test Site and virtually every one of them spread radioactive debris over parts of Utah, Arizona, Nevada, and beyond. The people who were directly in line with the wind-borne debris began to call themselves "downwinders." The name soon took on eerie associations for a people caught in the path of so many lethal pink clouds.

In 1955, local ranchers from St. George and other communities took the federal government to court, citing the atomic tests as the cause of death for over 17,000 sheep. They further claimed that the government had an obligation to protect its citizens, which meant that it should have at least warned the people of the dangers of nuclear fallout. Though it was too early to tell what the radioactivity had done to the people, it was obvious to the citizens of southwest Utah what it had done to the livestock. The A.E.C. argued that the livestock died from poor feed, infectious disease, and cold weather, but the downwinders knew otherwise. The feed hadn't changed and there had been severe winters before. There was little or no evidence of infectious disease. Nevertheless, in 1956 the courts ruled in favor of the government and dismissed the downwinders' case.

One of the more famous downwinders was actor John Wayne, who in 1954 was making the film *The Conquerors*. The movie was shot in Snows Canyon, Utah, just twelve miles north of St. George. The film was made during one of the A.E.C.'s test series in which a number of nuclear devices were detonated. Wayne's co-stars were Susan Hayward and Agnès Moore-head; the film's director was actor-director Dick Powell. After a day's shooting, all 200 members of the cast and crew would return from the canyon, often covered with radioactive dust and debris. The dust would collect in cakes around their eyes and mouths, and had to be spit out when the wind whipped it hard.

Like the people of St. George, the filmmakers wanted to believe the A.E.C. statements that the radioactivity falling on American citizens was well within safety limits. But the filmmakers, too, would suffer the dire consequences of being downwind.

By 1961, just a decade after the first test, people exposed to the fallout started to come down with leukemia and other forms of cancer. Prior to the nuclear tests, the four counties in Utah directly affected by the blasts experienced a cancer rate about 20 percent below the national average, since Mormons avoid alcohol and tobacco, and eat relatively simple diets. But in the early 1960s, the cancer rate among the four counties in line with the radioactive fallout was one-and-a-half times the national average.

In his book *Justice Downwind* (Oxford University Press, 1986), Howard Ball, a professor at the University of Utah, demonstrates that the A.E.C. systematically lied to the people downwind of the blasts. Using information only recently released under the Freedom of Information Act, Ball notes that the A.E.C. falsified documents and intentionally deceived the downwind communities, while internal A.E.C. memoranda expressed repeated concern for the dangerous levels of radioactivity raining down on Utah and other states and then further dispersed by the wind.

Eventually, whole families would be destroyed by cancer. Ball reports the testimony of one Utah man whose family had no prior record of cancer but, after being exposed to the fallout from blasts, later suffered nine cancer fatalities during a relatively short time period. Many downwinders who remember playing in the fallout as children later suffered bizarre combinations of leukemia and other forms of cancer. Ball recounts the story of one woman who regularly played in the radioactive debris, only to go home to eat dinner with the fallout still on her fingers. That woman was later diagnosed as having leukemia, and cancers of the skin, intestines, ovaries, and vagina. She died in 1983 at the age of forty-two.

Indeed, in one of the more graphic ironies, in 1979 John Wayne—the epitome of the patriotic and invulnerable American—died of cancer. Cancer also claimed the lives of Susan Hayward, Agnes Moorehead, Dick Powell, and nearly half of the 200 members of the cast and crew of *The Conquerors*. The ninety people from the set who contracted cancer numbered well beyond the national average of one-in-four people expected to contract cancer. What these figures do not describe is the untold amount of suffering, expense, loss of health and vitality, and time away from work and family that occurred between the initial exposures and the eventual deaths.

In 1984, U.S. District Judge Bruce Jenkins ruled in favor of ten Utah plaintiffs who charged that the federal government had negligently failed to warn or educate downwind residents of the hazards of nuclear fallout. The judge awarded the plaintiffs almost $2.7 million in damages for the fatal consequences of the government's deceit. But that ruling was struck down in 1987 by a federal appeals court which sided with federal authorities. The three-judge panel stated that it was within the A.E.C.'s discretionary powers to withhold such information, as provided by the Atomic Energy Act of 1946. The downwinders would have to appeal to the Supreme Court or the Congress to receive justice. The people of Utah say they will not give up the fight.

Meanwhile, biological problems caused by exposure to radioactivity will dramatically increase because of the increasing use of nuclear technology, and because all ionizing radiation, including the lowest level of x-rays, produces cumulative effects.

Studies have shown that the effects of radiation are felt for many years—and even generations—after the initial exposure. Research done on Japanese who were exposed to radiation from the atomic bombs dropped on Hiroshima and Nagasaki in 1945 has demonstrated that tumor incidence increases as the population ages. That is, the effects of radiation are more likely to manifest the longer one lives.

Even more alarming is the fact that the effects of radiation are most severe on the young, and especially on the growing fetus. Americans are only now coming to realize just how devastating the damage has been to children downwind from the blasts at the Nevada Test Site. Contrary to what was earlier believed, the effects of those explosions have gone far beyond Utah.

The wind drove the radioactive fallout as far away as Minnesota,

Michigan, New York, and into southern Ontario, Canada. In his book, *Secret Fallout: Low Level Radiation from Hiroshima to Three Mile Island* (McGraw Hill, 1981), Ernest Sternglass, professor emeritus of radiological physics at the University of Pittsburgh, demonstrates that the radioactive fallout caused dangerous levels of strontium-90, cesium-137, and iodine-131 to fall on these states, thus affecting the prenatal development of children. Sternglass and educational psychologist Steven Bell effectively correlated the effects of the radioactive clouds with infant development, intelligence quotients, and SAT test scores taken some seventeen years after exposure. For instance, accounting for such variables as socioeconomic status, educational quality in different geographical regions, and other factors, Sternglass and Bell showed that children who were gestating in their mothers' wombs and were in line with the radioactive fallout experienced dramatic declines in SAT scores many years later. However, children born in these same states before and after the nuclear tests achieved much higher scores. In other words, the differing degrees of proficiency on SAT tests corresponded closely to the concentration of radioactive fallout encountered prenatally by these children.

That radiation causes brain damage is well established in the medical literature. Research done on the island of Rongelap, 150 miles from the Marshall Islands where atomic bomb testing took place in the 1950s, showed that unborn children exposed to radioactive fallout suffered severe growth retardation, both in physical stature and brain size.

But it wasn't simply the downwinders or the states that were in the path of wind-borne fallout that have been affected by the radiation. Radioactive fallout descends from the sky when it rains or snows. These precipitations are then absorbed into the soil, plants, and water, and eventually ingested by humans and animals. Atmospheric air currents are capable of carrying fallout partway around the world, as occurred after the Chernobyl nuclear power plant accident.

According to physicists, virtually all of the radioactive plutonium and strontium released by the atomic explosions done at the NTS has descended to earth and been inhaled or ingested by the vast majority of people living in the Northern Hemisphere. Plutonium is the most carcinogenic radioactive element. It has been estimated that one pound of plutonium, divided into microscopic proportions, is enough to cause 42 billion cancers. Strontium is one of the most prevalent radioisotopes (a form of a radioactive element), thus causing significant contamination problems. Since the initial tests of the 1940s and '50s, many more nuclear devices have been set off both above and below ground, not only in the U.S. but by other nuclear powers including Britain, France, the Soviet Union, and China. In addition to fallout from nuclear tests, the construction over the past thirty years of hundreds of nuclear power plants worldwide has given rise to an ongoing nuclear fuel cycle. It begins with the mining, milling, and enrichment of uranium, and includes the creation of fuel rods, the consumption of radioactive fuels in the plant itself, the intentional release of radioactive byproducts from the fuel cycle, and the transportation and storage of nuclear waste. At any one of these steps, potentially disastrous accidents are possible. In 1986, the world witnessed the worst accident in the short history of nuclear power at the Soviet Union's Chernobyl utility. It may be decades before the full impact of that accident is felt by the world. And, despite the reassurances from the Soviet Union and from the U.S. government, no one knows for sure if or when a comparable disaster will occur.

But it isn't just the nuclear weapons and nuclear power industries that threaten us with radiation. Modern medicine is fast becoming a prolific purveyor of radiation with its use of radioactive diagnostic and therapeutic technologies. At the same time, radiation comes from many other less obvious sources: many household goods and consumer appliances; tobacco smoke; the radon gas often found in polluted indoor air; and natural sources, both within the earth and of cosmic origin.

I'll be looking in more depth at these sources of radiation, but it is important to note right away that there are many things we can do to protect ourselves. Research has shown that certain diets can be protective against the effects of radiation, and that certain foods, herbs, vitamin and mineral supplements, and miscellaneous substances can help our bodies counteract the toxic effects of radiation. After I review some common sources of radiation and chemical pollutants in Part I of this book, I'll provide a thorough discussion of the food substances that have been shown to be "protectants." Scientific evidence will be introduced that documents the effectiveness of each food substance as a means of protection against radiation and many common and dangerous chemical pollutants.

But first, let's get a better understanding of what radiation is.

WHAT IS RADIATION AND HOW DOES IT AFFECT US?

In its broadest definition, radiation is simply the process in which energy in the forms of, for instance, light or heat, is sent out through space. For our purposes, we'll be looking mainly at forms of electromagnetic radiation, ranging from radio and television waves to x-rays and gamma rays. These different types of radiation are classified according to the electromagnetic spectrum by their wavelength and frequency. That is, on one end of the spectrum are the "low energy" forms of radiation, such as radio and television waves, that have long wavelengths and low frequencies. As wavelengths become shorter and frequencies higher, the spectrum includes microwaves, infrared (which we feel as heat), visible light, ultraviolet light, x-rays, and gamma rays.

At the highest end of the spectrum, the radiant energies have a special power known as ionization. X-rays and gamma rays, when they pass through a cell, for instance, can actually separate electrons from their atoms and endow these runaway electrons with higher amounts of energy. The result may be damage to the tissue that could take a number of forms, from cancer to genetic defects.

While x-rays and gamma rays are the only forms of electromagnetic radiation that are capable of ionization, high-speed charged particles can also be ionizing. Two of the most common of these particles are known as alphas and betas, released during the decay of radioactive substances. To better understand radioactivity, it is necessary to take a closer look at the basic building block of matter, the atom.

Over the past fifty years, physicists have come to understand that atoms are mostly empty space, with tiny negatively charged electrons revolving in "clouds" around a positively charged central nucleus. The nucleus is positively charged because it is made up of at least one positively charged particle known as a proton, and at least one neutral, uncharged particle known as a neutron. These two "nucleons" are held together by what scientists call the strong nuclear force. This force is much more powerful than the attractive or repellent electric force over extremely short ranges, such as those involved in the atomic nucleus of most elements. Without this strong nuclear force, the like-charged protons in an atom's nucleus would repel each other and fly apart.

The number of protons in an atom is also always balanced by an equal number of electrons. This allows the atom to be electrically neutral and thus relatively stable. The atom's identity as an element, its "atomic number," is determined by the number of protons, from one proton in hydrogen to heavier elements such as lead with its eighty-two protons and the heaviest of all, lawrencium, with its atomic number of 103. The number of neutrons in an atom, however, can vary slightly and this allows for the process we know as radioactivity.

In the heavier elements, the greater number of protons in the nucleus results in greater electrical forces acting upon each proton. Though not as strong over very short distances, the electric force acts over a slightly larger distance than the strong nuclear force. An atom, for instance, that

ELECTROMAGNETIC SPECTRUM
WAVELENGTH IN METERS

| 10^{-16} | 10^{-15} | 10^{-14} | 10^{-13} | 10^{-12} | 10^{-11} | 10^{-10} | 10^{-9} | 10^{-8} | 10^{-7} | 10^{-6} |

X-RAYS

GAMMA RAYS

ULTRAVIOLET   VISIBLE

had ninety-two protons and only ninety-two neutrons in its nucleus would blow apart, with the strong force being overwhelmed by the electrical repulsion of so many positively charged protons. Nature compensates by supplying more neutrons in the nucleus of heavy atoms. The uranium found in nature, with its ninety-two protons, may have 142, 143, or 146 neutrons, and thus 234, 235, or 238 total particles in its nucleus. (Humans have produced a number of additional radioisotopes, or radionuclides, of uranium.)

The balance between the strong force and an atom's electrical charges can be delicate. Some elements, such as all forms of uranium, are unstable and will naturally go through transitions in which they lose energy. This process of unstable elements losing or emitting energy, without help from any outside energy source, is radioactivity.

One of the main types of radioactivity is gamma rays, which we've identified as a form of electromagnetic radiation. When protons and neutrons go through a process in which they rearrange themselves, a gamma ray may be emitted if the nucleus was in a high energy, "excited" state to begin with. Gamma rays, like x-rays, are not charged particles but forms of radiant energy. John W. Gofman, M.D., Ph.D., Professor Emeritus of Medical Physics at the University of California at Berkeley, and considered to be one of the foremost international authorities on the health effects of radiation, says in his encyclopedic book *Radiation and Human Health* (Sierra Club Books, 1981), "Our current understanding is that we can regard x-rays and gamma rays as identical in nature, except that in general x-rays are made in high-voltage machines, while gamma rays originate from the nuclei of atoms. (Not all x-rays are produced in machines, since some nuclear reactions are accompanied by x-ray emission.)" An element that emits a gamma ray does not change its identity, since it loses neither a proton nor a neutron.

The other two most common forms of radioactivity, alpha and beta

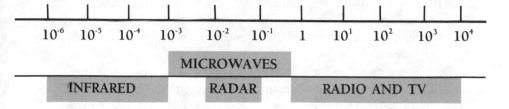

10^{-6}	10^{-5}	10^{-4}	10^{-3}	10^{-2}	10^{-1}	1	10^1	10^2	10^3	10^4

MICROWAVES

INFRARED   RADAR   RADIO AND TV

particle emissions, do result in a change in an element's identity. Alpha particles are compact clusters of two protons and two neutrons, while beta particles are energetic electrons. When either of these are emitted by an atom, the number of particles in the atom's nucleus changes. If the change is in the number of neutrons, a different form of the same element—an isotope—is the result. If protons are lost, a new element is formed.

For instance, let's look again at uranium-238, with its nucleus of 92 protons and 146 neutrons. The two protons and two neutrons that make up an alpha particle are also what make up the nuclei of helium. They are a stable grouping and will often be ejected from a heavy nucleus such as uranium-238's. Since uranium-238 when it decays loses two protons and two neutrons, it now has a nucleus made up of 90 protons and 144 neutrons. This is no longer uranium, but thorium-234.

But why should beta particles, which we've identified as electrons, also result in changes in an atom's nucleus? This is because these electrons come not from the cloud of electrons orbiting the nucleus, but from within the nucleus itself. As an excess neutron turns into a proton, it emits electrons in the process of beta decay. To continue our example above, thorium-234 will decay by emitting beta particles, and thus having one of its neutrons become a proton. The new element, protactinium-234, has 91 protons in its nucleus. When it also undergoes beta decay, it changes to uranium-234, with its 92 protons and 142 neutrons. Uranium-234 loses another alpha particle, and the new element is thorium-230. This process continues until a stable arrangement of protons and neutrons is achieved, in this case at lead-206.

Since radioisotopes are constantly decaying, eventually they will stabilize, having exhausted their ability to release energy. Different radionuclides have different time spans for achieving such stability, usually measured in terms of their half-life, the amount of time necessary for half of a radioactive isotope to decay. As any student of Zeno's paradox knows, one can keep dividing a substance in half for a very long time. Plutonium-239 has a half-life of 24,400 years, meaning that after 24,400 years, approximately half of the original plutonium is left. After almost 50,000 years, one-quarter is left, and so on. Strontium-90, a common radionuclide emitted from fallout, has a half-life of twenty-eight years; cesium-137, approximately thirty years.

Radiation is measured in a number of ways. The most basic measurement is used to determine the amount of energy emitted by a radionuclide in a given second. That measurement is called a *curie*, named for Marie Curie, who, along with her husband, Pierre, discovered radium. Though it was originally defined in terms of radium, a curie is today defined as the quantity of radionuclide disintegrating at a rate of 37 billion disintegrations per second. The curie is a standard measurement for all radionuclides, and for our purposes will be used to give the reader an understanding of the relative strength of a given radioactive element.

The *roentgen*, named for the discoverer of x-rays, Wilhelm Roentgen, is used to measure the amount of energy given off during ionization that is absorbed by a specific quantity of air. The roentgen is used primarily with x-rays and gamma rays and is tied directly to our next unit of measure, the rad.

The rad is short for radiation absorbed dose. It tells us how much radiation has been absorbed by some material after exposure to a certain number of roentgens. It turns out that in general human flesh absorbs about one rad for every single roentgen of radiation that bombards it.

Perhaps the most useful unit of measure is the *rem*, which is short for roentgen equivalent man. The rem incorporates both the amount of radiation and the "relative biological effect" from a dose of ionizing radiation. The health effects of radiation depend, of course, on the place of exposure on the body—the sex organs, lungs, and brain are highly sensitive to radiation—and the type of radiation one is exposed to. A single rad of alpha particle radiation can be ten times as harmful to sensitive organs as, say, a single rad of x-ray. We would say, then, that a rad of alpha particles to the sex organs or brain could cause ten rems of biological damage, whereas a single rad of x-ray might create only one rem of damage at these same sites.

In *Radiation and Human Health*, Gofman estimates that there are 3,771 fatal cancers for every million people exposed to one rem of radiation. Your chances of contracting a fatal cancer after being exposed to one rem are about 1 in 250. Since there is a higher risk associated with higher doses of radiation, ten rem exposures would pose a 1 in 25 chance of contracting a lethal cancer.

It is important to keep in mind that even seemingly small doses of radiation, measured in millirems or millirads (thousandths of a rem or rad), can be harmful, especially if exposure takes place over an extended period of time, or at a young age. Radiation has a cumulative effect; the longer the exposure, the greater the risk. Also, the young are far more vulnerable to radiation than the old. Moreover, there is no safe dose. Even the smallest dose of ionizing radiation can rip electrons free and set a cancerous cell in motion, lead to a genetic mutation in a future generation, and so forth.

I'll come back to the "no safe level" discussion, but first I should note that another important point to keep in mind when considering these measurements is that the biological effect of exposure is much different if, say, one's fingernail is exposed to a form of radiation compared to one's whole body. A single rad of radiation to the whole body can have a far more deleterious effect, since many sensitive areas are being assaulted by the radiation. Whole body exposure is rare, but it does occur at times when the body undergoes certain medical diagnostic tests in which a radionuclide, such as iodine-131, is injected into the bloodstream where it is carried throughout the body and absorbed by virtually every organ and cell.

Returning to the question of whether there is a "threshold" below which radiation has no harmful effect, we can see why this is not so by looking at how radiation interacts with organisms such as the human body. When ionizing radiation in the form of x-rays, gamma rays, or charged particles enters human tissue, it leaves destruction in its wake. The reason it is so devastating is because it possesses such enormous quantities of energy. When a "photon" (a packet of electromagnetic radiation) of x-rays, for example, interacts with the body, it can collide with an electron and rip it free from its orbit, thus giving rise to several potentially disastrous events. Some of the energy from the x-ray is used up in setting the electron free, but much of the remainder is transferred to the electron, giving it tremendous power to travel relatively great atomic distances. This newly freed electron can thus collide with other electrons, creating a billiard ball effect.

Other things happen, as well. When the x-ray interacts with the electron, it can often create a new x-ray of diminished energy. This new x-ray can thus set a whole new process in motion; that is, collide with an electron, transfer its energy, set the electron free to collide with other electrons, and produce a new x-ray of still further reduced energy. The process can go on and on until the x-ray finally gives up all its energy. But not until the real damage has been done: electrons have been set in motion to collide with other electrons in the tissue, creating havoc in the process. Besides setting electrons free, the introduction of such enormous quantities of energy excites other atoms, causing them to form new compounds with other atoms or molecules in the body. New chemical reactions take place that would ordinarily never occur.

Electrons normally orbit the nucleus in pairs and these pairs usually travel in opposite directions to one another. In this way, they create stability in the atom. When an electron is ripped from its orbit around the nucleus, the atom is suddenly imbalanced and unstable. It will then try to replace the missing electron by taking one from a nearby atom, thus causing a chemical chain reaction, whereby the instability of one atom is passed on to another, breaking old bonds and creating new ones in the process. This unstable atom is called a free radical and it is responsible for additional chemical chaos that takes place when electrons are knocked from their orbits.

The body carries on an immense number of chemical and biological functions every instant. Atoms of such elements as carbon, hydrogen, oxygen, and nitrogen combine to form compounds or molecules that facilitate life processes. Many of these are familiar: amino acids, proteins, hormones, hemoglobin, enzymes, sugars, and fats, for example. The cell does most of this work, and each cell is programmed to perform these tasks by a person's unique genetic code. Under ordinary conditions, the body is continually carrying on its chemical processes in the orderly and methodical way that nature has designed over millions of years of evolution. When electrons in human tissue are bombarded by energy from radioactive isotopes, however, they are set free to roam. In the process, they randomly change the biochemical balance, forming new compounds at specific sites in the body as they collide with other electrons.

Gofman provides an exhaustive analysis of the effects of radiation on human cells and tissue. He points out that a single photon of ionizing radiation may possess enough energy to break 14,000 to 20,000 chemical bonds in the body. "The introduction of an electron [with so much energy] can only be described as chemical and biological mayhem—a veritable bull in a china shop," he says in *Radiation and Human Health*.

Gofman points out that the body does manage to restore some of the original order after the ionizing radiation has spent its energy and its effects have finally come to a rest. "A particular carbon atom, broken away from a particular nitrogen atom to which it was attached, may reunite with its partner nitrogen atom," Gofman notes. "For *this* pair of atoms it can be said that no damage was sustained. But, unfortunately, this is not the general expectation. Rather, the general expectation is that chaos has been created out of order, chemically."

If ionizing radiation strikes the DNA, the genetic code, of a body cell, it can disrupt the functioning of the cell enough to cause it to go out of control and ultimately become cancerous. If ionizing radiation strikes a sex cell it can damage chromosomes. The damage will be passed on to future generations, possibly creating birth defects in people who were otherwise innocent of the initial exposure.

Radiation is particularly dangerous to young people because the radiation has a longer period to work on the child, thus enhancing its chances of causing deformity, disease, and injury to cells. The developing fetus, of course, is the most vulnerable to radiation, since cells are multiplying at their greatest rates.

Radioactive isotopes often collect at specific sites in the body, thus continually bombarding nearby tissue with ionizing radiation. Strontium-90, for example, goes directly to the bone and marrow, where many immune cells are produced. In this way, immunity is reduced or destroyed, thus leaving the body vulnerable to pathogens (microorganisms or substances that can cause disease) in the environment. Iodine-131 often collects in the thyroid gland, where it can cause cancer. As we will see later, this propensity of certain radioactive isotopes to collect at given sites in the body has encouraged the medical profession to increase its use of them to diagnostically examine specific organs or areas of the body. Once inside the body, however, there is little to control a radionuclide's behavior.

When x-rays penetrate the body, some of the photons pass through the body without interacting with electrons, thus causing no harm. As Gofman points out, however, alpha and beta particles will always interact with tissue. They are guaranteed to do harm. They immediately begin interacting with tissue and setting electrons free to collide with other electrons and upset delicate chemical bonds.

SOURCES OF RADIATION IN OUR LIVES

Humanity's exposure to radiation has undoubtedly increased within the past century, as the result of various applications and exploitations of the power of the atom. Nuclear power, nuclear weapons, nuclear medicine, nuclear consumer products—all of these are really experiments whose long-range implications are still being explored. This is not to say, however, that radiation—ionizing and otherwise—is a totally new, human-made development. As we've seen, radiation is a force of nature that is as old as the universe.

Natural and Background Radiation

Radiation in the form of cosmic rays, and from terrestrial sources such as from the uranium found in the earth, has always been a part of our environment. All people are being exposed to some ionizing radiation at all times. This radiation is no different and no less harmful for being "natural," and how much natural or background radiation you are exposed to will depend upon a number of factors.

One factor is simply the altitude at which you spend most of your time. Our atmosphere acts as an absorber of radiation, and the closer to sea level you are the less radiation will reach you. If you live in Denver, though, or you are a pilot or flight attendant and thus spend many hours a day at 25,000 or 30,000 feet, you are slightly increasing your exposure to cosmic radiation. Gofman calculates in *Radiation and Human Health* that just from the extra cosmic radiation associated with living in Denver (which also has higher-than-average terrestrial levels of radiation because of uranium in the local soil), we can expect approximately eighty extra cancer deaths per year there.

The terrestrial radiation we are exposed to can irradiate us from both within and outside our bodies. The most prominent ion found in human cells is the potassium ion, which irradiates us at a level of about 17 millirads per year. The radioisotopes most commonly found in the earth's minerals are rubidium, uranium, and thorium. It has been calculated that they contribute about 32 millirads per year on average to human exposure, but in some western states such as Colorado and New Mexico with higher concentrations, especially of uranium, local citizens may be getting a dose of up to 100 millirads per year.

A dose of such proportions can often be greater than that received from many of the typical human-made sources of radiation, such as, for instance, fallout from weapons tests or routine emissions from nuclear plants. This fact is often seized upon by nuclear advocates as reason enough to be nonchalant about low levels of human-made radiation. As Gofman points out, however, "There exists no reason whatsoever to dismiss as negligible any radiation dose from a man-made source simply on the grounds that the dose it delivers is lower than the dose from some combined sources of natural radiation. Most natural sources of ionizing-radiation exposure cannot be avoided by man . . . Adding doses of man-made radiation equal to the total received from natural sources is *public health in reverse*."

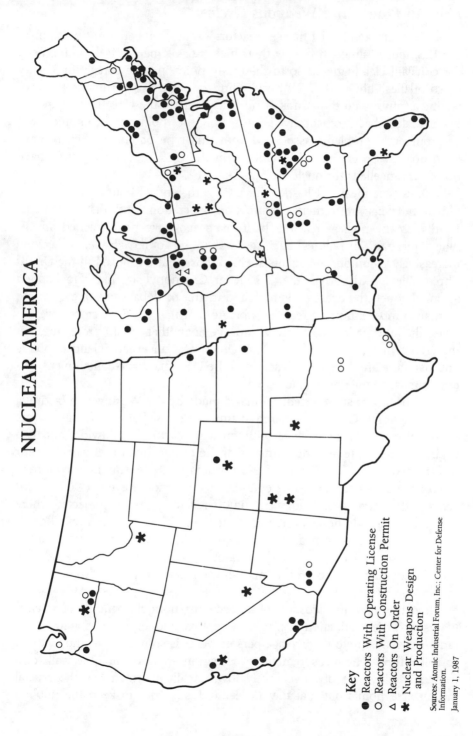

NUCLEAR AMERICA

Key

● Reactors With Operating License
○ Reactors With Construction Permit
△ Reactors On Order
✳ Nuclear Weapons Design
   and Production

Sources: Atomic Industrial Forum, Inc.; Center for Defense
Information.
January 1, 1987

Nuclear Power and Weapons Cycles

There are about 110 nuclear reactors capable of being in operation in the U.S. today, although due to their high rate of mechanical failure, need for constant cleaning, and so forth, at any point in time usually only sixty or so of these are working. At one point the federal government was projecting a future with thousands of nuclear plants in the U.S. This figure has been scaled back drastically because of the political, economic, and environmental problems associated with this type of energy. There have been no new orders placed by utilities in the U.S. (that subsequently have not been cancelled) for nuclear plants since 1974.

Does that mean we'll soon have little to worry about with regard to radiation levels from their construction, operation, and dismantlement? Hardly. Many nuclear reactors built years ago have now reached an age when mechanical failures such as leaks and other accidents become increasingly common. Accidents such as those that happened in the U.S. at Three Mile Island and in the U.S.S.R. at Chernobyl are likely to happen again, although the exact odds remain a matter of debate. Also, even more so than at most European reactors, operators of many U.S. reactors have not made the kind of low-cost safety improvements that would protect against the effects of a severe accident. The Union of Concerned Scientists points out that there are thirty-nine reactors in the U.S. that have containment systems similar to the one at Chernobyl.

According to some recent estimates made by the Worldwatch Institute, a Washington, D.C.-based research institute, we now have some thirty years of actual operating experience with nuclear reactors worldwide, and can begin to make more realistic estimates of the frequency of accidents. Senior researcher Christopher Flavin of Worldwatch says, "Assuming a continuation of the accident rate of one core-damaging accident every 1,900 reactor years and assuming an additional 6,000 reactor-years as projected, there would be three additional accidents by the year 2000." Even after Chernobyl, over a dozen workers at the Tennessee Valley Authority's nuclear utility tested positive for drug use, and operators at a plant in Pennsylvania were found sleeping in the control room with the reactor at full speed. It doesn't inspire confidence.

Even without the prospect of an accident, normal operation of nuclear plants, and the production of nuclear weapons, add appreciable amounts of radiation exposure to the average person. This is so in spite of the fact that so-called fence-line measurements of radiation—right outside the walls of a nuclear facility—are often relatively low. Again, Gofman has the crucial insight. He points out that the nuclear industry tries to keep the public's focus on fence-line gamma radiation figures for various reasons. "With enough steel and concrete between a person and a gamma-ray source," Gofman says, "it is no miracle that the dose received from direct gamma radiation is very small. The fence-line gamma dose has to be trivial, if the workers inside the plant are going to avoid acute radiation sickness." He points out that such measurements are misleading, however, because they fail to take into account the entire cycle of a plant's use of nuclear materials. There are liquid effluents, waste shipments, burial site leakages, mining exposures, reprocessing factors, and so forth. Gofman has calculated that even if only .1 percent of cesium-137, a single isotope used in the nuclear power cycle, is being lost to the environment at some point, this represents enough radiation to account for thousands of deaths from premature cancers in the U.S. alone. This figure becomes even more ominous when you consider that there are already over 200 technologically produced radionuclides in our environment, and that 99.9 percent containment may be an unrealistic goal given the nature of human and mechanical failures.

Many critics of nuclear power think that the industry has consistently understated the amount of high- and low-level nuclear waste it generates, and that nuclear advocates too easily dismiss the technical problems and difficulties of disposing of radioactive waste. Even with the passage of the Nuclear Waste Policy Act of 1982, the federal government has shown little progress in finding a permanent solution to our growing nuclear waste problem. Assuming no new nuclear plants are built, by the year 2000 there will be an estimated 40,000 metric tons of nuclear waste in need of permanent storage. Our nuclear weapons program also produces large amounts of highly radioactive waste, with 340,000 cubic meters of it now being temporarily stored at sites in South Carolina, Idaho, and Washington State.

The government's failure at solving the long-term problem of storing nuclear wastes is compounded by its inability to even store this stuff safely over the short-term. At the Hanford Nuclear Reservation in Washington, above-ground waste storage tanks designed to last fifty to 100 years routinely fail after as little as a decade. And three of the six commercial "low-level" waste landfills in the U.S. (in West Valley, N.Y., at Maxey Flats, Kentucky, and in Sheffield, Illinois) have had to be closed due to radioactive contamination of adjacent property. How is one to feel, then, about government scientists' attempt to find a permanent solution for spent fuel that is going to take approximately three million years to decay, according to the National Academy of Sciences, to the point of posing the same level of risk as the uranium ore from which it came?

In the latest development, the government has abruptly terminated the process of searching for the best long-term waste site, and announced that Yucca Mountain, Nevada, will be the site of the nation's first nuclear waste repository. Yet, as the Safe Energy Communication Council of Washington, D.C., has pointed out, a Nevada Bureau of Mines and Geology study of the site suggests that within the lifetime of the waste site there is a chance of fault shifting that could be accompanied by volcanic eruption. As the SECC sanely concludes in its *Mythbuster* series on nuclear waste disposal, "In the long run, there is only one solution: the production of nuclear waste must be phased out in an orderly and economical manner."

Radon

Humans have long regarded the home as the most private and safest of places. Unfortunately, it is fast becoming one of the most radioactive. Clearly the most dangerous source of radioactivity in the home—and the worst indoor pollutant—is radon gas, a radioactive byproduct of uranium decay that seeps up from the ground. Radon was only recently recognized as a threat to health, but National Cancer Institute officials now say that it may be responsible for at least 30,000 lung cancer deaths each year.

Radon came to the public's attention shortly after December, 1984 when Stanley Watras, a nuclear engineer at the Limerick Generating Station in Limerick, Pennsylvania, began to set off the power station's radiation detection alarms due to high levels of radioactive particles on his skin and clothing. Watras had absorbed an alarming amount of radiation—not from the power station, but from his own home. The Watras family lived above an enormous strip of granite, called the Reading Prong, that runs through three states. The prong, which contains a large deposit of low-grade uranium, runs well below ground through parts of New York State, northwest New Jersey, and eastern Pennsylvania.

After studying the Watras house, Environmental Protection Agency (EPA) officials determined that the family was breathing in the radon which had accumulated in the home by seeping up through the basement. The EPA says that the Watrases were receiving the equivalent of 45,000 chest x-rays per year, or the equivalent toxicity from smoking 150 packages of cigarettes a day.

The EPA had long believed that the only people at risk from radon were uranium miners who breathe the radon gas in the closed quarters of the mine. Until Stanley Watras set off the alarms at the Limerick Power Station, no one at the EPA thought that radon had any effect on those living and working above ground.

Since December, 1984, EPA officials have reinvestigated the potential threat of radon and discovered that it is formidable. In the first place, radon is everywhere, though it is concentrated in certain areas of the country where granite formations, phosphate rock, or dirt contain deposits of uranium. Places of particular concern—aside from the Reading Prong deposit—are parts of Maine, where it has contaminated well waters; in the Appalachian Mountains; sections of Montana, South Dakota, and Colorado; and parts of Florida. There are potentially high concentrations in Utah, California, Missouri, Arkansas, Tennessee, Wisconsin, and Michigan as well.

In 1987, the EPA stated that radon may pose a serious threat to eight million of the nation's homes. According to 1988 EPA estimates, approximately 20 percent of all homes in the U.S. contain potentially toxic levels of radon gas. Naomi Harley, professor of environmental medicine at New York University, says, "Nothing approaches the magnitude of this, not asbestos or formaldehyde. Radon is a major cancer causer and certainly leads the list of indoor-pollutant problems in the nation."

Although radon gas is now being recognized as a major health threat, the gas itself is not as worrisome as are the products of its decay. Because it's a gas and a relatively inert one at that, it passes into and out of our lungs quickly without the opportunity to do much damage. Radon decays, however, into particles called radon daughters, radioactive isotopes of polonium, bismuth, and lead. These three elements are heavy metals, not a gas like radon, and as radon decay products they act like ultrafine particles in the air. Generally short-lived, they don't pose much of a threat attaching themselves to trees or furniture, for instance, but when inhaled they stick inside the lungs and bombard nearby tissue with gamma rays and alpha and beta particles, as they continue the decay sequence from uranium to lead.

Thus, radon and its daughters are a problem primarily when radon is confined in concentrated amounts in the home. In addition to seeping up through the basement, radon is often stored in certain building materials, such as brick and cinderblock, from which it is emitted. Homes that are particularly at risk are those that are well-insulated, since the house doesn't "breathe" or allow air to circulate from outside. Also sump pumps, which open basement floors to the ground below, and basements that have cracks or no concrete floor, all pose an increased health risk.

Certainly the solution to the radon problem is not for 20 percent of all homeowners in the U.S. to attempt to sell their homes. EPA officials have been encouraging people to circulate the air inside their houses by installing well-placed fans and to seal cracks in basement floors. There are radon monitors for the home that can be purchased by contacting local EPA or public health representatives (see Appendix Three for resources). These monitors accurately measure the radon within the home.

After taking these steps, one should deal with radon—and all forms of radiation—by following the dietary advice provided in this book. As you will see, there is a great deal that can be done to protect yourself against radon and other sources of radiation.

Radon is now viewed as an alarming threat to health. Many mortgage lenders are requiring radon tests before providing home loans. The federal government has also begun taking the same steps before it guarantees home mortgages. Unfortunately, there are many other sources of ionizing and non-ionizing radiation in the home which only makes matters worse—and all the more difficult to deal with.

Consumer Devices

Aside from radon, the source of radiation in the home that has been most widely publicized are the luminous (or "radio-luminous," because it is the use of radioactive isotopes that provides the glow) dials on watches and clocks. These dials used to be painted with radium, another byproduct of uranium decay, but the U.S. now prohibits the use of radium because of the health threat it poses. Today, most luminous dials that are radioactive are painted with two other radionuclides, tritium and promethium, which emit beta particles, in contrast to radium, which emits alpha particles and gamma rays.

Gofman points out, however, that in order to obtain the equal brightness emitted by one microcurie (one-millionth of a curie) of radium, watch manufacturers are now using 11,000 microcuries of tritium and 390 microcuries of promethium. The large quantities of such radionuclides are potentially hazardous to those who wear watches or own clocks in which they have been used. This is especially true of watches, since one need only drop one's arm to waist-level to bring the watch into close proximity to vital internal organs and the genitals.

The United Nations provides a lengthy list of consumer products that make use of radio-luminosity, including timepieces, aircraft instruments, compasses, thermostat dials and pointers, automobile lock illuminators and shift quadrants, fishing lights, marine navigation instruments, public telephone dials, and light-switch markers. The list goes on. Not only do such devices pose an immediate threat in the home, but once they are disposed of they can allow ionizing radiation to seep into water, soil, food, and air.

At the very least, it would be wise to check out anything in your home that glows in the dark, find out if it emits ionizing radiation, and ask yourself if you can do without it. Chances are, you can.

Of course, the list of consumer products that contain ionizing radiation by no means ends with radio-luminous dials and markers. The majority of smoke detectors, which now number in the millions, depend upon ionizing radiation for their operation. Such detectors contain between 1 and 100 microcuries of americium-241, an alpha and gamma ray emitter; up to 15 microcuries of radium-226; and up to 20 microcuries of plutonium-238, depending on the make.

There are photoelectric smoke detectors available which do not contain radionuclides yet are equally effective in detecting smoke in the home, office, workplace, or public building. They usually cost a little more, but the health benefits outweigh the costs.

Certain ceramics and glazes contain ionizing radiation because of the presence of radioactive elements used in manufacturing the product. For instance, some early Fiestaware pieces, now sought after as collectibles, contain uranium. Acidic foods can leach the uranium from the glaze. The food is then ingested and thus transports the radiation-emitting elements throughout the body. David Poch, author of *Radiation Alert* (Doubleday, 1985), estimates that by using such plates three times per day, exposure levels can reach 5 to 10 millirems per hour.

Some manufacturers of eyeglasses also use certain radioactive elements to enhance optical quality. Eyeglasses thus may contain uranium and thorium, both of which emit gamma rays and alpha and beta particles. One study, done by McMillan and Horne, found that some eyeglass lenses emit one millirad per hour, giving rise to the threat of cataracts and cancer.[1]

Jewelry may also contain uranium and thorium to enhance its attractiveness and give a luminous quality. Dental porcelains sometime contain uranium and cerium to give them a fluorescent quality similar to natural teeth. Radioactive metals have been found to be recycled into some cast-iron frying pans. The list goes on—potentially radioactive objects commonly sold for use in the home and office today number in the thousands, and any one of these may now be emitting ionizing radiation in your vicinity.

The Other Smoking Hazard

Most people are already familiar with such potential sources of radiation as fallout and radon. You may be startled to find out, however, that recent research points to cigarette smoke, which is all too prevalent, as another common source of exposure to radiation.

Until recently, scientists had been unable to explain why cigarette smoking is directly associated with several forms of cancer in addition to that of the lungs, such as cancer of the bladder, cervix, pancreas, and prostate. This causal connection with cancers away from the lungs could not be linked to the presence of tars and nicotine in cigarette smoke. Now, some researchers report that cigarette smoke contains radioactive isotopes that affect the lungs and other parts of the body as well.

After almost two decades of research, several respected scientists have filed reports in the *New England Journal of Medicine* and other journals showing that when cigarette smoke is inhaled, two dangerous alpha-emitting radioisotopes enter the body. Particles from radioactive polonium-210 and lead-210 affect not only the lungs but many other sites throughout the body, including various organs and lymph nodes. Polonium-210 and lead-210 are daughter products, or decay derivatives, of radium-226, which is found in the phosphate fertilizers used in commercial tobacco farming.

According to Michael Castleman, managing editor of *Medical Self Care* magazine and the author of two excellent articles reviewing this research,

> For the past sixteen years, a small group of scientists . . . has gathered evidence they claim solves the major riddle of the cigarette/disease mechanism. They call their idea the 'warm particle theory,' [which] asserts that insoluble low-level alpha-emitting radioactive particles in cigarette smoke trigger the majority of diseases associated with smoking. Or, more succinctly: Cigarettes are radioactive.
>
> The scientists who support the warm particle theory admit that their numbers are small at the moment, but they include some of the nation's leading authorities on the health effects of radiation . . . .
>
> Everything is slightly radioactive. Our soil, food, water and bodies all contain trace amounts of naturally occurring radioactive isotopes. Significantly, however, the vast majority of these background radioactive particles are soluble in water. When they enter the body, which is more than 90 percent water, they go into solution and are quickly excreted, resulting in no long-term internal build-up of radioactive sludge.
>
> Tobacco, like everything else, contains trace levels of radioactivity, most of which is also soluble in water. Most tobacco-related radioactivity washes out of the lungs. But some radioactive particles in tobacco are insoluble. They don't wash out of the lungs; they accumulate there and bombard delicate lung tissue with low-level alpha radiation, the same kind of radiation emitted by plutonium.[2]

Polonium-210, which has a half-life of 138 days, was first isolated in cigarette smoke, in minute but significant amounts, by Dr. Edward P. Radford, professor of environmental epidemiology at the University of Pittsburgh and chairman of the Biological Effects of Ionizing Radiation (BEIR) Committee of the National Academy of Sciences, and Dr. Vilma Hunt. Further research was done by Dr. Edward Martell, a radiochemist with the National Center for Atmospheric Research in Boulder, Colorado, and the author of some seventy-five research papers. Using funds provided by the National Science Foundation, whose research grants, he said, are less influenced by the tobacco interests than those of the Department of Health, Education, and Welfare (now HHS), the nation's largest supporter of health research, Martell took a fresh look at the work begun by Radford and Hunt. He summarized his own findings and those of many other researchers working in related areas in an article entitled "Tobacco Radioactivity and Cancer in Smokers," published in *American Scientist*.[3] In the article, Martell noted that:

• Lead-210, which has a half-life of twenty-two years, is another insoluble radioactive particle in cigarette smoke. Lead-210 accumulates in the lungs, becomes highly concentrated there, and some of it decays into polonium-210.

• Phosphate fertilizers used in commercial tobacco farming contain significant quantities of radium-226 and its nine primary decay products, including lead-210 and polonium-210.

• When tobacco smoke is inhaled, radioactive particles subject the lungs to "hits" of alpha radiation that are hundreds of times greater than naturally occurring background radiation levels.

• Unexpectedly large amounts of the 210s are found in smokers' lung tumors and in lymph nodes adjacent to the sites of smokers' secondary cancers. Smokers' secondary cancers "almost invariably occur at sites immediately adjoining lymph nodes with visible accumulations of insoluble particles and measurable radioactivity."

• Fatty arterial deposits that characterize atherosclerosis also show abnormally high concentrations of alpha activity. Martell suggests that insoluble radioactive smoke particles at the plaque sites may be directly related to the high incidence of early coronaries among cigarette smokers.

Medical researchers have suggested that, because polonium-210 and lead-210 contribute to tobacco-related cancer, the number of cigarettes smoked may be more important than their tar and nicotine content. Two features of low-tar, low-nicotine cigarettes may have little effect or even an adverse effect on the amounts of polonium-210 and lead-210 inhaled in smoke. That is, the use of higher-porosity paper and perforated filters may cause the smoke to contain higher levels of lead-210, and cigarette filters have been shown to have no noticeable protective effect against polonium-210 inhalation. One estimate of smoking's radiation threat puts the smoking of twenty-nine cigarettes as equal to a single chest x-ray. For the pack-a-day smoker, the amount of radiation exposed to is thus estimated to be equal to approximately 300 chest x-rays per year.

Many people may be surprised at the small amount of research and publicity on cigarette radiation. Part of the reason is that researchers are still focusing almost exclusively on the potential chemical carcinogens in tobacco smoke. According to Martell, "There are many chemical carcinogens there, but the chemical approach does not explain the big picture. Today, most cigarette cancer researchers are still working on the chemistry of smoking, not on its radiochemistry."

"It's no accident," says Radford about the lack of attention being paid to the radiation hazards of smoking. He points out that, "The tobacco lobby and the nuclear lobby are two of the largest and most powerful in Washington. They don't control research funding, but I'd say they have disproportionate influence over it. The nuclear industry does not want the warm particle theory to gain credibility because it would prove once and for all that low-level radiation is very dangerous. That would mean substantial downward revisions in radiation exposure limits, revisions the nuclear industry cannot afford. And the tobacco industry certainly doesn't want cigarettes labeled radioactive. It's a case where two major lobbies have parallel interests."

Cigarette smoke also contains several chemical pollutants, such as cadmium and lead. (See Chapter 2.)

An issue that has received even less research attention is the potential radiation and chemical pollutant hazard associated with tobacco smoke inhaled, not by the smoker, but by bystanders, either from the tip of the burning cigarette or after the smoke has been exhaled by the smoker. Certainly, the tendency of recent research on the chemical carcinogenicity of secondhand smoke has been to find it more of a hazard than previously thought, and future studies may lend even greater ammunition to anti-smoking advocates by showing the radiation and chemical hazards to be considerable both for smokers and for anyone exposed to their habit.

Nuclear Medicine

So far, the emphasis of this chapter has been on the hazards of radiation and how to avoid them. The information that will follow will therefore be all the more ironic in view of the medical profession's use of radiation—often in shockingly high quantities—as a diagnostic and therapeutic tool. Modern scientific (allopathic) medicine's use of ionizing radiation, or what is being called nuclear medicine, is by far the largest purveyor of human-made radiation in our world, exposing more people to ionizing radiation than both the nuclear power or weapons industries together. Unfortunately, conventional allopathic medicine is not the only form of medicine in the West that regularly uses ionizing radiation. Chiropractic, osteopathy, and dentistry also commonly employ x-rays, for instance.

In fact, the history of medicine's use of radiation reads like a dark melodrama in which human sacrifices are made in pursuit of knowledge. Many researchers believe that the medical use of x-rays, especially in some of the diagnostic procedures such as mammography, has caused more disease than it's uncovered. This is not to say that the use of ionizing radiation has been without benefit to humanity. On the contrary, it has helped to save the lives of countless people. But radiation's harmful effects have been consistently underestimated.

The medical use of radiation goes back to the first human-made production of x-rays by Wilhelm Roentgen in 1895. X-rays were seen from the very beginning as a breakthrough in medical therapy. Like a ray gun that could be used to kill "enemy" diseases (an attitude that has characterized the way modern medicine views illness even today), x-rays were fired upon tumors, skin diseases (including acne), arthritis, and even hypertension. The initial results sometimes seemed miraculous: tumors shrank to normal size, skin problems cleared up, arthritis mysteriously disappeared, and hypertension seemed somewhat alleviated. These early results propelled the development of radiation therapy with an almost boundless enthusiasm.

At the turn of the century, the inventor Thomas Edison began development of his fluoroscope machine, an x-ray device that provided a continuous picture of the interior of the body. Edison's assistant was one Clarence Dally, who served as Edison's experimental "patient," posing behind the fluoroscope by placing his hand or his entire body in the beam of x-rays while Edison carried on his experiments. Dally died of radiation-induced cancer in 1904, the first person known to be killed by overexposure to x-irradiation.

The death of Clarence Dally did not reduce the general excitement about radiation, a fact that seemed to ensure continued overexposure. By the time Dally died, the medical literature was already turning up numerous cases of radiation-induced sicknesses and abnormalities, such as burns and skin ulcers.

Still, the use of x-rays only increased. In the 1930s, chest x-rays were widely used to diagnose tuberculosis, giving rise to a sizable increase in breast cancers. The 1930s also saw the terrible rise of birth defects and childhood leukemias resulting from the indiscriminate use of x-rays on pregnant women. No example better illustrates human capriciousness with regard to x-rays than the use of fluoroscopes in shoe stores during the 1950s. The stores provided x-ray machines so that people—especially children—could see their feet when they tried on a new pair of shoes. Little did the customer realize that he or she was probably getting a high dose of x-rays to the gonads, causing untold numbers of genetic defects and cancers.

During the 1970s the American Cancer Society (ACS) and the National Cancer Institute (NCI) launched a major campaign to have women undergo mammograms, an x-ray examination used to detect the presence of breast cancer. From the ACS and NCI point of view, the campaign was an enormous success, resulting in 250,000 women being irradiated for detection of breast tumors. Through much of the 1970s, the mammograms used an enormous amount of radiation, exposing each woman to an average dose of 10 rads per test. Soon, the medical literature was replete with reports showing breast cancers in women after they had had mammograms, forcing medical authorities to wonder if the mammograms weren't causing more cancers than they detected! The average radiation dose for mammograms was soon dramatically lowered. Today, mammograms are generally set at 0.1 rad.

The human cost in deformity, disease, and death from excessive use of ionizing radiation has caused the so-called "safe" exposure levels to be lowered throughout the twentieth century. In 1900, U.S. safety standards for occupational exposure were set at 10 rems per day! In the early 1920s, the limits were lowered to 50 rems per year, and later that decade lowered again to 25 rems annually. From there, the so-called safety standards have been consistently reduced until they reached the levels they are today: 5 rems per year for people working with ionizing radiation, such as nuclear power plant personnel or medical workers who specialize in radiation-related medical techniques; and 0.17 rems per year for the general public and for pregnant women working with ionizing radiation.

These levels should not be misconstrued as safe. Indeed, as we've seen, experience has shown that no safe exposure to radiation exists. Safety levels will likely be adjusted downward in the future. And, most importantly, since the effects of radiation are cumulative, all ionizing radiation is potentially hazardous, no matter what the amount.

Despite the short, dangerous history of radiation, the medical profession continues to use it as if it were safe. The use of radioisotopes and x-rays in the diagnosis and treatment of disease is a growing industry within western medicine. And studies have shown that too many doctors, dentists, and radiologists administer x-rays and isotopes without the slightest evidence of caution.

The United Nations reported that 130 million Americans received one or more x-rays in 1970. Since that time, the number of Americans being x-rayed each year has increased. No one knows how many Americans are annually x-rayed today, but some authorities estimate that at least 100 million people now receive dental x-rays each year. Gofman, in *X-Rays: Health Effects of Common Exams* (Sierra Club Books, 1985), estimates that the number of actual x-ray exams, for medical and dental reasons, performed annually in the U.S. is *300 million*.

In addition to these x-rays, there is an increasing use of radio-pharmaceuticals, or radioisotopes used in the diagnosis and treatment of disease. These radioisotopes migrate to specific organs—the bones, thyroid, or brain, for example. Once collected inside the organ, the radioisotope can be monitored by sensitive x-ray equipment to determine whether the organ is functioning properly. The procedure is generally referred to as a scan. Examples of these are barium scans, used in upper and lower gastrointestinal (G.I.) tract exams; iodine-131, used to monitor and treat the thyroid and to scan the lungs and blood; technetium-99, used in brain scans; gold-198, used to monitor the liver; mercury-197, used to scan the spleen; and cobalt-60, used in the treatment of cancer. Gofman reports that the use of radio-pharmaceuticals has been doubling every three years since the early 1970s.

Because of variations among x-ray machines, and among the technicians who operate them, it is impossible to give a figure in roentgens or rads for an "average x-ray." One Canadian study, however, done by K. W. Taylor et al., surveyed thirty hospitals and laboratories in Toronto and found that the same x-ray examinations and treatments varied by as much as a factor of ten.[4] The researchers surveyed three different laboratories that provided lateral view chest x-rays, for example, and found that the dose of x-rays to the skin varied from 24 to 150 milliroentgens.

The use of barium meal in upper G.I. tract examinations was equally varied among three different facilities. At the first lab, they found that the average upper G.I. test exposed patients to a 1.6 to 4.8 roentgen dose at the skin; the second facility gave a dose of 12.8 to 15 roentgens at the skin; the third facility, 50 to 90 roentgens. Note that these were not milliroentgens being administered, but full roentgens!

The same was true for the use of barium enemas. Of two facilities' tests, the first administered a dose of 16 to 20 roentgens at the skin, the second 56 to 128 roentgens at skin level. Taylor et al. noted that many of the people who undergo these examinations are young—still in their reproductive ages—and are commonly found to have no serious diseases.

The United Nations Scientific Committee on the Effects of Atomic Radiation (UNSCEAR) in 1977 ranked the medical procedures that provide high, medium, and low doses of ionizing radiation. According to the UN report, a high dose gives an exposure of between 3 and 26 rads at the skin. The procedures that provide a high dose were: barium meal (upper G.I. fluoroscope exam), barium enema (lower G.I. fluoroscope exam), whole chest fluoroscope, lumbo-sacral spine, lumbar spine, and cardiac catheterization.

Those procedures that provided a medium skin dose of 0.3 to 5.0 rads were: head, cervical spine, clavicle, shoulder, dorsal spine, thorax, gall bladder, abdomen, abdomen-obstetric, urography (from kidney down) and urography retrograde (from bladder up), Fallopian tube fluoroscope, placenta exam, bladder exam, pelvis, hip and upper femur, dental, angiography-head and -abdomen, tomography (chest), and mass survey of chest.

Those that provided a low skin dose of 0.07 to 1.7 rads were: arm and hand, chest (not fluoroscope, but a single picture), femur (lower two-thirds), and leg and foot.

In his book *X-Rays: More Harm Than Good* (Rodale Press, 1977), P.W. Laws lists mammograms as providing an average skin dose of 1,500 millirads per film (with two films taken, one for each breast). The average skin dose for an x-ray to the skull is 670 millirads, according to Laws. He points out that x-rays taken of the abdomen provide not only skin doses of radiation, but also administer high levels of ionizing radiation to the sex organs. He says that the x-ray procedures that administer radically high doses of ionizing radiation to the sex organs are lumbo-sacral spine, lumbar spine, and intravenous pyelogram.

Once inside the body, x-rays and radio-pharmaceuticals can do great damage to organs that are not the primary targets of the radiation. X-rays can bounce off their primary sites and scatter; radio-pharmaceuticals spread to other parts of the body through the bloodstream, thereby posing a risk to sensitive organs that were never meant to be irradiated.

Each examination using radiation poses a different degree of cancer risk, depending on the size of the dose. Gofman has calculated that a twenty-five-year-old man who undergoes a barium meal examination has a cancer risk of between 5 in 10,000 to 2 in 100, depending on the amount of radiation administered in the test. Since the dose depends upon the machine and the x-ray technician involved in its administration, your life literally rests in the hands of those who are responsible for nuclear medicine.

While the figures from UNSCEAR and Laws are over ten years old, and the growing awareness of the hazards of radiation to human health has resulted in some improvements by lowering average radiation doses for medical tests, wide variations in exposure are still possible. *The Los Angeles Times* reported in April, 1987 that there were more than 8,400 medical and dental x-ray machines that were overdue for inspections by state safety officials in California alone. *The Times* revealed that for every device that is overdue for inspection, there is at least an equal number of x-ray machines that have gone uninspected because they have never been registered with the state (a misdemeanor offense). When inspections of facilities are done, however, health officials discover that doctors and radiologists are uniformly overexposing patients to radiation.

"Los Angeles County health physicists have found that virtually every facility they inspect is exposing patients to higher doses of radiation than needed for a good x-ray because of violations of one or more radiation safety regulations governing the equipment and its use," *The L.A. Times* reported. They added, "But records indicated that some Los Angeles County machines have not been checked for twenty-five years." There is no reason to assume that California is atypical of the situation regarding safety inspection procedures throughout the nation. Actually, California, which has some of the toughest consumer-advocacy laws in the U.S., probably monitors such safety procedures more closely than most other states.

In addition to hospitals and laboratory facilities, industrial uses of x-ray machines are equally under-inspected. These x-ray devices are often ten times as powerful as diagnostic machines and can administer lethal doses of x-rays to workers.

The nuclear medicine industry is replete with shoddy inspection procedures, cavalier administration of x-rays to patients, and careless handling of nuclear waste materials. *The San Francisco Examiner* also reported in April, 1987 that California state inspection files revealed a laundry list of abuses, including:

• "Careless storage of radioactive material, often in refrigerators that also contain food."

• "Hundreds of gallons of radioactive materials are poured down drains into San Francisco Bay every year— sometimes legally, sometimes illegally."

• "Radioactive spills are common."

Right now, the information is there to judge the risks of nuclear medical procedures, especially if institutions were more forthcoming with information on their particular machines and more vigilant about safety and inspection procedures. As Gofman has said, "We need to have a

31

tremendous amount of education of the radiologist, the public, and physicians. Right now the risk ought to be made for these procedures so you can make a decision if you want to have it."

Although x-rays are certainly overused and sometimes irresponsibly monitored, they have at times no doubt produced more benefit than harm, and have even proved life-saving. Thus, it is not necessarily a question of whether to use x-rays, or nuclear medicine, at all. Rather, it is a matter of learning to use them in a wise, humanitarian manner. Equally important, since all radiation has the potential for hazardous, cumulative effects, we need to learn how to safely and reliably counteract its side effects. Then, when people are voluntarily or involuntarily exposed to some aspect of nuclear medicine, they can take advantage of safe and effective self-help remedies.

Non-Ionizing Radiation

So far, we have been talking about ionizing radiation – that is, radiation that can strip electrons from atoms – but there is another threat that has only recently come to the attention of researchers and public health officials. That threat is from non-ionizing, low-level forms of radiation emanating from a range of devices, including microwave ovens, computer video display terminals (VDTs), television sets, high-voltage power lines, radio transmitters, and other sources. In fact, our atmosphere is permeated by microwave, television and radio waves, and other low-frequency electromagnetic radiation. For years, scientists have maintained that such electromagnetic waves are harmless, but a growing body of evidence is now proving otherwise. New research suggests that what is being called "electronic smog" is far more harmful than previously thought.

In 1971, a presidential advisory council warned that the environment was being saturated by non-ionizing electromagnetic radiation, all of which posed a "critical problem to public health." It is now estimated that the current level of non-ionizing radiation is 100 to 200 million times greater than the natural non-ionizing radiation in the environment.

Studies conducted during the 1970s and 80s indicate that these low-level forms of energy can cause cataracts, cancer, birth defects, brain damage, and cardiovascular disorders. In addition, many health professionals fear that such forms of energy have subtle effects on the immune, nervous, and endocrine systems, giving rise to behavioral problems, nervous disorders, and a range of diseases.

For many years, people have been concerned that television sets and VDTs produce x-rays, which give rise to a whole range of biological problems—from cancer to birth defects. The amount of ionizing radiation from either of these sources usually is low, however, and exposure levels must be extreme in order to produce effects that manifest soon after exposure.

The vast majority of VDTs operate at the voltage level of a black and white television set and do not produce x-rays in measurable quantities. Low-level x-rays are possible, however, if the machine is not operating according to specifications. Also, older, poorly maintained terminals can emit measurable quantities of x-irradiation, indicating that VDTs should be checked regularly. In addition, color monitors operate at higher frequencies and, in some cases, may produce measurable amounts of x-rays. For the most part, however, VDTs do not produce measurable amounts of ionizing radiation.

But that does not necessarily make them safe. Indeed, many studies have shown that regular operation of a VDT has resulted in eye strain, blurred vision, fatigue, nausea, irritability, insomnia, birth defects, cataracts, and cancer.

The real threat from VDTs and television sets probably lies not in their production of x-rays, but in their capacity to produce non-ionizing, "pulsating fields" of energy. When these forms of radiation hit the skin, they cause atoms and molecules to become excited and vibrate, thus creating friction and heat. The body reacts by transferring the heat to the bloodstream and then to the surface of the skin, where it can dissipate. However, as the electromagnetic energy increases, the body's capacity to dissipate the heat diminishes. The excitation of atoms and molecules and the resultant heat can give rise to a chain of biological events, beginning with destruction of tissue, altered immune function, cell breakdown, and possible chromosomal damage. In fact, this process of molecule vibration is precisely how a microwave oven cooks food: by causing atoms and molecules to vibrate, resulting in friction and heat production which then cooks the food.

U.S. regulations allow 1 milliwatt per square centimeter of leakage from a microwave oven at the time of manufacture. However, that allowable leakage increases to 5 milliwatts per square centimeter after purchase. Often, food gets trapped in the doors of the oven and microwaves can leak out. Any cracks in the door, or a poor fit caused by wear, will increase the leakage of the radiation.

Researchers at the University of Washington in Seattle found that rats exposed to long-term, low-level microwave energy suffered a fourfold increase in malignant tumors compared to rats left unexposed. Other studies have found increased levels of leukemia among high power and telephone linemen, power station operators, and shipyard electricians. Researchers in Poland have discovered a threefold increase in the incidence of cancer in military personnel regularly exposed to microwave and radio frequency radiation, compared to soldiers who were unexposed.

As with all safety regulations, the setting of so-called "tolerable" levels are arbitrary, and like those set for ionizing radiation, will likely come down as more studies demonstrate the risk. Indeed, the American "safe" standard for microwave emissions is 1,000 times higher than the Soviet Union's, which allows only 0.01 milliwatt per square centimeter. In fact, the Soviets warned the world decades ago of the dangers of non-ionizing radiation, but the U.S. refused to heed the warnings. Critics have charged that the reason the U.S. refuses to acknowledge the harmful effects of non-ionizing radiation is because the military-industrial complex sees microwaves and other low-frequency radiation as essential to weapons and satellite development.

This book deals at great length with dietary factors and food substances that can be used to protect us against the adverse effects of radiation, both ionizing and non-ionizing, and chemical pollutants. In dealing with the problems associated with the various forms of radiation discussed in this chapter, particular attention should be paid to the following substances:

aloe
bee pollen
calcium
chaparral
chlorophyll
iodine
iron
lecithin
magnesium
fermented foods
oils
potassium
sodium alginate and sea vegetables
selenium
Siberian and panax ginsengs
vitamins A, B complex, C, and E
zinc

These foods and food substances will enhance the immune system and protect against the dangerous side effects of radiation. The scientific evidence supporting the use of these substances is provided in Part II.

CHAPTER 2

The Chemical
Pollutant Hazard

I n 1965 I gave a speech at my high school in which I described the environmental dangers reported by Rachel Carson in her moving book, *Silent Spring*. Back then, people liked to brand Carson as an alarmist or crackpot, though even some skeptics admitted that she was brilliant and perceptive. Now it is frequently stated by many scientists that the escalation of toxins in our environment has reached a critical level: we are being exposed to a continuous and almost overwhelming assault of toxins that cannot be avoided. No matter how ideal our lifestyle, no matter how remote and clean our environment, all of us are now exposed to dangerous levels of chemical pollution.

Like radiation, most of these toxins are trapped in the body and produce cumulative, long-term effects. Unfortunately, there is no one set of symptoms that specifically can be attributed to exposure to chemical and radioactive toxins. Some symptoms, such as changes in behavior, changes in metabolism, and altered resistance to disease, to name just a few, manifest early but easily can be interpreted as caused by something other than toxicity. Other symptoms, such as cancer, genetic changes, and organ and glandular disturbances, may take years to manifest and thus are even more likely to escape correlation with previous exposure to chemical or radioactive toxins. Moreover, studies show that exposure to any toxin—radiation, environmental pollutants, and drugs—weakens the immune system and damages other body systems, thereby making us even more vulnerable to other toxins to which we are both routinely and occasionally exposed. Exposure to radiation makes one more sensitive to environmental pollutants, and vice versa. And, adding to the hideous implications, some people are more vulnerable or sensitive to certain toxins, while other people are sensitive to others.

Industrial discharging of toxic wastes, and their collection at dumping sites, constitutes just one of several major environmental pollution problems that now affect everyone. In 1980 the U.S. Surgeon General declared the toxic waste mess "an environmental emergency." Even the EPA, which within the past few years has been widely regarded as slow to respond to potential public health hazards, warned that toxic waste dumping is "a ticking time bomb primed to go off."

Why is the concern about toxic wastes and environmental pollution growing so rapidly across the U.S. and in other countries? According to the Office of Technology Assessment, a research department of the U.S. Congress, as of 1985, "There are at least 10,000 hazardous-waste sites in the U.S. that pose a serious threat to public health and that should be given priority in any national cleanup." According to the federal General Accounting Office, there are more than 378,000 toxic waste sites that may require cleaning up. This figure means that there are more than 7,500 toxic waste sites per state, or *at least* several in every county throughout the country.

Currently, the situation does not seem to be getting much better. The EPA has managed to clean up only six sites since Congress created a $1.6 billion "Superfund" program to deal with toxic wastes. Another congressional research organization determined that, of the 1,246 hazardous-waste dumps it surveyed, nearly 50 percent were polluting nearby groundwater. They charged the EPA with "inaccurate, incomplete, and unreliable monitoring of these sites." Lee Thomas, the third director of the EPA during the Reagan terms, admitted, "We have a far bigger problem than we thought when Superfund was enacted. There are far more sites that are far more difficult to deal with than anybody ever anticipated." Basically, even where the EPA has initiated cleaning up of toxic wastes, the pollutants are frequently stored in what have already proved to be inadequate storage facilities.

Unfortunately, toxic waste dumps are not the only serious environmental problem. In addition to the many hazards associated with radioactive substances just described, other potentially ominous environmental risks include acid rain, smog, polluted drinking water, chemical toxins in our home and work environments, polluted soil and waterways, and noxious gases and other contaminants discharged from industrial sources.

How dangerous are these chemicals that now permeate our environment? According to the EPA itself, there are over 70,000 chemicals being used in commercial production in the U.S. The EPA has already classified almost 65,000 of them as potentially, if not definitely, hazardous to human health.

All told, more than 6,000 new chemicals are tested in the U.S. each week. Since 1965, well over seven million distinct chemical compounds have been described in the scientific literature. A basic problem is that government agencies frequently allow chemicals to be used and marketed commercially long before they have been adequately tested, if tested at all, for possible toxicity.

According to Zane R. Gard, M.D., writing in the April 1987 issue of *The Townsend Letter:*

> Three thousand [chemicals] have been identified as intentionally added to food supplies and over 700 in drinking water. During food processing and storage, more than 10,000 other compounds can become an integral part of many commonly used foods. . . . Ninety percent of toxic waste is improperly disposed and may end up in our water supplies, beaches, or abandoned in open fields. . . . Directly or indirectly this toxic residue invariably works its way into the human body. Add to the list potential body toxins, radiation, petrochemicals, industrial waste, medical and street drugs, tons of pesticides, herbicides and insecticides, and the result is an incredible chemical avalanche to have befallen the human race in a comparatively short time of evolutionary history.
>
> Currently clinical, scientific, and governmental studies indicate a staggering increase in the incidence of environmentally-induced illnesses. Four major factors responsible for this outbreak are (1) discrepancies in established "safety" standards for "allowable" contamination, (2) inadequate toxicity data, (3) approved use of many toxic substances in this country which have been banned in other countries as known threats to public health, and (4) the lack of formalized training of physicians in medical toxicology. While many of these chemicals have unequivocally saved lives, property, and entire industries, we cannot ignore the risks involved. The toll on human suffering is incalculable at present, as current statistical data does not accurately reflect non-occupational exposures, nor cumulative, interactive, or long-term chemical effects.

Medical researcher Alan Levine, M.D., has stated that, "The vast increase of chemicals in our environment, foods and medicines has greatly altered the body's ability to rid itself of toxins . . . the average citizen of the 1980s is biochemically and genetically different from the average citizen of the 1950s . . . ordinary text and training are geared to treat people who no longer exist."

The federal government, for various reasons, has been extremely slow to clean up environmental pollutants. Even if citizens' action groups, such as those listed in Appendix Six, were able to stop the introduction of all new toxic chemicals, our environment will be severely affected for many generations by the level of current toxins. In this and other chapters, I'll present information on the most common and dangerous of these pollutants. More importantly, you will find reliable, safe, and effective self-help natural remedies that counteract these toxins.

The self-help information and the natural remedies in this chapter are for the most common chemical, environmental, or drug toxins. Fortunately, the antidotes to these common toxins are the same as for radioactive toxins. This information will be beneficial if you have been subjected to toxins (and most people have been), if you currently are exposed to toxins (and most people are), or if you will be exposed to toxins (and most people will be).

At the end of the chapter you will find other general self-help guidelines for the prevention and treatment of chemical toxicity. Part III presents an integrated preventive and therapeutic program for optimal health, and offers specific dosage suggestions for the use of various supplements.

LEAD

Lead is a toxic trace element that affects almost everyone. It is considered very dangerous both because it is so pervasive in our environment and because, like radioisotopes, it is a cumulative poison. Unfortunately, early symptoms of lead poisoning, such as nervousness, irritability, headaches, fatigue, muscular problems, constipation, and indigestion, are hard to pinpoint as caused by lead. As it continues to accumulate in our bodies, lead creates widespread damage. Its chronic toxicity has been implicated in a sweeping range of physical, mental, and emotional disorders from occasional "everyday" aches and pains and irritability to serious degenerative disease and insanity. (See Chemical Toxins Table, page 48.)

Dr. William Strain, director of the Trace Element Laboratory at Cleveland Metropolitan General Hospital, calls lead pollution "the greatest neurotoxin [a substance that damages nerves] threat to all mankind. It is a damn epidemic."[1] Strain and several other noted scientists cite ample evidence to indicate that lead was a factor that contributed to the fall of both the Greek and Roman Empires. During their heydays, the Greeks and Romans began to smelt and use lead in a variety of ways, which produced wide-ranging and unmanageable physical and behavioral disorders throughout their populations.

Experts agree that health threats due to lead today far exceed those the ancient Romans and Greeks contended with. Airborne lead levels are more than two hundred times greater now than they were three thousand years ago. The amount of lead in our oceans has increased more than tenfold since ancient times. Sediment from the bottoms of lakes in the U.S. contains an average of twenty times more lead now than it did just less than one hundred years ago.[2, 3] According to Dr. Clair Patterson, a geochemist at the California Institute of Technology and a leading lead researcher, the average American has more than one hundred times as much lead in his or her blood as the average person did before smelting began.[4] The lead content of bones is now five hundred to more than two thousand times higher.[5, 6] Although lead is now found throughout the world and already affects everyone, inhabitants of industrialized nations contain six times the amount of lead in their blood as do inhabitants of remote areas.[7, 8]

In their excellent book *Trace Elements, Hair Analysis and Nutrition* (Keats Publishing, 1983) Drs. Richard A. Passwater and Elmer M. Cranton state that, "Scientists at the American Association for the Advancement of Science meeting in 1981 agreed there is a growing body of evidence to suggest that modern civilization—at least in a clinical sense—may be slowly going the way of the Roman Empire."

Dr. Ellen K. Silbergeld of the U.S. National Institutes of Health reported to scientists at this meeting, "We know that lead is one of the most ubiquitous and persistent neurotoxins in the environment. The laboratory evidence shows that adverse effects occur at very low levels, but the biochemical bases of lead toxicity do not support the notion that there is any safe threshold for lead exposure."

After testing 35,504 people, Dr. Emanuel Cheraskin, professor emeritus at the University of Alabama, and Dr. Gary Gordon, chairman of the board of the American Academy of Medical Preventics, concluded that more than 38 million Americans are currently being slowly and silently poisoned by lead.[9] According to Dr. J. Blosser, one out of four American men and 10 percent of American women suffer from lead poisoning. The percentage of women will increase as more enter the workplace, with pregnant women especially at risk.[10]

Children are extremely vulnerable to lead because they absorb 30 to 50 percent of ingested lead, whereas adults absorb 5 to 10 percent. According to Blosser, more than 40 percent of all urban children in American have health problems due to lead poisoning.[11] Lead causes a wide range of disorders in children, including nerve damage, brain dysfunction, skeletal retardation, and behavioral and learning problems.

In 1972, Dr. Oliver J. David, a child psychiatrist, and his associates at the State University of New York Medical School reported in *Lancet*, the prestigious British medical journal, that there is a definite link between lead absorption and hyperactive behavior in children.[12] Four years later David and his associates showed that lead chelating agents successfully treated hyperactive and learning-disabled children whose blood and urine lead levels were in a "nontoxic" range.[13] Those levels were, however, in the upper ranges of "normal." The children studied had no brain damage or other apparent cause of their hyperactivity and learning disabilities except for lead.

In 1979 Dr. Herbert L. Needleman, professor of pediatrics at Harvard Medical School, reported in the *New England Journal of Medicine* that every child probably to some degree is affected by lead, and that the threshold for safety has long since been exceeded.[14] The areas of behavior or learning that Needleman correlated to lead absorption were: ability to follow simple directions and sequences, ability to organize, propensity for daydreaming, distractibility and excitability, degree of frustration tolerance, hyperactivity, and impulsiveness, level of independent work and persistence with a task, and in general the ability to function well.

Lead can be both ingested and inhaled. Common sources of lead pollution are the 1,300,000 to 1,400,000 tons of lead used annually to make such products as solders, the anti-knock substance in leaded gasoline, batteries, pottery, and pigments. Smelting, fabricating lead, and burning leaded gasoline exposes workers to high lead levels, and releases more than 600,000 tons of lead into our atmosphere each year, which we routinely inhale. We also ingest it after it has settled on our food crops and in our water supply. Moreover, as researcher L. R. Ember notes, "Food also can be contaminated by lead from the solder in tin cans, pesticide sprays, and cooking utensils. In older homes, where the plumbing consists of lead pipes and the water is acidic and low in mineral content, lead may leach into the water supplies. Weathering of lead-laden paint and putty in older homes contaminates dust with lead, which can be inhaled or ingested; chipping, peeling, and flaking paint in these homes may offer a child a tempting but dangerous morsel."[15]

Patterson's research group reports that the standard tin-plated can containing food at a supermarket is sealed with solder that is 97 percent lead. Patterson states that whether the cans are varnished or not, the lead content of foods in lead-soldered cans is consistently much higher than the lead content of the same foods in fresh or frozen forms.[16]

Exposure to cigarette smoke can significantly increase our daily intake of lead. Lead is used in tobacco fertilizer, and airborne lead from cigarette smoke is readily absorbed.

Lead is not only absorbed through our air, food, and water, it is also absorbed through our skin. For example, people absorb lead when they take hot baths, especially when the hot water comes through old, leaded pipes.

Lead can be absorbed from many other sources. Lead and cadmium are leached, especially by acidic foods such as tomatoes and fruit, from improperly glazed ceramic food containers, dinnerware, and utensils. Consumption of alcohol allows high levels of lead and other toxic heavy metals and chemicals to settle in soft tissues, including the brain. Fruits and vegetables grown in roadside gardens are likely to contain higher levels of lead than those grown further from roads and highways.

As stated in *Trace Elements, Hair Analysis and Nutrition*, "Moderate lead levels can cause kidney damage and suppress the immune system, thus increasing one's susceptibility to many diseases including cancer. . . . Blood is not a good indicator of lead poisoning because lead quickly departs from the bloodstream and enters the skeletal tissues and hair. Hidden in the skeletal tissue, lead interferes with red blood cell production. . . . A better technique of screening for lead is hair analysis."

Although the risk of lead toxicity poses a serious threat to all citizens, rich or poor, urban or rural, the good news is that fortunately there are several natural remedies that have been documented as protecting against the toxic effects of lead. Foods and their nutrients protect against radioactive and chemical toxins in a variety of ways which we'll look at in the next chapter. Many of the same nutrients counteract the effects of lead, also through several different mechanisms. Some prevent or at least decrease the absorption of lead, others remove lead from body tissues, and some block lead from interfering with metabolic functions.

Lead competes with and replaces certain minerals, primarily zinc, iron, and copper, when there is a deficiency of those vital nutrients. (This tendency for the body to absorb similarly structured elements, referred to as "selective uptake," will be covered in more detail in Chapter 3.) Excess lead then causes a wide range of problems, including abnormal brain functions, especially in children.

Through the principle of selective uptake, optimal amounts of zinc,[17-20] iron,[21-24] and copper[25-28] protect against the absorption of lead and remove it from the body. Two other minerals, calcium[29] and chromium,[30] help to protect against lead toxicity. Calcium has both a preventive and a curative effect, and it helps to eliminate the pain sometimes associated with lead toxicity. Optimal levels of calcium prevent the absorption of lead from the intestinal tract. Deficiencies of calcium result in higher levels of lead in the blood, bone, and soft tissues. In acute cases of lead poisoning, calcium and vitamin D administered together either orally or intravenously have effectively hastened recovery.

The B vitamins, taken together as a whole B complex, protect against the toxic effects of lead.[31-38] Several health therapists have used additional megadoses of vitamin B1 (thiamine) along with a high-potency whole B complex, to counteract lead. Dr. G. R. Bratton of the University of Tennessee reported that thiamine removed lead from body tissues and also reduced the symptoms of lead toxicity.[39] Daily dosages of additional B1 have ranged from 25 mg. to 100 mg., together with high-potency whole B complex.

Vitamin C is a powerful anti-toxin. It neutralizes the toxic effects of lead, increases the elimination of lead in general, and specifically protects muscle tissue from lead damage.[40] In order to protect against lead toxicity, the recommended adult dosage range of vitamin C is 1,000 to 3,000 mg. per day. For acute lead poisoning, up to 10,000 mg. per day of vitamin C can be used.

A diet that contains appropriate amounts of fiber has been shown to protect against the toxic effects of lead.[41] Algin, or sodium alginate, is a form of fiber found abundantly in the family of sea vegetables known as kelp. As we'll see in Chapter 4, algin is a natural chelating agent, one that can attach to the lead in the intestinal tract and carry it harmlessly out of the body. Algin decreases lead absorption as it increases lead elimination from the body.[42, 43]

Pectin, another form of fiber, performs the same functions.[44, 45] It is found in sunflower seeds and just beneath the skin of apples. Pectin can be obtained in the form of a food supplement at natural foods stores, or as a gelling agent for jams, jellies, and preserves from some supermarkets.

The herb Siberian ginseng (*Eleutherococcus senticosus*) also counteracts the side effects of lead, especially damage to conditioned nerve and muscular reflexes.

Preliminary evidence indicates that a number of other foods and specific nutrients help protect against lead. Legumes and beans, when used generously in the diet, are considered to help eliminate lead from the body. Bee pollen, one of the most nutrient-rich foods, helps protect against and detoxify from lead poisoning. A mineral-rich diet and supplement program help the body detoxify and protect against the heavy, toxic metals. Vitamin A helps to activate enzymes that are involved in neutralizing lead and other toxins. Vitamin D, when given simultaneously with calcium, helps speed recovery from lead toxicity. Lecithin is another important detoxifier of poisons in the body. It also protects and repairs the myelin sheaths of nerve fibers from damage due to lead and other toxic chemicals and heavy metals. The sulfur-containing amino acids cysteine and methionine, found in the cabbage family of vegetables, aid detoxification, as do other chlorophyll-rich vegetables.

CADMIUM

Cadmium now rivals lead as the heavy metal which causes the most widespread and serious health problems. Cadmium, like lead, is dangerously pervasive in our air, food, and water and is also a cumulative poison that can cause a wide range of toxicity symptoms. Cadmium toxicity decreases the immune response due to its effect on the kidneys and liver and on T cell production, thereby being the culprit in nearly as sweeping a range of disorders as is lead. Japanese pathologists suspect that a painful disorder in bone metabolism and also some types of kidney damage may result from ingestion of cadmium-polluted water. Because it alters delicate balances in the body's relationships with other trace minerals and nutrients, such as disrupting calcium absorption and copper metabolism and depleting necessary zinc, iron, and copper, cadmium poisoning leaves a subtle trail that is as insidious as it is difficult to follow. It causes cardiovascular disease, kidney damage, and hypertension. Blood tests for cadmium toxicity are not reliable because cadmium rapidly leaves the blood and is absorbed by the tissues. When humans ingest excess cadmium, the blood level of the toxin remains extremely low, yet the tissue level becomes high and dangerous.[46-49]

Cadmium is released into the air as an industrial contaminant and is inhaled or ingested after it settles on our soil and food and in our water. Unfortunately, most of the cadmium that is inhaled is fully absorbed by the body. For example, researchers at Tufts University demonstrated that 70 percent of the cadmium content of a cigarette passes into its smoke, most of which is absorbed by humans exposed to that smoke. Cadmium absorbed from cigarette or cigar smoke has been shown to cause serious or deadly kidney damage, emphysema, and bronchitis.[50] Other common sources of cadmium pollution are smoke (from burning of wastes, wood, garbage, etc.), industrial effluents, plastics, fertilizers, auto exhaust, refined foods, coffee, and many others. Even our water contains cadmium— especially soft water or acidic water that leaches cadmium, the first water out of the faucet each day, hot tap water, and water from galvanized or black plastic pipes.

Cadmium and zinc are structurally similar. Through the principle of selective uptake, optimum amounts of zinc prevent the absorption of cadmium. Both cadmium and lead are absorbed more readily and are much more toxic when there is a zinc deficiency. When the regular intake of zinc is high, the zinc is stored and cadmium is expelled. Cadmium competes with zinc for binding sites in various enzymes and other proteins. The kidneys have an abundance of zinc-containing enzymes; thus cadmium, during a zinc deficiency, inhibits those enzymes and drastically interferes with kidney functions and blood pressure.

Until recently, high blood pressure, or hypertension, has been associated primarily with high salt intake. Some research indicates, however, that a high cadmium to zinc ratio in the kidneys causes high blood pressure in various populations around the world.[51] It has also been found that humans dying from disorders related to high blood pressure have a high cadmium to zinc ratio in their kidneys, and that the urine of hypertensive patients contains up to 40 percent more cadmium than does the urine of those who have normotensive (normal tension) scores.[52] Studies conducted in several American cities show that there is a direct correlation between environmental cadmium and death rates due to high blood pressure.[53]

High blood pressure more often is associated with men, yet women are also at significant risk from cadmium toxicity, especially women with zinc, calcium, iron, or other mineral deficiencies, vitamin D deficiencies, older women, and women with osteoporosis.[54] Pregnant and nursing women, who are generally more apt to be mineral-deficient, may absorb cadmium at a rate of two to three times greater than usual.[55, 56]

The amount of cadmium we routinely ingest is rapidly increasing because more is being released into the air and is falling onto our water, soil, and food. High-phosphate fertilizers, sewage sludge, and irrigation water are copiously contaminated with cadmium. Some foods seem to concentrate this toxin more than other foods. Even food from gardeners and farmers who use organic growing techniques have tested high in cadmium when the air, soil, or water have high levels.

Processed grains have much greater concentrations of cadmium than whole grains. More than 77 percent of the zinc naturally occurring in whole wheat is removed with the bran and germ during the milling process. Refining or milling whole wheat produces white flour, which is high in cadmium and deficient in zinc. Unfortunately, even organically grown whole grains, and some vegetables, often contain significant amounts of cadmium because these foods easily absorb cadmium from toxin-laden air, soil, and water. Other foods that especially concentrate cadmium are dairy products; meats, particularly liver and kidney; fish, especially those high on the food chain such as the large ocean fish tuna, flounder, cod, and haddock, and shellfish such as oysters and clams; poultry; potatoes; and tomatoes.

Some research indicates that sodium alginate, derived from sea vegetables, may act as a binder of some heavy metal pollutants such as cadmium and barium. In one study, sodium alginate prevented the death of rats exposed to a toxic dose of cadmium.[57]

There are several other foods and food nutrients in addition to zinc and sodium alginate that effectively protect against cadmium assimilation, reduce cadmium retention, and remove cadmium from the body.[58-69] See Chemical Toxins Table, p. 48.

MERCURY

Mercury, one of the oldest common pollutants, is another toxic heavy metal prevalent in our environment. It is found in a natural state in soil and has been processed and used in a wide variety of industrial applications from the manufacture of wood pulp to agricultural fungicides. The European expression "mad as a hatter" came into existence during the last century when workers in hat factories frequently went insane due to the mercury used in making felt hats.

Sir Isaac Newton is considered to have had a short bout with insanity while using mercury "quicksilver" in his experiments. Indeed, in Newton's time, mercury quicksilver was often called "quacksilver," and those who used it, especially to make synthetic drugs, were the original "quacks." Newton finally stopped experimenting with heavy metals, but he never fully recovered his former brilliance and vitality.[70, 71] High school chemistry students are now taught that the silvery liquid is a serious health hazard.

Mercury concentrates as it makes its way up the food chain. When found in fish at levels of more than one part per million it can cause severe problems for the humans who eat them. In Minamata, Japan in the 1950s, commercial mercury residue concentrating in the flesh of fish was found to be the cause of one of the most infamous calamities related to mercury poisoning. Minamata fishermen and their families developed blurred vision and numbness that progressed into severe paralysis and birth defects and abnormalities. In northern Minnesota's waters, fish have been found whose methyl mercury contamination nearly rivals that of the fish from Minamata. Minnesota's contamination might be the product of air-borne metallic particles from copper smelters, coal-burning power plants, and chemical factories from as far away as Texas and Missouri.

Mercury, like most of the other toxins, is a cumulative poison that can produce a range of disorders as wide in scope as that of the other heavy metals. It especially results in neurological and behavioral disruptions. One of its many possible cumulative effects is to inhibit the immune response by decreasing the production of white blood cells, including T cells, which eliminate harmful foreign substances.[72]

There are two forms of mercury: methyl mercury (organic mercury) and inorganic mercury. Both forms are toxic. Some of the most common sources of contamination are from pesticides, pharmaceutical medicines, cosmetics, dental substances such as silver amalgam fillings, and large ocean fish such as swordfish and tuna. We ingest or inhale inorganic mercury through our air, food, water, and soil—our bodies can even absorb it through our skin from cosmetics and pesticides—and then our bodies convert it into the even more highly toxic methyl mercury.

Fortunately, there are several natural substances that help protect against and detoxify mercury. Of these, the nonmetallic element selenium stands out because it binds both forms of mercury and helps counteract their toxic side effects.[73-76] Other substances and nutrients that are helpful in dealing with mercury are listed in Chemical Toxins Table, p. 48.

ALUMINUM

Aluminum has only recently been recognized as a toxic metal. Unfortunately, it is still used in a wide variety of common products including food additives, antacids and other over-the-counter drugs, some baking powder, and pots and pans. Some plant foods and gardening substances contain aluminum, as do many animal feeds. Tap water often contains an aluminum additive that is not fully filtered out, and white flour is often bleached with potassium alum. Table salt "pours when it rains" because of an aluminum additive that prevents caking. Processed junk foods contain aluminum, and last but by no means least are the ever-present "tin" can and "tin" foil.

Not only is its production energy-wasting and expensive, but since aluminum is processed from bauxite ore found on the surface mainly in tropical forests it is also extremely disturbing to the ecology. The processing of aluminum also creates other severe pollutants, such as fluorine gas.

The list of potential effects of aluminum toxicity rivals that of the other heavy metals in breadth and scope. It runs the gamut of physical, neurological, genetic, and behavioral disruptions and has been implicated in everything from Alzheimer's disease and depression to constipation and schizophrenia. (See Chemical Toxins Table, p. 48.)

Like many of the other environmental toxins, aluminum has cumulative effects in the human body—what started out at age fifteen as occasional headaches may by fifty be Parkinson's disease. Also, like the other heavy metals, aluminum increases in concentration as it proceeds up the food chain. People who eat animal foods such as meats, poultry, and dairy are regularly ingesting higher concentrations of aluminum.

There are several natural substances and foods that prevent the assimilation of aluminum or counteract its side effects. They are calcium, fiber, lecithin and other choline-containing substances, magnesium, vitamin C, and zinc.[77-79]

SOME BASIC PREVENTIVE SUGGESTIONS

Since it's not possible to live totally protected from these and other common industrial pollutants, we can try to minimize their effects. I'll be going into greater detail later on many of the following basic suggestions.

1. Try to maintain an optimal diet and holistic health program.

2. Try to breathe fresh air regularly and take vacations in areas with fresh air and wholesome foods.

3. Drink high-quality bottled water or efficiently filtered water. Tap water may contain up to 600 different chemicals from industrial and agricultural sources. Many cities add on the average approximately seventy chemicals to tap water to bleach, disinfect, or deodorize it. Consider using a shower filter because you absorb as many pollutants from shower and bath water as from drinking and cooking water.

4. Eat organically grown foods whenever possible. These contain less contaminants.

5. Have a small backyard garden away from the road.

6. Take time to thoroughly wash supermarket or commercially grown fruits and vegetables.

7. Avoid processed foods and junk foods. Eat whole, natural foods, as free of hormones, radiation, and other contaminants as possible.

8. Chew your food long enough both to savor it and to liquefy it, thereby aiding digestion, metabolism, and elimination.

9. Enjoy frequent aerobic exercise.

10. Decrease the use of toxic chemicals in your home, work, and recreational environments.

11. Bless your food—a common practice among traditional societies—and try to be grateful and enjoy whatever you do and whatever you eat so that your immune and other bodily protective systems will function better. The spirit is a powerful factor in influencing the body.

CHEMICAL TOXINS TABLE

Metal	Common Sources	Toxicity Symptoms	Counteracting Nutrients

Aluminum	cans
	foil
	antacids
	pots and pans
	baking powder
	some cheeses
	cooking utensils
	deordorants
	plant foods and
	  gardening
	  additives
	refined junk foods
	tap water
	bleached white
	  flour
	buffered aspirin
		Alzheimer's disease
		colitis
		constipation
		headaches
		hyperactivity
		irritability
		learning disorders
		loss of appetite
		  energy or hair
		memory loss
		neurological
		  disorders
		numbness
		skin ailments
		thyroid disorders
			calcium
			fiber
			lecithin
			magnesium
			vitamin C
			zinc

Cadmium	batteries
	cigarette smoke
	coffee
	gasoline
	metal pipes
	plastics
	refined foods
	solders
	steel
	some water
		anemia
		dry skin
		hair loss
		headaches
		immune disorders
		kidney/liver
		  damage
		low blood
		  pressure
		protein/sugar
		  in urine
			cabbage family
			  vegetables
			calcium
			copper
			fiber
			iron
			manganese
			pectin
			selenium .
			vitamins C
			  and D
			zinc

Carbon Monoxide	auto exhaust
	cigarette smoke
	smog
		anemia
		angina
		asthma
		bronchitis
		emphysema
		headaches
		memory loss
		respiratory disorders
			eleuthero
			vitamins A, B
			  complex, C
			  and E
			cysteine
			bee pollen
			nutritional
			  yeast

Chlorine	water disinfectant	vitamin deficiencies	vitamins C and E

Metal	Common Sources	Toxicity Symptoms	Counteracting Nutrients
Copper	tap water plumbing	mineral deficiencies, esp. zinc, magnesium, iron, manganese and molybdenum gastrointestinal tract irritations mental disorders	manganese molybdenum vitamin C plus bioflovanoids zinc
Fluoride	tap water beverages bottled with tap water fertilizers fluorinated hydrocarbons mouthwashes toothpastes dental fluoride	abnormal hardening of bones and teeth accelerated aging cancer brain damage genetic damage immune disorders vitamin deficiencies kidney disorders Mongolism mental dysfunctions thyroid damage tumors	calcium magnesium vitamins C and E
Hexavalent Chromium	air and water tobacco smoke	cancer gastrointestinal disorders	vitamin C
Industrial/ Agricultural Chemicals (DDT, PCBs, dioxin, etc.)	plant and animal tissues air, water, soil, and food	vitamin depletions	bee pollen lecithin vitamins A, B complex, and C fermented foods sauna therapy and/or short juice fast
Lead	dyes gasoline insecticides paint plumbing pottery solder insecticides	cramps anemia fatigue headaches insomnia nausea vomiting weakness	chlorophyll cysteine eleuthero iron legumes and beans pectin lecithin phosphorus

Metal	Common Sources	Toxicity Symptoms	Counteracting Nutrients

Lead (cont.)	scrap metal
	tobacco
	  smoke
	textiles
		cancer
		nerve
		  disorders
		brain damage
			cabbage family
			  vegetables
			selenium
			sodium alginate
			vitamins A, B1,
			  B2, B complex,
			  C, D, and E
			zinc

Mercury	amalgam fillings
	fish
	soil
	fungicides
	some cosmetics
	pesticides
	film
	plastics
	paint
		allergies
		arthritis
		birth defects
		cataracts
		depression
		dizziness
		epilepsy
		fatigue
		fever
		headaches
		insomnia
		kidney damage
		memory loss
		nervousness
		paralysis
		seizures
		vision loss
		weakness
			cabbage family
			  vegetables
			calcium
			fiber
			lecithin
			pectin
			selenium
			sodium alginate
			vitamins A, B
			  complex, C,
			  and E
			cysteine
			nutritional
			  yeast

Nitrates and Nitrites	processed meats
	fertilizers
	tap water
		cancers of
		  bladder, liver,
		  stomach and
		  other organs
		heart disease
		high blood
		  pressure
			bee pollen
			lecithin
			vitamins A, B
			complex, C,
			and E
			nutritional
			  yeast

Nitrogen Dioxide and Ozone	smog	cancer
		emphysema
		respiratory disorders
			bee pollen
			eleuthero
			Panax ginseng
			vitamins A,
			  PABA with
			  B complex, C,
			  and E

The Chemical Pollutant Hazard

Metal	Common Sources	Toxicity Symptoms	Counteracting Nutrients
Polynuclear Aromatic Hydrocarbons	smoke from tobacco, wood, coal, oil, and most commercial incense	cancer	calcium pantothenate cysteine iron selenium vitamins A, B1, B2, B complex, C, and E zinc
Synthetic and Chemical Drugs	antibiotics, painkillers, barbituates cocaine, heroin, crack, etc.	birth defects cancer vitamin and mineral deficiencies metabolism disruptions liver damage mental disorders sexual disorders kidney damage	bee pollen eleuthero multiple minerals vitamins A, B complex, C and bioflavonoids and E fermented foods lecithin
Tobacco Smoke	cigars, cigarettes, pipes	various cancers immune disorders lung problems	selenium vitamins A, C, and E zinc

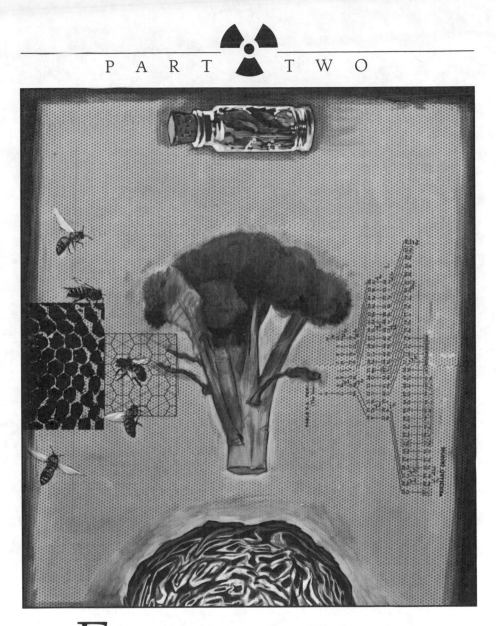

FOODS, HERBS, VITAMINS & MISCELLANEOUS SUBSTANCES THAT PROTECT YOU FROM RADIATION & CHEMICAL HAZARDS

How Foods, Herbs, Supplements, & Miscellaneous Substances Protect & Heal the Body

Despite the pervasiveness of radiation and environmental pollutants, there is nonetheless a great deal you can do to protect yourself from their toxic side effects. There is an impressive array of foods, herbs, vitamin and mineral supplements, and miscellaneous substances that combat the effects of these toxins. By reading on, you will find that diet can do a great deal to protect you every day from invisible toxic enemies.

The substances I'll discuss function in a variety of ways. Indeed, the body has a number of defense mechanisms that protect it from the insults of the environment. Among these mechanisms are the body's ability to "selectively uptake" certain nutrients and to chelate or bind other substances and thus eliminate them from the body. There is also the body's action with regard to how free radicals or oxidants are handled, and its highly complex and remarkably effective immune system—a multifaceted web of defenses that attack and eliminate pathogens when they invade the body.

Healthy functioning of the immune system is dependent to a large extent on proper nutrition. Zinc, for example, helps to promote and regulate immune response. Many other minerals, vitamins, and foods promote immune function, while, conversely, inadequate amounts of certain nutrients deplete our most vital defense against radiation and other harmful substances.

In fact, diet and nutrition seem to play a major role in virtually every defense our body has against the effects of radiation and chemical pollutants. Let's take a closer look at some of the ways diet protects us.

THE BODY'S "CHOICE" MECHANISMS

The human body is both choosy and adaptable. It prefers quality, but it will settle for less. That, in a nutshell, is the law of selective uptake.

For example, the body needs calcium for bones, teeth, and tissue, but in the absence of calcium-rich foods, the body will absorb something that is atomically similar to calcium, but slightly different: strontium-90. Once strontium-90 has been consumed, the body will attempt to utilize it as it would calcium. It will send the radioactive isotope to the bones and teeth, where it will collect and, over many years, release radioactive particles. Strontium-90 not only resembles calcium, but it too can be found in high quantities in many dairy products. Strontium-90 occurs in other foods as well since plants and animals, similarly to humans, also absorb it when deficient in calcium.

Here is a case in which the body has been poisoned because it wasn't given adequate amounts of calcium. Other elements work in the same way, as can be seen by the following chart.

Radioactive Element	Absorbing Organ	Preventive Element
cesium-137	liver, reproductive organs, muscles, kidneys	potassium
cobalt-60	liver, reproductive organs	vitamin B-12
iodine-131	thyroid, reproductive organs	iodine
plutonium-238, -239	lungs, liver, reproductive organs	iron
strontium-90	bones	calcium
sulfur-35	skin	sulfur
zinc-65	bones, reproductive organs	zinc

Elements are grouped together in "families" on the periodic chemistry chart. The grouping is done according to the number of electrons that orbit the nucleus of each atom, and particularly by the number of electrons in the outermost shell—the valence electrons— of the atom. Strontium-90 and calcium are in the same family. One big difference, however, is that strontium-90 is radioactive.

The same situation exists for iodine—necessary for healthy functioning of the thyroid—and iodine-131, a radioisotope. If the body is deficient in iodine, it will absorb iodine-131 if such an isotope is available in the food, air, or water supply. Once inside the body, iodine-131 will collect in the thyroid and have a devastating effect on this organ that supervises metabolism.

The law of selective uptake describes not only the body's attempt to choose quality, but also its willingness to settle for less in order to survive. Of course, when it settles for radioactive elements, long-term survival is very much in jeopardy.

Calcium and iodine are by no means the only two elements with radioactive isotopes in their families. Cesium-137, which, like strontium is a common byproduct of nuclear power plants and fallout, is chemically related to potassium and will be absorbed by the body when potassium deficiencies exist. Once absorbed, cesium-137 will collect in muscles and reproductive organs, where it will play havoc with reproductive cells and DNA. Cesium also collects in the kidneys and liver, two organs that are constantly cleansing the blood. Once in the liver and kidneys, cesium can go anywhere in the body since the entire blood supply passes through these organs.

Plutonium, another common byproduct of fallout and nuclear power plant emissions, is similar in atomic structure to iron. As a result, plutonium collects in the blood and it too travels throughout the body. Secondary sites, of course, are the blood-cleansing organs such as the lungs, liver, and kidneys. Plutonium, whose half-life is 24,400 years, like other long-lived radionuclides has a devastating effect on reproductive organs and sex cells, thus threatening future generations.

Cobalt-60, a common radionuclide used in nuclear medicine and, as is cesium-137, in the process of food irradiation, shares some common structural characteristics with cobalamin or vitamin B_{12}. Cobalt-60 collects in the liver and reproductive organs. Sulfur-35, a byproduct of reactors, is similar to sulfur, and zinc-65 is similar to zinc.

In the absence of these nutrients, or when inadequate amounts are consumed, absorption of their radioactive "sisters" becomes all the more likely. In other words, the less nutritious our diets, the more susceptible we are to the effects of radiation.

We do not yet know the exact degree of protection afforded by selective uptake of stable elements before, during, and after contamination by their radioactive sisters. Humane considerations make extensive testing on humans unfeasible. Enough information and research exists, however, to support the general validity of selective uptake for all the radionuclides mentioned above. It is crucial that further research be done with patients receiving radiotherapy, at known sites of radioactive contamination (such as at Chernobyl or among the population of Hanford, Washington), and with those who suffer accidental exposure, such as nuclear plant workers. Until more is known, we can protect ourselves to a significant degree by following the optimal diet plan presented in Part III and by avoiding unnecessary contact with sources of ionizing radiation.

Chelation is another way that food and specific nutrients protect against radiation and chemical pollutants. Some food substances bind with a radioisotope and eliminate it from the body through digestion. Sea vegetables—or, more specifically, the sodium alginate found in sea vegetables—and pectin have a powerful binding effect on radionuclides and chemical pollutants. These foods actually serve to neutralize the effects of radiation by leaching it from the bones and other tissues and causing it to be eliminated from the body as waste. I'll go into more detail on how this mechanism works when we talk about the research supporting sea vegetables' radioprotective abilities in Chapter 4.

CONTROLLING FREE RADICALS

I described free radicals earlier as atoms that have lost electrons because of the effects of radiation or chemical pollutants. These free radical atoms are unstable; as a result, they cause chemical chaos in the surrounding tissues. They can break old chemical bonds that formerly existed and form new ones that under normal healthy circumstances would never exist.

In addition to exposure to radiation or environmental pollutants, the consumption of unhealthful fat substances can lead to the formation of harmful free radicals within the body. By joining with fat compounds in the tissue, they can cause fat molecules to oxidize and turn rancid, which results in even more free radical production.

Free radicals can also disrupt DNA and RNA functioning, leading to the production of protein molecules which are treated as foreign substances by the body. The immune system mobilizes to attack these proteins, but the constant battle of the body against itself tends to be a weakening force. Numerous scientific researchers cite free radical formation as a primary cause of various health disorders and accelerated aging.

Most free radicals in the body are damaging byproducts of oxygen metabolism. In his book *Maximum Life Span* (Avon, 1983), longevity expert Roy Walford, M.D., describes free radicals as "great white sharks in the biochemical sea." He says, "These short-lived but voracious agents oxidize and damage tissue, especially cell membranes." Certain vitamins and food substances, because they have the ability to neutralize oxidants or combine with free radicals, are called antioxidants. In effect, antioxidants sacrifice themselves to free radicals by donating electrons, or combining with these unstable atoms, thus causing the free radical to stabilize. Antioxidants are also called free radical "scavengers" because of their ability to "gobble up" wandering free radicals and restore stability to tissues.

Antioxidants occur naturally in many foods and act to prevent the fats in foods from oxidizing either before or during digestion. Oxidation occurs when oxygen, or its chemical equivalents, directly attacks fat molecules in the absence of control enzymes such as superoxide dismutase (SOD). The attack of oxygen upon "unprotected" fat molecules produces oxidized fats commonly called rancid (peroxidized) fats. These peroxidized fats are highly toxic carcinogenic substances, capable of causing mutation. Upon further breakdown, peroxidized fats form the highly reactive molecules that are free radicals. As noted previously, free radicals are strongly implicated as causative agents in some of the side effects of radiation. Free radicals can cause a serious weakening of the immune system. They also contribute to aging, cardiovascular disease, cancer, arthritis, cataracts, senility, and a host of other conditions including such common ones as bruises and dandruff.[1]

Dr. Denham Harman of the University of Nebraska originated the theory that free radicals are the primary cause of aging. He referred to free radicals as "internal radiation." That is an apt description of them because radiation sickness is a pure form of free radical disease. External radiation kills because it creates free radicals. "Internal radiation," free radicals created chemically within the body, can kill too.

And, just as the prudent person avoids excess external radiation, he or she can minimize unnecessary internal radiation (exposure to free radicals) by decreasing consumption of fats, especially fried foods or fats and oils cooked at high temperatures, stored for long periods of time, or exposed to air or light. At the same time, he or she can increase the consumption of foods, herbs, and supplements containing antioxidants. Common antioxidants include vitamins A, E, C, B_1, B_5, B_6, PABA (a member of the vitamin B complex), the amino acid cysteine, the minerals zinc and selenium, the SOD enzymes, and the herbs aloe vera and chaparral.

Some of these substances have yet to be researched as possible radioprotectants. For example, no scientific research has been conducted on the herb chaparral regarding radioprotection. However, chaparral has been used effectively by traditional herbal healers for health problems, including some tumors and cancers (which are frequently an eventual side effect of exposure to "excess" radiation or to some chemical pollutants). Chaparral contains a substance called NDGA, which is a powerful antioxidant. See Chapter 6 for more on chaparral.

According to Sister Rosalie Bertell, a biostatistician who specializes in the relationship of radiation to cancer and the author of *No Immediate Danger* (The Book Publishing Company, 1986), "It seems that there are precise radiation dose cut-offs such that exposures below this dose cause damage to the cell but still leave it intact and able to function in a faulty way and to reproduce itself. Above this cut-off point, the cell dies. It is the living damaged cell which gives us the long-term problems such as leukemia and other cancers, heart diseases, etc. My research shows that the rise in leukemia usually associated with radiation exposure can be considered a secondary effect. By this I mean that the exposure causes one to age at a faster than normal rate, probably causing damage to one of the bioregulatory systems which under normal conditions break down more gradually with the passage of time. This model predicts a whole syndrome of problems usually associated with natural aging occurring at an earlier age for persons so exposed. Information needed to monitor this effect is not even being gathered."[2]

The relationship among free radicals, antioxidants, tumors, cancers, radiation, chemical pollutants, and aging is still a new and provocative subject area. Dr. Harry Demopoulos of New York University's Medical School Department of Pathology has said, "Free radical pathology is as great a breakthrough in medicine as Pasteur's germ theory of disease."

BOOSTING YOUR IMMUNITY

We are currently seeing a sharp increase in immunological dysfunctions and diseases. Cancer, tumors, AIDS, Epstein-Barr virus (which especially affects older or less healthy people), mononucleosis, hepatitis, herpes, yeast infections, and other bacterial and viral problems are just some of the manifestations of a compromised and weakened immune system. We have also seen a dramatic rise in the number and variety of chronic degenerative diseases. Because these trends are happening at a time when we are beginning to experience the cumulative effects of toxins, evidence suggests that there is a direct relationship between many modern diseases and the pollutants that pervade our air, water, soil, and food.

Radiation, environmental pollutants, drugs, and other common toxic substances severely strain our immune system, leaving us vulnerable now and in the future to a wide range of acute and chronic disorders. We cannot efficiently cope with toxins without a strong immune system.

Dr. J. A. Bellanti, author of *Immunology* (W. B. Saunders, 1978), defines immunity thus: "The immunologic response may be viewed as an adaptive system in which the body attempts to maintain homeostasis [equilibrium] between the internal body environment and the external environment." Scientific studies published in various medical journals confirm that deficiencies and imbalances in nutrients can disrupt the proper functioning of the immune system. Excesses in certain substances such as fats, or prolonged, extreme excesses in a few nutrients such as the fat-soluble vitamins A, D, and E, and the minerals copper and iron, can also diminish immunological response.[3,4]

Optimum nutrition is the primary determinant of a person's ability to maintain a healthy immune system. Common factors can prevent individuals from obtaining adequate, let alone optimum, levels of nutrients. Those factors include:
- inadequate nutrition
- excessive dieting
- poor dietary habits
- physical stress such as exposure to toxins
- emotional stress
- illness and chronic disease
- drugs
- surgery

Vitamins, minerals, and other food substances that significantly strengthen the immune system have been extensively documented in numerous scientific studies. Much of the following information on immunity has been gathered from the investigative reports of the Nutritional Advisory Group of the American Medical Association (a group that until recently has been skeptical about the effectiveness and safety of natural therapies). Refer to Chapters 4-7 in Part II for a thorough discussion of each specific nutrient, including recommended dosage levels.

Vitamin A is fat-soluble and occurs naturally in two forms: 1) that which is known as carotene, beta-carotene, or pro-vitamin A, which is derived from plant sources and then converted in the body into vitamin A; and 2) that which is commonly known as vitamin A or pre-formed vitamin A because it is derived from animal sources that have converted carotene into vitamin A.

Both forms of vitamin A tone the mucous membranes, which are the first lines of defense against foreign toxins. Both forms also have proven instrumental in strengthening the immune system. However, pro-vitamin A beta-carotene is the more beneficial.

Optimum levels of either pre-formed or carotene vitamin A stimulate several immunological responses, including production of lymphocytes (T cells, which are involved in rejecting foreign tissue, regulating cellular immunity, and controlling the production of antibodies) and five classes of antibodies or immunoglobulins produced by B cells (lymphocytes that mature in the bone marrow).[5] Deficiencies of either form of vitamin A lead to a reduction in size and/or amount of T cells and B cells. This reduction in T cells and B cells resulting from vitamin A deficiency has been shown to increase the frequency and severity of immunologic disorders ranging from infections to cancers.[6]

In tests where prolonged, excessives doses of pre-formed vitamin A were given, the T cell response was affected negatively.[7] Such doses of pre-formed vitamin A can lead to toxicity. Pro-vitamin A carotene cannot be converted by the body into vitamin A quickly enough to cause toxicity. Hence, carotene is now being used by more clinicians in place of pre-formed vitamin A in order to eliminate toxicity.

Not all of the B vitamins have been adequately researched regarding their effect on the immune system. However, the B vitamins riboflavin (B2), pyridoxine (B6), pantothenic acid (B5), cyanocobalamin (B12), and folic acid have been conclusively shown to markedly benefit immune system response. See Chapter 5 for a thorough discussion of the B vitamins, how they counteract toxins and aid optimal health, their dosage levels, and food sources.

A riboflavin deficiency reduces the ability of animals to manufacture B cells and also decreases the production of antibodies, or immunoglobulins.[8-10] Riboflavin aids in the scavenging and neutralization of free radicals.[11]

A pyridoxine (B6) deficiency markedly reduces the production and efficacy of both B cells and T cells. A deficiency of pyridoxine causes atrophy of the lymph tissue, poor antibody production, diminished activity of the thymic hormone, and other basic disruptions of the complex immune system.[12, 13] B6 deficiency also disrupts the synthesis of protein and DNA. Protein and DNA counteract toxins, and their disruption causes further abnormalities in lymphocyte and immunoglobulin production.[14-17]

Pantothenic acid is sometimes known as vitamin B5. A pantothenic acid deficiency has a similar diminishing effect on the immune system as a riboflavin deficiency. A deficiency in pantothenic acid reduces the ability of mammals to manufacture B cells. A pantothenic acid deficiency also inhibits the production of antibodies, or immunoglobulins.[18]

An inadequate amount of vitamin B12 has several harmful effects upon the immune system. A B12 deficiency markedly inhibits the response of lymphocytes (leukocytes formed in lymphatic tissue). The deficiency causes a reduction in the ability of neutrophils (another form of white blood cell) to ingest and neutralize harmful foreign bacteria and cells. A B_{12} deficiency also decreases the bactericidal capacity of these white blood cells. Both lymphocytes and neutrophils act as scavengers for harmful foreign agents.[19, 20]

Folic acid is another B vitamin very important in regulating the immune system. A folic acid deficiency will depress immune functions in both humans and animals and can increase allergic reactions.[21-23]

Of all the essential nutrients, vitamin C has gained the most respect worldwide for its ability to stimulate and improve immune response. In 1970, two-time Nobel laureate Dr. Linus Pauling showed that vitamin C significantly increased the competence of the human immune system.[24]

Medical studies show that the body manufactures more antibodies when given high amounts of vitamin C.[25, 26] According to a 1976 study reported in the *New England Journal of Medicine*, vitamin C significantly improves the ability of white blood cells to scavenge for and ingest harmful toxins.[27] This is a process referred to in medicine as the "phagocytic white blood cell function of the immune system."

Vitamin C has been proven to stimulate the immune system's ability to neutralize free radicals.[28, 29] It has proven helpful in treating cancers and other chronic degenerative diseases[30-32] and viral infections such as hepatitis.[33]

Numerous studies show that vitamin E improves the immune system's response to a variety of foreign, harmful substances, including toxins, bacteria, viruses, and pollens, when given in amounts larger than the general RDA.[34-47] Vitamin E stimulates production of antibodies.

In one test-tube study, when vitamin E was given in megadoses for a prolonged period of time, inhibition of the immune system was reported in a few subjects.[48] However, this observation was based on only one set of test-tube experiments, and the doses were massive amounts over a prolonged period of time. Although vitamin E is fat-soluble, as are vitamins A and D, it is relatively nontoxic compared to those vitamins. It is an important antioxidant that both aids the immune system's scavenging of free radicals and helps prevent some chronic degenerative diseases.[49, 50] From the findings of a wealth of scientific research, it is obvious that vitamin E, in recommended amounts, is essential to optimum functioning of the immune and other systems.

Calcium has been documented as improving several functions of the immune system, some of which include regulating lymphocyte and neutrophil function, and the synthesis and functioning of prostaglandins.[51-54] (Prostaglandins are hormone-like substances, formed in blood platelets, that boost production of T cells.)

Copper is a trace element found in all body tissues. It is an element essential to a wide range of normal metabolic activity. It is present in many enzymes that both break down or build up body tissue. Copper is involved in protein metabolism and thus in immunologic and healing processes. It aids in the formation of hemoglobin and red blood cells by facilitating iron absorption.

It is important to take in appropriate amounts of copper; both deficiencies and excesses can have adverse effects on the immune system. Abnormal copper levels were found in humans with immunodeficiency disorders,[55] and imbalances increased the severity of infections in laboratory animals.[56-59] A copper deficiency caused rats to have an inadequate immune response during infection. They were unable to produce the phagocytic cells needed to ingest and neutralize harmful substances.[60] Excessive copper has been documented as a contributing factor in free radical tissue damage, heart disease, lymph tumors, arthritis, leukemia, Hodgkin's disease, and several other degenerative diseases.[61, 62]

Cobalt, a component of vitamin B12, is involved in the maintenance and function of enzymes and enzymatic and other metabolic functions, red blood cells, and many other body cells. Because cobalt and B12 are so closely connected, the two terms are often used interchangeably. In a series of experiments, cobalt was shown to increase the ability of neutrophils to devour harmful invaders. Cobalt also increases the capacity of comparatively large macrophages in the white blood cells to gobble up, or phagocytize, foreign harmful substances.[63] In order to be of benefit, cobalt must be ingested as a form of vitamin B12.

An appropriate amount of the mineral iron is important for a vital immune response. Like copper, however, both deficiencies and excesses in iron can produce adverse effects on the immune system, resulting in increased susceptibility to infectious diseases and chronic degenerative disorders. An iron deficiency increases the number and severity of infections while it decreases the amount and effectiveness of white blood cells, T cells, and the capacity of phagocytic cells to eliminate harmful intruders.[64-71]

On the other hand, prolonged, excessive intake of iron has been linked to bacterial infections, free radical tissue damage, cancer, heart disease, and other degenerative diseases.[72-74] Extremely malnourished individuals from poor Third World countries have developed severe infections, many dying, from excessively high initial doses of iron. Their bodies had not been given time to adapt to metabolizing iron.[75-80]

Iodine likewise aids the immune system.[81] However, according to one study, iodine fed to cattle in excessive amounts produced decreased

antibody response, lowered lymphocyte response, and diminished phagocytic activity of neutrophils, the first of the white blood cells to reach an
invader.[82]

Mammals given a diet deficient in magnesium developed leukocytosis,
a persistent increase in white blood cells.[83-88] If the magnesium deficiency
was not corrected, the leukocytosis continued and developed into leukemia
and lymphoma (lymph tumor).[89-91]

According to one study, manganese stimulates macrophages in white
blood cells to more efficiently search out and destroy invaders during the
immune response.[92] Good sources of manganese are brown rice, brown rice
polishings, wheat bran, whole-grain cereals, egg yolks, nuts (especially walnuts), seeds, green vegetables, and spices. A significant percentage of the
manganese in food is lost, however, during any milling and processing; and
the manganese content of foods will vary depending on the amount present
in the soil in which they are grown. Soils that are very alkaline have abnormally low amounts of manganese. The recommended amount of manganese for adults is three to nine milligrams daily. The optimal diet recommended in Part III supplies approximately six to eight milligrams.

Selenium has been shown to be an immunostimulant[93] and to augment
the effects of vaccines.[94] When there is a deficiency of selenium, the
important anti-bacterial activity of neutrophils is disrupted.[95] When
ingested in appropriate quantities, selenium has a protective and therapeutic
action against a variety of carcinogenic agents.

It has been documented that a deficiency in zinc impairs the functioning of the immune system. There are no major body storage areas for zinc,
and only about ten percent of the zinc in food is absorbed by humans;
deficiencies in zinc can therefore develop rapidly.

Studies show that a deficiency in zinc has adverse effects on lymph
tissue, on T cell and B cell production, and on the number of
lymphocytes.[96-101] Other studies demonstrate that a zinc deficiency
decreases the scavenging activity of cells.[102, 103] Conversely, optimum levels
of zinc in humans were shown to increase the phagocytic capacity of white
blood cells to neutralize toxins.[104] As with several other vital nutrients, both
prolonged deficiencies and excessive amounts can produce adverse effects.
Abnormal zinc levels have been found in patients with immunodeficiency
disorders.[105]

Several studies document the need for adequate protein in the diet to
maintain a healthy immune system.[106] Proteins are composed of amino
acids. Amino acids may be divided into two categories, essential and non-
essential. Essential amino acids are those which the human body cannot
make on its own, and which, therefore, must be derived from food sources.

Non-essential amino acids can be manufactured within the human body.

The importance of balancing the essential amino acids in order to obtain the best possible protein from foods cannot be over-emphasized. The ability of the immune system to produce antibodies is adversely affected by either deficits or excesses of single essential amino acids.[107] Continued deficiencies of the sulfur-containing amino acids, such as cysteine and methionine, lead to reduction of cells in lymph tissues.[108, 109] The amino acid cysteine also improves the scavenging of free radicals.[110]

A balanced essential amino acid treatment was shown to substantially stimulate the immune systems of seriously infected monkeys. The amino acids effected a significant increase in lymphocyte production and thus catalyzed recovery.[111]

Research indicates that essential amino acids can affect the B cells in the immune system since antibodies are formed from proteins.[112] Unfortunately, there is little research on the effects of non-essential amino acids on the immune system.

The National Research Council recommends that adults consume 0.42 grams of protein per day for each pound of normal body weight, and children a slightly higher ratio. Second only to water, protein is the most plentiful substance in the human body. Proteins make up many of the substances the human body uses in its complex immune response. For example, interferon, which recently drew widespread interest in the medical community, is an antiviral protein. Obviously, more research is needed on the effects of amino acids on immunity.

It is important to remember that radioactive and chemical toxins frequently lodge in the fat cells of our food sources and in our bodies. When we consume excess fats we also ingest more harmful toxins; and the more we store excess fat throughout our body, the more we store those dangerous toxins, which have widespread deleterious repercussions. In Part II, I'll describe how radioactive and chemical toxins harm the whole body, including the blood, lymph, organs, and glands, and the immune, reproductive, nervous, and skeletal systems.

Numerous studies have demonstrated that an excess of fats, or lipids, in the diet markedly diminishes immune functions. The first research to indicate that excess fats could have an adverse effect on the immune system took place in 1914. That study showed that cholesterol injected into animals depressed the phagocytic function of white blood cells.[113] Increased cholesterol levels have subsequently been shown to have adverse effects on several immune functions. High cholesterol suppresses "host resistance," B cells, T cells, and the activity of phagocytes.[114-119]

Cholesterol levels can be increased by the overconsumption of foods high in saturated fats such as coconut oil, butter, cheese, beef fat, lard, eggs, and milk chocolate. Saturated fatty acids are usually hard at room temperature and, with the exception of coconut oil and a few other foods, come primarily from animal sources. Lecithin, however, apparently decreases cholesterol levels in some individuals and therefore frequently improves immunological response.

Several later studies confirmed that high levels of fats in the blood weaken the immune system and the capacity for phagocytosis.[120, 121] Obese mammals developed more severe infections and smaller-than-normal spleen and thymuses as compared to normal and slightly underfed control animals.[122, 123] When researchers investigated different kinds of fats, they found that both the type and amount of individual free fatty acids influenced lymphocytes and phagocytic cells.[124-126]

On the other hand, in appropriate amounts polyunsaturated fatty acids had a positive influence on the health of the immune system.[127-130] Polyunsaturated fatty acids are most commonly derived from seeds, vegetables, and nuts. Good sources include the oils made from sesame seeds, olives, sunflowers, wheat germ, soybeans, safflower seeds, corn, and cottonseed. Ocean fish are also an excellent source. Polyunsaturated fatty acids are usually liquid at room temperature.

It has been well documented that a deficiency in polyunsaturated fatty acids is potentially harmful to the immune system's important B cells and T cells.[131-134] Optimum levels of them have a healthy influence on scavenger white blood cells and lymphocytes.[135-137]

One study showed that excessive ingestion of fatty acids can impair a wide range of immune responses.[138] Again, taking in balanced amounts of polyunsaturated fatty acids is a key consideration, as both deficiencies and excesses can be harmful to the immune system.

As I noted in the previous chapter, research and documentation have shown that heavy metals and other environmental pollutants have highly toxic effects. Cadmium, lead, and mercury, three common heavy metals, have been shown to have a harmful effect directly on the immune system. Excess cadmium in the body severely reduces the formation and activity of antibodies.[139-142] It suppresses the phagocytic activity of the white blood cells[143, 144] and increases the susceptibility to and severity of infections, while increasing vulnerability to other toxins.[145, 146] Lead's harmful and varied effects on the immune system are similar to cadmium's. Oral ingestion of even minute, subtoxic (below common toxicity levels) amounts decrease immune responses to infectious bacteria, viruses, and toxins.[147, 148] Lead reduces the response of certain antibodies[149, 150] and also disrupts the immune response of splenic lymphocytes.[151] Mercury can adversely disrupt formation of lymph tissue,[152] and even minute amounts of it decrease the resistance of the immune system.[153, 154]

For information on how several herbs strengthen and stimulate the immune system and detoxify the blood and lymph, refer to the discussion of *Panax ginseng* and *Eleutherococcus* in Chapter 6, and Herbal Formulas One, Two, and Three in Chapter 9.

CHAPTER 4

Fighting Radiation
& Chemical Toxins
with Food

What follows in this chapter and the three subsequent ones is an abundance of scientific evidence to support the use of food and food substances in the prevention and treatment of ill effects due to radiation and environmental pollutants. However, the research available on the subject is still very much in its infancy. A great deal of work still needs to be done if science and medicine are to ever fully understand the powerful and multifaceted role diet plays as a radio- and chemical protectant.

As the studies reported in the following sections indicate, food can play a key role in our ability to withstand and overcome the effects of radiation and chemical toxicity. And it works in a wide variety of ways: by strengthening the immune system, by preventing assimilation of toxic substances, by scavenging for and joining with free radicals, by binding with contaminants already in the system, and by cleansing the tissues and stimulating the organs of detoxification. The studies show that certain foods and food substances can both prevent and treat the effects of radiation and chemical pollutants. They are powerful weapons in the fight against a devastating worldwide problem.

In reporting this research, I have had to rely heavily on animal data. Obviously, it would be unconscionable to expose humans to radioactive or chemical toxins merely to test various food substances for their protective qualities. Aware of this ethical and scientific dilemma, researchers have used other mammals in their studies. (The ethical considerations of animal studies also deserve more attention.) Such research demonstrates that humans and animals usually react similarly to radiation and chemical pollutants, and to the remedies that counteract these toxins. Where human research has existed, it is mentioned. Significantly, well over one-third of all the studies reported in this book have been conducted on humans, and the results are most encouraging.

I have tried to avoid reporting product-sponsored research, since it can be biased. The preponderance of the research mentioned here is from American scientists; yet I frequently have cited studies done in other parts of the world, especially from countries in Europe and the Far East, where traditional remedies and a reliance upon nutritive therapies are still part of the cultural fabric of society. Scientific concern about radiation and environmental pollutants, and the desire to find safe and reliable remedies, have become worldwide issues.

Where possible, I have given recommended quantities for prevention and therapy. For the most part, the healthful diet described in Chapter 8 will provide an abundance of the necessary nutrients and can protect against absorption of radiation and environmental pollutants under normal conditions. Such a diet alone would probably have protected most humans before the twentieth century, when a more active lifestyle and an often more healthful environment were more common. Today, from the time of fetal development through the golden years, our food, air, water, soil, and indoor environments are infused with radiation, chemical pollutants, and drugs. Our immune and detoxification systems are weakened to varying degrees. There are few among us who can claim full health and optimal vitality while living today's lifestyle.

Even if we could claim a consistent and satisfactory degree of health and vitality, unavoidable, daily, "low-level" exposure to radiation and other toxins is a highly stressful event for the human body and such trying conditions may well warrant preventive doses of certain nutrients, herbs, and supplements. Certainly in the event of an intensive exposure—such as certain x-rays and radiotherapy, regular cigarette smoke, routine exposure to a more highly polluted or radioactive environment, or increased toxins in what we consume—one may safely take the therapeutic dosages recommended. In the event of an emergency, such as a nuclear reactor accident or a spill during the transportation or storage of a chemical toxin, one could take 20-25 percent more than the therapeutic amounts described, though not for more than two weeks. The dosages I recommend are conservative to be on the safe side.

There are some readers who would prefer not to rely on any pills, supplements, or even herbs, which are really just potent wild plants and should be viewed as medicinal vegetables, to enhance their health. I have observed during my two decades of clinical experience that most people's health is improved with the wise use of selective natural supplements, or therapeutic herbs. Traditional natural healing systems from around the world have relied upon concentrated natural substances to improve health. For readers who do prefer to rely only on diet, exercise, and a religious/spiritual practice, let me suggest an experiment. During a period of your life that is typical for stress levels and other factors, try the preventive program outlined here for three to six months, or the therapeutic program for one to two months. Then evaluate, with an open mind, the changes in your health. If you don't feel healthier, drop most of the program and keep what feels right.

If you feel healthier, continue with the program or modify it slightly. Use the preventive program as a transition diet, the optimal program as what it is--an optimal dietary and health program. Once you have been on the optimal program for several months or more and you feel consistently healthy and vital, feel free to experiment again by reducing or changing the amounts of supplements.

When using supplements, it is essential to keep in mind that the increase of one vitamin or mineral will require increases in other complementary nutrients. The body is a symphony of chemical reactions. Nutrients work together to bring about healthy metabolism. For example, calcium cannot be metabolized without adequate amounts of vitamin D and phosphorus. The same considerations apply to other nutrients. These nutrients are noted where necessary.

Supplements and herbs have obviously proven quite helpful, but even their benefits are enhanced by a healthful diet--whole foods as they have been used since the dawn of humanity. It is a basic premise of this book that protection against radiation and chemical pollutants begins with a healthful whole foods diet, one that is rich in all essential vitamins, minerals, amino acids, carbohydrates, fats, and fiber. Supplements are regarded as just that—supplemental to a healthy way of eating and living.

What follows in Part II is important because you will learn how each food, herb, or supplement specifically protects you and affects different bodily processes, how to use these natural substances, the correct dosage, and possible contra-indications, and some of the other major health benefits of these substances. Equally important, you will learn which foods, herbs, and supplements effectively counteract each specific common radioisotope and chemical pollutant. Moreover, you will learn how these substances generate resistance, detoxification, and optimal health and well-being.

SEA VEGETABLES

There is no family of foods more protective against radiation and environmental pollutants than sea vegetables. All sea vegetables contain radioprotective properties. And as we will see, specific sea vegetables can prevent assimilation of different radionuclides, heavy metals such as cadmium, and other environmental toxins.

One of the more powerful protective elements in sea vegetables is sodium alginate, found in the family of sea vegetables known as kelp, which includes arame, wakame, kombu, and hijiki. Sodium alginate reduces the amount of strontium-90 absorbed by bone tissue by 50 to 83 percent, according to studies done by Yukio Tanaka and other scientists at the Gastro-Intestinal Research Laboratory of McGill University in Montreal.[1-3] Research also indicates that sodium alginate helps protect humans from the damaging effects of other common radioactive and environmental contaminants.

Radioactive strontium-90 is one of the more prevalent sources of radiation. It is a key element of fallout and low-level radiation due to worldwide atomic bomb testing, nuclear power plant leaks, and routine emissions. Strontium-90 and cesium-137 were two of the more plentiful radioisotopes released during the Chernobyl accident.

Today almost everyone has significant amounts of strontium-90 in their bones. It stays in the body throughout the lifetime and, like most other radioisotopes and chemical pollutants, it does not produce one unique symptom or disease associated with its long-term effects. Rather, its effects show up as statistical increases in the incidence of already known conditions and diseases. Among the serious problems caused by strontium-90 are leukemia, sarcoma of the bones (bone cancer), Hodgkins disease, anemia, and decreased production of red and white blood cells.

When analyzing the probability of bone cancer as a result of exposure to strontium-90, researchers S. C. Skoryna et al. found that strontium-90 closely parallels radium in that the greater the dose of radiation, the greater the probability of developing bone sarcoma, and that even the smallest possible dose of strontium-90 is capable of producing sarcomas.[4] They concluded that even minuscule amounts of strontium-90 would, over the years, certainly cause an appreciable increase in the frequency of death from bone sarcoma.

Radioactive strontium in the human diet enters the small intestine, is absorbed into the bloodstream, and then is deposited primarily in the bones. The sodium alginate in sea vegetables binds, or chelates, with the radioactive isotope in the gastrointestinal tract, forming an insoluble gel-like salt called strontium alginate, which is then safely excreted in the feces.

An experiment conducted by J. F. Stara at the Environmental Toxicology Laboratory of the Environmental Protection Agency showed that sodium alginate significantly reduced the amount of radioactive strontium absorbed in the bones of cats.[5] Stara observed that radioactive strontium in the bones is re-secreted into the intestines where it is bound by alginate, neutralized, then excreted in the stool. Both Stara and Tanaka have concluded that alginate can be used not only as a preventive but also as a therapeutic measure against radioactive strontium poisoning. The researchers have also studied other forms of hazardous environmental pollutants, and in 1971 reported, "The chemical pollution in air, soil, and water is particularly serious, since the pollutants find their way into the food chain and their absorption into the body can be hazardous. We have been interested for several years in metal pollution, including radionuclides. . . Our investigation has shown that alginate can bind radioactive strontium, one of the most hazardous pollutants, effectively in the gastrointestinal tract, thus preventing its absorption into the body, and it now shows that alginate binds with other metal pollutants such as excess barium, cadmium, and zinc."[6]

Although Tanaka used rats and other mammals in his early research,[7] he tested human volunteers in latter experiments.[8] All of these experiments produced similar results—showing that alginate is an effective preventive and therapeutic substance against radiation and heavy metals.[9]

In two experiments using rats, sodium alginate decreased, by a factor of up to twelve, the uptake of several radioactive isotopes—including strontium-90, strontium-85, barium, radium, and calcium.[10, 11] And in a British study, sodium alginate was shown to reduce, by at least fourfold, absorption and retention of both strontium-85 and strontium-90.[12]

In a 1965 study, Skoryna, et al., concluded that the ingestion of small but regular doses of alginate is effective in preventing the daily absorption of small doses of radioactive strontium and other contaminants that are present in the environment. For protection against higher doses of radioactive strontium, the researchers suggested that people could temporarily increase their intake of alginate to produce more effective results. Brown sea vegetables, such as kelp, were the most effective sources of sodium alginate for reducing the danger from radioactive strontium.[13]

In another experiment, the addition of 2.5 percent sodium alginate to the total diet of leghorn hens produced a 20 to 45 percent reduction of radioactive strontium-85 in bones, muscles, and egg shells.[14] When sodium alginate intake was doubled, there was no significant improvement in results compared to the 2.5 percent diet. This experiment illustrates the importance of finding optimal therapeutic dosages of protectants to avoid unnecessary overdoses of some substances. A few substances, such as vitamins A and D, can have toxic side effects if overused.

Alginate is nontoxic and is not reabsorbed into the rest of the body from the gastrointestinal tract. Alginate is specific and consistent in its reaction, is resistant to stomach acidity and the enzymes present in the gastrointestinal tract, and it is inexpensive. It has also been shown to have no adverse effect on the ability of humans—both adults and children—to assimilate calcium and other natural minerals.

In 1964 D. Waldron Edward, et al., reported that sodium alginate, derived from brown sea vegetables, suppressed the absorption of radioactive strontium from ingested food material, while permitting calcium to be available to the body.[15] In later experiments, Skoryna and other researchers investigated the possibility that long-term feeding of sodium alginate might eventually cause a calcium deficiency because of its chelating or binding effects.[16] They exposed young rats to varying intensities of radiation and gave them different dosages of sodium alginate. Even at the highest dosage levels of sodium alginate (20 percent of the total diet), a very large amount of calcium was still available for absorption from the intestine. For over three months at this highest dosage level, the physical appearance and general condition of the exposed rats were excellent. The growth of the young rats was only slightly less than that of the control group. Calcium uptake by the bones of young rats fed at the lower sodium alginate level (1.4 percent of the total diet) for three months was not significantly different from control values. This is of particular relevance to children and people with bone disorders because the experiments were conducted on growing rats at a formative period in their skeletal development.

Besides binding with several radioactive isotopes, sodium alginate attracts, bonds with, and helps remove many of the metallic environmental pollutants, including lead, cadmium, barium, strontium, excess iron, plutonium, and cesium. After attracting and reacting with these pollutants, sodium alginate transforms them into harmless salts for safe elimination from the body.[17]

Other research indicates that different sea vegetables have a propensity to bind with and neutralize various heavy metals. Brown sea vegetables, such as hijiki, arame, kombu, and others bind excess strontium and iron. Red sea vegetables, such as dulse, are the most effective at binding plutonium, and green algae bind cesium most effectively.[18]

Beckmann demonstrated that sodium alginate does not bind the important electrolytic minerals sodium or potassium and therefore does not reduce the supply of these ions to the metabolism.[19] Electrolytes, substances in the body that produce electrical charges, are involved in many basic bodily functions, such as nerve impulses, muscle activity, heart function, and metabolism.

The United States Atomic Energy Commission has recognized the efficacy of sodium alginate for reducing radiation toxicity. According to the Division of Biomedical and Environmental Research of the A.E.C., maximum protection against radioactive poisoning for humans requires taking a minimum of two to three ounces of sea vegetables a week or 10 grams (two tablespoons) a day of alginate supplements. During or after direct exposure to radiation, the dosage should be increased to two full tablespoons of alginate four times daily to insure that there is a continual supply in the gastrointestinal tract. A somewhat less precise dosage recommendation would be to double the amount of sea vegetables suggested in the optimal diet in Chapter 8.

The important point is that the regular use of sodium alginate in one's diet will help counteract the effects not only of radiation but of many environmental pollutants. If taken as a supplement, alginate—whether in powder or tablets—is more effective when mixed with sufficient fluids to make a gelatinous substance.

Several experiments indicate that sodium alginate is completely safe to ingest.[20] Sodium alginate preparations have been used in the food and pharmaceutical industries without evidence of ill effects. The only adverse effect from sodium alginate was an occasional delay in transit time (elimination of feces) or even constipation, probably due to the gelatinous, nonabsorbable nature of alginate. However, there is rarely a problem with constipation if sodium alginate is made into a fruit gelatin (see recipes, Chapter 8). Sodium alginate was equally effective whether injected directly into the intestines, introduced by tubes into the stomach, or administered in the more traditional manner of ingestion with food.[21]

The normal recommended daily dosage of kelp is one to two teaspoons of the dried granules sprinkled on food as a salt substitute, or five to ten tablets daily, or a small handful of whole kelp which has been presoaked and cooked.

Agar, which is derived from the sodium alginate in kelp, is a safe, nontoxic substance that can be used as a thickening agent or gelatin. It can be purchased at most health or natural foods stores. This form of alginate can be made into tasty fruit gelatins.

It is best not to increase the recommended dosage of kelp or other sea vegetables unless you have been or will be exposed to more-than-usual levels of contaminants. There is a risk of assimilating too much iodine, which will be discussed next. In appropriate amounts, however, iodine is an important protector against a common radioactive isotope.

Radioactive iodine-131 is a byproduct of fission reactions. It is released during nuclear power plant emissions, both routine and accidental, and nuclear weapons tests. It is one of the most pervasive radioactive isotopes in our environment. Iodine-131 is used with x-rays for diagnosing the thyroid, lungs, and blood. Both iodine-131 and iodine-125 are used in radiotherapy. Gofman in *X-Rays: Health Effects of Common Exams* estimates that the use of radioactive iodine in the treatment of thyroid disorders, including cancer, increases the chances of contracting cancer of the thyroid by 25 percent.

If sufficient amounts of natural iodine are available, radioactive iodine will not be absorbed. If the supply of natural iodine is deficient, however, radioactive iodine is very readily absorbed by all mammals, especially humans. It concentrates primarily in the thyroid gland and secondarily in the reproductive organs. It is a very toxic, carcinogenic substance.

Fallout containing radioactive iodine settles on grazing land and, like strontium-90, becomes concentrated in milk products. Anyone who drinks milk or eats dairy products is therefore at a greater risk of being exposed to this dangerous isotope. However, radioactive iodine also can be inhaled from the air, or ingested with other foods.

Natural iodine is one of the abundant minerals present in sea vegetables, and it is necessary for healthy functioning of the thyroid. The thyroid gland directs metabolism, and therefore is essential to the healthy functioning of virtually every system of the body. Inadequate amounts of iodine will reduce production of thyroid hormones, thus decreasing metabolism and, among other things, causing diminished absorption of nutrients. The result is reduced energy, weight gain, chronic lethargy, and a depleted immune system.

Iodine is also necessary for healthy functioning of the nervous system. Because iodine affects metabolism, nerves, and circulation, optimal amounts of iodine are necessary for a wide array of biological functions.

Though radioactive iodine has a comparatively short half-life of eight days, this does not mean it is less dangerous than other common radioactive isotopes. On the contrary, its short half-life causes it to emit radiation more rapidly than long-living isotopes. And despite its short half-life, the time it takes for iodine-131 to cause cancer can be deceptively long—twelve years or more. You should not be lulled into thinking that the possibly long delay in manifestation of symptoms means this is not a dangerous radioisotope. Iodine-131 is both a common and potentially lethal radioactive isotope.

According to Dr. Helen Caldicott, M.D., author of *Nuclear Madness*

(Bantam Books, 1979) and founder of Physicians for Social Responsibility, once a radioisotope lodges in a target gland, it will irradiate nearby tissue and can disrupt functions and possibly eventually cause cancer. All the blood in the human body passes through the thyroid every seventeen minutes, thus exposing all the blood to radiation. Radioactive iodine in the thyroid can cause severe, and potentially lethal, metabolic and other functional disorders in areas that were not initially irradiated.

Other serious problems can arise. Iodine-131 can accumulate in the ovaries of women or testicles of men, potentially leading to genetic disorders or mutations among children. Pregnant women, developing fetuses, and infants are most vulnerable to radioactive isotopes. Iodine-131 can accumulate in the thyroid of a developing fetus, where it concentrates a hundred times more than in the thyroid of an adult. As Caldicott notes, this intense concentration of radioactive iodine in the fetus can lead to a wide range of metabolic problems including reduced rate of growth, low birth weight, and increased infant mortality.

Natural iodine does more than both feed the thyroid gland so it can produce certain hormones and help prevent the assimilation of radioactive iodine. Once radioactive iodine is absorbed by the thyroid, taking natural iodine helps offset the side effects of exposure to and assimilation of radioactive iodine. According to the late Dr. Russell Morgan, who served as chief radiologist at Johns Hopkins University, one mg. of iodine for children and five mg. for adults taken daily will reduce by about 80 percent the radioactive iodine accumulated in the thyroid.[22-28]

Danish researchers found that iodine had a radioprotective effect in rats that were exposed to a single dose of 1,000 rads of gamma rays.[29] In this study, the effects of the radiation were observed on three groups of rats. The first was given iodine plus a calcium compound ($Ca2+$ or gluconolactobionate) for thirteen days prior to irradiation and twenty-one days after irradiation. The second group was given only the calcium compound during the same period. The third group was given nothing. Sixty-seven percent of the iodine-treated rats remained alive after thirty days, in contrast to 36 percent of the rats that received only $Ca2+$. Rats that received neither iodine nor $Ca2+$ died within three to five days after irradiation.

Another result from these studies was that renal calcification developed in 85 percent of the rats that received $Ca2+$, but in only 16 percent of the rats that had iodine added to the $Ca2+$. The researchers concluded that iodine has a significant radioprotective effect.

Preventing the absorption of radioactive iodine is a far more effective solution than trying to stockpile iodine compounds for (hopefully quick) distribution in the event of an emergency. The optimal diet for protection against fallout and radioactive isotopes supplies appropriate amounts of natural iodine.

Whole foods are the best source of iodine. The minerals in whole foods act synergistically in the body—each mineral reinforces the beneficial effects of the others. Sea vegetables contain iodine, sodium, potassium, calcium, magnesium, phosphates, sulfates, chlorides, bromides, and other nutrients in a well-balanced form. Moreover, many natural nutrients are usually easier to assimilate than ones that are artificially produced.

Inorganic iodine, such as is found in iodized salt, or iodine artificially made or separated from organic matter, can sometimes act as a local irritant, according to Edward Shook's *Advanced Treatise in Herbology* (Trinity Center Press, 1978), possibly producing or contributing to various forms of dyspepsia, indigestion, decreased ability to assimilate food, severe gastric pain, and other gastric disorders.

Unfortunately iodine is leached from the thyroid gland when we drink chlorinated tap water. Most cities in the U.S. now add chlorine to their drinking water. Our bodies are over 70 percent water, and our health is directly influenced by the quality of our drinking water. Because of the many radioactive and chemical pollutants in tap water, I strongly recommend that you consider drinking good quality bottled, filtered, or purified water. The cost is negligible compared to the health benefits. Excessive use of table salt also produces a similar effect of iodine depletion.

Another reason to avoid iodized salt is that salt, which contains excessive sodium and no potassium, is known to contribute to high blood pressure and hypertension. Humans need the mineral sodium, but only in a proper balance with potassium, calcium, and magnesium. These minerals, especially potassium and sodium, are important electrolytes. A favorable amount of these minerals offers significant protection from radiation. One can obtain all the sodium and potassium one needs, and in a proper balance, by eating whole, unprocessed foods.

Sea vegetables are rich in vitamins, contain all fifty-six minerals and trace elements identified as bodily requirements, plus they have other nutrients, many of which are known to offer protection against radiation or chemical pollutants. By weight of edible portion, sea vegetables as a group rank first among all foods in amounts of magnesium, iron, iodine, and sodium. They rank second in amounts of calcium and phosphorus. Sea vegetables are about 25 percent protein and 2 percent fat. They also contain beta-carotene, B_1, B_2, possibly some B_{12}, niacin, pantothenic acid, and vitamin E, as well as proteins, carbohydrates, the mineral selenium, and virtually all other minerals and trace elements required in human nutrition. The vitamin C (ascorbic acid) content of sea vegetables compares favorably with that found in green vegetables. Traces of vitamin D have also been found in a number of sea vegetables. In some instances, their vitamin, mineral, and trace element content is comparable to or greater than the richest land vegetable sources. Sea vegetables are highly nutritious while extremely low in calories. Many of the nutrients in sea vegetables will be discussed in later chapters as counteractants of radiation and chemical pollutants.

Another benefit of eating sea vegetables is that they help dissolve fat and mucus deposits. The body frequently stores environmental contaminants in fat or adipose tissue because they are not essential to life. By helping to dissolve fat deposits and by pulling some contaminants out of the body, sea vegetables can help detoxify from different types of radiation and industrial pollutants.

Sea vegetables—a traditional source of iodine throughout history—have been enjoyed as a daily food by the Japanese, Chinese, Icelanders, Scots, Irish, French, Welsh, Russians, Native Americans, and peoples of the South Pacific. Currently, certain sea vegetables and marine plants are widely used by the commercial food industry as food additives, and in their whole form sea vegetables are an important product category in the natural foods industry. They are available in several forms: dried whole leaves, powdered, or flaked. Sea vegetables present a new variety of flavors for the palate. If one is just beginning to eat sea vegetables, it might be better to start with the milder-tasting dulse, kombu, and arame, and then experiment with the more flavorful kelp, wakame, and hijiki.

Sea vegetables are macroscopic varieties of marine algae. They feed crustaceans and fish and ultimately support the whole life cycle of the oceans. Along with bee pollen, sea vegetables are one of the most concentrated food substances. As such, they are extremely valuable medicinally. However, their recommended daily dosage should not be exceeded or bodily balance may be further disrupted instead of being restored.

One-half ounce of kelp provides 21 mg. of iodine, and one-half ounce of dulse provides 1.12 mg. of iodine. The U.S. Recommended Daily Allowance (RDA) of iodine for adult women is 0.1 mg., and for pregnant or nursing women and adult men it is 0.15 mg.

Besides sea vegetables, other good sources of iodine include Swiss chard, turnip greens, wild garlic and onions, watercress, squash, mustard greens, watermelon, cucumber, spinach, asparagus, kale, egg yolks, seafoods, fish liver oils, and citrus and pineapple. However, foods grown in the Great Lakes area or Pacific Northwest are sometimes deficient in iodine due to variations in the soils' mineral content. If you garden, test your soil for iodine content and other important minerals such as calcium and magnesium.

If you are currently using a concentrated source of iodine for medical reasons, you should check with a physician or nutritional therapist before adding sea vegetables to your diet to avoid overstimulation of the thyroid gland. Overconsumption of iodine in any form should be avoided by people who are hyperactive or have cardiovascular problems, because the possible glandular overstimulation might also overstimulate the heart. More important is controlling the amount of fat and cholesterol in the diet, both of which are the underlying causes of most cardiovascular diseases.

Sea vegetables offer the nutrient resources of the sea in a wide spectrum of tastes and colors. Sea vegetables promote health, help prevent absorption of various toxins, and are highly concentrated, nutritious foods.

BEE POLLEN

Radiation exposure adversely decreases a number of bodily substances. These include antibodies, red and white blood cells, and levels of vitamins C and E in the blood. Fortunately, there's a powerful food substance—bee pollen—that has been proven to counteract the effect that radiation has on these important barometers of health. According to several respected European and Soviet gerontologists (researchers who study the factors relating to longevity and aging), bee pollen has been shown to be able to rejuvenate the body, stimulate organs and glands, enhance vitality, and bring about a longer life span.[30]

Bee pollen should not be confused with the pollen that is blown by the wind and is a common cause of allergies. Allergy-causing pollen is called anemophiles; it is light and easily blown by the wind. Bee pollen is heavier and stickier, and is collected off of bees' legs by special devices placed at the entrance to hives. It is called entomophiles or "friends of the insects," and will usually not cause allergy symptoms.

Human consumption of bee pollen dates back to ancient times. The practice of eating bee pollen is praised in the Bible, and has long been prescribed by traditional health practitioners for its healing properties. In herbal traditions, wildflowers and pollen are considered among the more potent and pure forms of medicine.

Bee pollen's ability to consistently and noticeably increase energy levels makes it a favorite substance among many athletes, and this current practice is also a tradition that can be traced back to the earliest Olympic Games in Greece. Interestingly, bee pollen contains most of the known nutrients, including all of those necessary for human survival. Several common nutrients in bee pollen, such as proteins, appropriate fats, vitamins A, B, C, and E, calcium, magnesium, selenium, nucleic acids, lecithin, and cysteine, will be discussed individually in subsequent chapters for their ability to counteract the effects of radiation and chemical toxins.

Imported pollen is usually older than domestic, has been fumigated during entry into the U.S., and is sometimes collected from bees that frequent sprayed flowers, or flowers grown in poor environmental conditions. For these reasons, imported pollen, if used initially in large quantities, has been observed to trigger an allergic response in a small percentage of people. One exception is pollen from Cernitin, a Swedish company, which produces high-quality bee pollen. Domestic or local pollen from unsprayed flowers has been used effectively to prevent and treat many allergies.

In a study conducted at the University of Vienna Women's Clinic, Dr. Peter Hernuss and his colleagues found that bee pollen significantly reduced the usual side effects of both radium and cobalt-60 radiotherapy in twenty-five women who had been treated for inoperable uterine cancer.[31] Hernuss took extensive blood samples from the patients at the beginning and end of the treatments. Each patient also completed detailed questionnaires. A number of blood tests designed to measure the various indices of general health revealed that the women who took the pollen were considerably healthier and had stronger immunological responses. These women registered beneficial increases in a number of areas, including red and white blood cell count, and serum protein level. The women also reported feeling an improved sense of well-being. When compared to women who received the same treatment but did not receive bee pollen, the researchers found that the bee pollen group suffered half as much nausea; one-fifth as many suffered from poor appetite after radiation treatments; half as many showed sleep disorders; half as many suffered urinary and rectal disorders; and one-third as many manifested general decline and weakness after treatment. The dosage of bee pollen received by these women was twenty grams, which is about three-quarters of an ounce, or approximately two tablespoons, taken three times per day.

Similar results were obtained by Izer Osmanagic, M.D., Ph.D., and his colleagues at the University Radiological Institute of Sarajevo, Yugoslavia. In 1973, they reported on a series of four experiments on humans and noted that bee pollen successfully corrected radiation sickness after massive abdominal x-rays, and that it improved the immune response.[32] They also found that x-rays break down some of the body's proteins, thus producing histamine, which then causes several allergic responses. Various laboratory analyses, and the patients' subjective reports, confirmed the therapeutic effectiveness of bee pollen.

In a 1948 issue of the *Journal of the National Cancer Institute*, William Robinson, a researcher at the U.S. Department of Agriculture, described a series of tests in which cancerous tumors were induced in mice.[33] One group of mice were fed bee pollen, after which the proliferation of cancer cells stopped. A control group of mice not fed the bee pollen experienced continued growth of cancer cells.

Researchers have also found that bee pollen protects mice against x-ray treatments. Researchers William Shipman and Leonard J. Cole at the Life Science Division of Stanford Research Institute (whose work was supported in part by grants from the American Cancer Society and the National Center for Radiological Health) found in 1971 that bee pollen strengthened the immune systems of mice and improved their resistance to x-rays. The researchers also reported that bee pollen has antibacterial properties.

In addition, bee pollen has been demonstrated to offer substantial protection from many common pollutants (including components of smog such as carbon monoxide and nitrogen dioxide, lead, mercury, DDT, cadmium, nitrates and nitrites) and the toxic side effects of many drugs. Bee pollen promotes healing of a wide variety of health problems. It has been shown to have both antibacterial and antiviral properties.

A common adult dosage of bee pollen is initially one-quarter teaspoon three times per day. The dosage is gradually increased to one-to-three teaspoons, three-to-four times per day. Adults suffering from allergies are best advised to start off at 1/32 of a teaspoon daily and then to increase very slowly, usually over a period of two weeks, to higher doses. Bee pollen is usually taken on an empty stomach in a variety of ways: by itself, mixed with water, or added to vegetable juice, soup, or other foods. It should not be cooked.

Bee pollen, and another food soon to be discussed, nutritional yeast, could have profound and worldwide ecological importance. They are inexpensive sources of protein and many other nutrients. Vast quantities can be produced with little use of soil compared to land used for crops.

BEE PROPOLIS

Bee propolis is another substance from the bee kingdom that has radioprotective, antibacterial, and antiviral effects when eaten. Like bee pollen, it is being rediscovered and put to use by athletes and other health-conscious people today.

What is bee propolis? It begins as a resinous material, gathered by bees from the leaf buds and bark of trees, especially poplars and conifers.

The final propolis is a mixture formed by the bees from this bee resin and wax, plus pollen, beebread, and other bee materials. It is a sealant and tightener for the hive, and it acts to protect bees from bacterial or viral infection and dangerous toxins.

In fresh condition, propolis is sticky, aromatic, soft, and tastes burningly bitter. It has a peculiarly pleasant aroma similar to birch or poplar buds, or sometimes to honey or vanilla. To be taken internally, propolis is usually administered in the form of a purified alcohol or water extract. Externally, it can be applied either as a solution or a salve.

According to researchers at the Second Leningrad Scientific Conference on the Application of the Products of Apiculture [bee culture] in Medicine and Veterinary Medicine in 1960, "The bee pollen of propolis is rich in pro-vitamin A [carotene], B$_1$, B$_2$, C, E, H [biotin], niacin, P [bioflavonoids], and others. It also contains up to .40 percent albumin substances."[34]

Bee propolis also contains a large number of protective minerals and trace elements, including calcium, magnesium, iron, copper, zinc, manganese, cobalt, and silica. There are many other substances and derivatives found in propolis, and several scientific tests show that it contains a whole complex of not-yet-identified components.

Like vitamin A, bee propolis has a tonifying and healing effect upon the important epithelial tissue of the body. Epithelial tissue is a membrane-like protective tissue that covers free surfaces such as the outer layer of the skin. It also forms the surface layer of mucous and serous membranes, lining the body's organs, glands, cavities, and ducts from the mouth to the gastrointestinal and genitourinary tracts. In other words, these nutrients fortify and protect internal and external "castle walls" of the body. Considered the body's first line of defense, epithelial tissue is involved in all infections, inflammations, and immunological problems due to internal or external harmful agents. It serves the general functions of enclosing and protecting, producing secretions and excretions, and acting to absorb nutrients. It also has specialized functions such as movement of substances through ducts, production of cells, and reception of stimuli.

Drs. F. C. Porchum and A. J. Borovaja have conducted clinical investigations into the use of bee propolis. They researched both its bactericidal properties and the effect propolis has on radioepithelitis (inflammation of epithelial tissue due to radiation).[35] They found propolis to be effective at the clinical stage of radioepithelitis. Alcohol solutions of propolis produced a therapeutic effect mainly in the first three stages of epithelitis. Propolis salves were therapeutic in more advanced cases of confluent epithelitis (conditions of merging sores) and in the stage of inflamed epithelial erosions.

Besides toning and healing epithelial tissue, bee propolis immobilizes infectious bacteria, viruses, and other harmful foreign agents. Propolis acts by surrounding the agent, sealing it up, and making it useless. In the human body, the propolis-wrapped virus can be destroyed and eliminated. Unlike penicillin and other drugs, propolis is consistently effective because bacteria and viruses cannot build a tolerance to it. Also, propolis does not seem to have any side effects.

Bioflavonoids are natural substances found in foods and function as companions to vitamin C (see Chapter 5). The rich concentration of bioflavonoids in propolis helps to protect against infections. How? Think of toxins as being enclosed in a protein coat. As long as the coat remains unbroken, the infectious and dangerous material remains imprisoned and is harmless to the organism. Bioflavonoids act to inhibit an enzyme which normally removes the protein coat, and thus the dangerous material is kept locked in. Bioflavonoids from such substances as propolis thus help strengthen immunity.

Bent Havsteen, M.D., formerly of Cornell University and now with Kiel University in West Germany, has made a thorough study of propolis and bioflavonoids. According to Havsteen, bee propolis also stimulates interferon production. Interferon is a natural protein substance that has been shown to combat many diseases. Havsteen notes that bioflavonoids stimulate white blood cells to produce interferon. And with this substance in the body, there is increased resistance to many infections.

Bee propolis appears to be a remarkable antibiotic that helps fight disease reactions within the body. It even helps control runaway cell breakdown, a condition symptomatic of cancer. Because propolis is still a newly rediscovered product containing a wide variety of substances and their derivatives, one should be cautioned against its excessive use—especially internally. Propolis's documented healing properties, however, definitely should be the subject of further research. I have used small amounts of bee propolis for several years in an "Immune System Building Tincture" I've developed (see Chapter 9, Herbal Formula Three).

FERMENTED FOODS

Radioactive fallout and chemical pollutants rain down on our food supply, or make their way into our food via waterways, underground wells, or through the very soil itself. Eventually, they are ingested by humans and lodge in the intestines, where they can damage sensitive tissues and cause far-reaching problems, including cancer.

Because of their especially beneficial effect on the intestines, fermented foods help to counteract these toxins in a number of important ways: They stimulate production of friendly intestinal bacteria, which promotes healthy digestion, and they assist the assimilation of nutrients, in particular the B vitamins. These functions act to directly counteract toxins, and equally important, to improve the immune system and help the body to detoxify.

A healthy intestinal environment promotes production and assimilation of B vitamins, which have been shown to help counteract radiation and environmental pollutants (see Chapter 5). Improvement in digestion also encourages the elimination of these harmful radioactive particles and chemical pollutants. Some forms of natural bacteria in fermented foods are said to metabolize, break down, and neutralize more than a hundred kinds of chemicals.

There are many health-promoting fermented foods that are widely available in natural foods and health food stores, including fermented soybean products such as miso, tempeh, tamari, and shoyu. Other fermented foods include popular condiments such as pickles and sauerkraut.

The human use of fermented foods goes back thousands of years, when due to the lack of refrigeration ancient peoples of necessity included naturally fermented foods in their diets. They also used seeds and grains to make fermented drinks, including beer and wine.

Yogurt is a fermented food that contains many beneficial bacteria and enzymes. It has been heavily promoted during the past decade as a healthful food, though in its frequently sweetened, additive-laden form it bears little resemblance to the traditional food that earned it its reputation. In addition, the problems associated with all dairy products may outweigh the benefits. This is particularly true when considering radiation, since cows' milk can contain comparatively high quantities of strontium-90 from fallout and nuclear power plant emissions. Also, the fat content of most dairy products can be a problem. Fat is a leading cause of heart disease, cancer, adult-onset diabetes, and other disorders. Studies have shown that fat also has a weakening effect on the immune system in general.

A dramatic anecdote for the use of fermented foods in the prevention and treatment of radiation sickness comes from Japanese medical doctor Shinichiro Akizuki, director of Saint Francis Hospital in Nagasaki and author of the book, *Physical Constitution and Food*. Akizuki was director of Saint Francis Hospital when the U.S. dropped the atomic bomb on Nagasaki in 1945. His hospital was only a mile from the center of the blast.

According to Akizuki, the staff at Saint Francis treated hundreds of people for radiation sickness in the aftermath of the explosion. He and his hospital staff remained at St. Francis, well within the fallout. However, none of his staff members became ill—a remarkable occurrence since they were so close to the epicenter of the explosion and were exposed to enormous doses of radioactivity. Akizuki hypothesized that it was the daily consumption of miso soup (miso is a fermented soybean paste) taken by him and his staff that protected them from the effects of the radiation.

Clearly, miso warrants further study. Because it is beneficial to intestinal health—which would provide indirect protection against many toxins, including radiation and chemical pollutants—it can be recommended on the basis of the scant but promising evidence. Certainly if you have taken antibiotics—either synthetic or a natural herbal antibiotic—which kill most forms of internal bacteria, both harmful and beneficial, it would be advisable to follow a course of treatment that included fermented foods such as miso.

Interestingly, a study done by Japan's National Cancer Center in the late 1970s found that Japanese who consume miso on a daily basis suffer 33 percent less stomach cancers than non-consumers of miso, and 18 percent less than occasional consumers.

Many varieties of misos are available through natural foods stores and mail order markets throughout the United States. Some of the misos that are mass-produced and packaged are pasteurized, which raises the question of whether important bacteria are still alive in the miso. Unpasteurized miso is available, as well, and is recommended over the pasteurized varieties.

There is a drawback to miso of which consumers should be conscious. Miso contains sodium, and some misos, especially the ones that are aged for two years, such as hatcho, contain as much as 17 percent sodium. High sodium consumption is among the causes of high blood pressure. As long as one does not overindulge in miso, and one consumes a diet low in fat and cholesterol, miso can be a highly beneficial food in anyone's diet.

Making one's own fermented foods is not that difficult and can be well worth the effort. Instructions can be found in many natural foods cookbooks and holistic health magazines. It is best to eat small amounts of fermented products at first, as their introduction into the diet may cause temporary digestive upset in some people. Since fermented foods are living, cultured products, they are most beneficial when not heated above 130 degrees F., which kills many friendly bacteria.

GRAINS

There is promising research being conducted on the radioprotective qualities of the grains millet and buckwheat by Hansgeorg Weidner of Germany, who reports that the whole buckwheat plant, including seeds and blossoms, offers protection. Buckwheat contains rutin, a bioflavonoid, which Dr. P. V. Atkins has shown to offer some radiation protection and to stimulate the renewal of bone marrow.[36] The rutin in buckwheat also helps strengthen capillary walls.

Buckwheat and even more so millet are more complete proteins than the other grains. However, all whole grains contain nutrients and properties that protect against radioactive and chemical toxins. These nutrients include calcium, iron, magnesium, potassium, selenium, zinc, and vitamins B and E. Grains contain fiber and phytic acid (phytates) that, it may be implied from a number of studies, bind with and neutralize radioactive and chemical toxins.[37-42] Grains also help promote a neutral metabolic pH, which has been shown to help diminish the malignancies resulting from x-irradiation.[43]

Despite popular misconceptions, grains are nourishing while being low in fat and calories. Many traditional cultures from around the world have made grains the mainstay of their diet. Cooked grains help regulate energy and blood sugar levels. Unlike sugary foods and even fruits, cooked whole grains digest at a moderate rate producing a normal blood sugar level over a long period of time. Consequently, many progressive nutritionists now recommend that cooked whole grains be the basis of an optimal diet.

BEETS

Traditional healers and naturopaths have long used small amounts of beet root as a natural remedy for inflammation of nerve cells, anemia, several liver, kidney, and blood disorders, and other diseases. Beets are thus a promising protectant food since, in addition to diminishing both red and white blood cell production, and thereby causing anemia and other blood disorders, radiation also disrupts nerve cell function and causes disturbances in the stomach, liver, and intestines.

Beets are rich in nutrients, especially iron and other minerals. Studies done in Germany have demonstrated that beet juice, raw or fermented, is helpful in a variety of blood conditions, including anemia, which are often associated with iron deficiencies. Because of their beneficial effects on the blood and circulatory system, beets have long been considered a regenerative food by traditional and folk healers.

Beets have been shown to rebuild hemoglobin of the blood after exposure to radiation.[44] Rats fed a diet of 20 percent beet pulp were able to prevent cesium-137 absorption 97 to 100 percent more effectively than rats exposed to the same radiation but given no beets.[45]

Since beets are rich in iron, according to the principle of selective uptake they can help prevent the absorption of plutonium-238, iron-55, iron-59, and plutonium-239. The roots are preferable to the beet greens because of the presence of oxalic acid in the greens. Oxalic acid, which at high levels can prevent absorption of minerals, can also adversely affect people suffering from kidney stones and other kidney-related problems.

DRIED, PRIMARY-GROWN, NUTRITIONAL YEAST

Nutritional yeast is a tiny, one-celled plant, 1/4000th of an inch in diameter or about the size of a human blood corpuscle. Grown specifically for human consumption, nutritional yeast (*Saccharomyces cerevisiae*) is, like bee pollen, a high-powered and concentrated food that can protect against radiation and environmental pollutants.

Nutritional yeast contains an abundance of protein (some brands of dried yeast contain as much as 50 percent protein), a good balance of essential amino acids, and a rich supply of vitamin B-complex (it contains all of the B vitamins, in fact, except B_{12}, which is now included in some brands of yeast). Nutritional yeast has a much higher percentage of protein and B-complex vitamins than eggs, milk, liver, or beef. Nutritional yeast also contains at least eighteen minerals, including many key trace minerals. One of these minerals, selenium, is an important antioxidant which protects the body against radiation and pollution damage. Selenium also provides some protection of the body's genetic material (DNA) from destruction or mutation resulting from exposure to radioactive or chemical contaminants. In addition, selenium prevents the oxidation of vitamin E, an important vitamin which counteracts radiation and toxic chemicals. Nutritional yeast also contains the nucleic acids DNA and RNA, both of which have been shown to have radioprotective qualities.[46]

In 1963, researchers in the U.S.S.R. reported that a dried, edible, food-grade yeast of the strain *Saccharomyces cerevisiae* significantly helped to build and regenerate cells damaged by radiation.[47] In Linda Clark's book *Are You Radioactive?* (Pyramid Books, 1973), the German researcher Dr. Holger Metz notes that this strain produced the following relief from radiation damage in human beings: "No redness of skin, very little loss of hair, no mucous membrane inflammation, no depression, quick recovery of physical condition, and good blood picture."

In a study done at New York's Montefiore Hospital, human cancer patients were given three tablespoons of yeast daily for one week before receiving heavy doses of irradiation. Those patients receiving yeast remained free of symptoms. Patients not given yeast developed severe vomiting, a decrease in hemoglobin, and marked anemia.[48]

Sometimes exposure to radiation or strong chemical pollutants produces a delayed tumor growth which can be cancerous. However, a survey made by Miller, et al., of thirty-four diets, demonstrated that dietary supplements rich in both protein and B vitamins, particularly riboflavin (B_2), inhibit tumor formation.[49] Yeast is rich in both protein and the B vitamins. Similar findings have been reported by K. Sugiura, who induced liver tumors in rats by feeding them a brown rice diet containing yellow dye. The animals were then transferred to dye-free rations of either brown rice alone or brown rice supplemented with yeast. The incidence of liver tumors was significantly lowered in the rats given the rice with yeast.[50]

Some brands of nutritional yeast have a good balance of important protective minerals such as calcium, magnesium, iron, zinc, chromium, and potassium. Yeast can be a good source of iron in a natural, bioavailable form. (Synthetic iron sulphate, the type usually found in drugstore supplements, can cause constipation, and may decrease or prevent the assimilation of vitamin E.)

Anemias frequently result from exposure to radiation or chemical pollution. Most anemias are best treated with iron, B_{12}, folic acid, and B_6— taken with the whole B-complex. Nutritional yeast contains a good amount of all these nutrients and is therefore excellent for treating the anemia side effects of radiation or chemical toxicity.

Primary-grown yeasts bond with and absorb heavy metals such as uranium, lead, and mercury.[51] Besides heavy metals, yeasts also protect against other common pollutants including carbon monoxide, DDT, nitrates, nitrites, and against the side effects of many drugs.

Most brands of nutritional yeast have a pleasant, nutty flavor, superior to that of brewer's or torula yeasts. Indeed, nutritional yeasts are commonly referred to as "good-tasting yeasts." Individuals and stores would be well advised to request that the yeast companies they purchase from state how their nutritional yeast has been produced. Until recently, most commercial nutritional yeasts were either brewer's yeast, a byproduct of the brewing industry, or torula yeast, a byproduct of the paper industry. Both of these yeasts are now considered inferior by nutritional therapists, since they may pick up some of the many chemicals and other undesirable materials used during the brewing or wood pulping processes. Although brewer's yeast is de-bittered to remove the contaminating oils, the recovered end product is the barely edible, awful-tasting powder that alienated some people from "health foods." Also, this de-bittering process results in the loss of some protein, minerals, and trace elements from the product.

Nutritional yeasts that are "primary-grown" are cultivated on food media that are of higher quality than the ones used to grow torula or brewer's yeasts. The media are often enriched as well, so that the resulting nutritional yeast contains more nutrients than brewer's yeast or torula yeast.

Some nutritional yeast companies add nutrients to their finished product in order to artificially boost or fortify the yeast after it is grown. Unfortunately, this practice produces inferior yeast. Most companies now grow their yeast on a rich medium such as sugar beet molasses, or by adding nutrients while the yeast is growing. These two processes bind the nutrients into the yeast cells as the yeast grows, thereby simulating the natural process whereby edible plants take up nutrients from the soil. The resulting yeasts are rich in easily assimilated, natural nutrients.

Dried yeasts have no leavening power; they contain no live cells. Drying does not diminish the supply or absorption of B vitamins, including thiamin. These nutrients are readily available when dried yeasts are digested in the human stomach and upper intestine.

Dried nutritional yeasts should also be differentiated from baking yeasts, which are intended for baking but are not to be ingested in their raw form as a food supplement. After nutritional yeasts are grown, they are dried with heat, which renders the yeasts inactive, so they cannot continue growing in the consumer's stomach or cause gas, like uncooked baking yeast can. A small percentage of people may suffer from gas or flatulence even when taking nutritional yeast. This can usually be remedied by initially taking smaller amounts, less than one teaspoon, mixed with water or juice, on an empty stomach. Then, the amount of yeast can gradually be increased. Taking yeast in liquid solution on an empty stomach will also allow the user to experience the quick energy that it often provides.

Gout sufferers should use nutritional yeast cautiously, if at all, using minimal doses until the symptoms of gout have been overcome. Yeasts are high in nucleic acids, which is one reason they effectively protect against radiation and environmental pollutants. Nucleic acids form organic compounds known as purines in the body. Normally, the purines are filtered out through the kidneys and excreted through the urinary tract. Gout sufferers have difficulty eliminating purines. Gout is caused by a diet rich in animal food proteins, fat, and cholesterol. The painful symptoms of gouty arthritis can often be alleviated by following the healthful diet outlined in Part III.

The appropriateness of nutritional yeast for sufferers from candidiasis is a matter of continuing debate in the health field. The strain of yeast usually cited for causing candidiasis is *Candida albicans*, not *Saccharomyces cerevisiae*. Candidiasis is a controversial disease that has been surfacing in greater numbers during the past decade. It arises when *Candida albicans* yeasts dominate intestinal flora and secrete toxins into the system, thus giving rise to a wide variety of symptoms, including eating disorders, intestinal problems, lack of vitality, problems of reproductive organs, skin diseases, and emotional and psychological imbalances.

Some nutritionally oriented physicians recommend strict dietary restrictions for candidiasis sufferers. They recommend temporarily avoiding any food with nutritional or baking yeast in it, even if the food has been cooked. The theory is that these foods further irritate the already unbalanced, irritated, infected, less-resistant mucous membranes.

Saccharomyces cerevisiae is a genus and species of yeast completely different from *Candida*. Also, it has been inactivated through drying. Normally, most people can safely consume *Saccharomyces cerevisiae*. However, if candidiasis is suspected, then it is advisable to approach the consumption of *Saccharomyces cerevisiae* with caution.

Nutritional yeast assists the liver in detoxifying the blood, which is extremely important for counteracting radiation and environmental pollutants. Yeast has also been shown to reduce cholesterol levels and, according to Walter Mertz, a biological chemist at the Walter Reed Army Institute, it helps normalize glucose utilization and blood sugar levels because of the abundance and bioavailability of the mineral chromium. These and other characteristics make nutritional yeast especially useful for weight-watchers, diabetics, hypoglycemics, and heart patients.

A concern about consumption of yeast—as with all supplementation of the diet—is the need for complementary nutrients. Consumption of yeast should be accompanied by regular ingestion of calcium and magnesium supplements because yeast is high in phosphorus, which needs calcium and magnesium to be metabolized.

The usual recommended dosage of nutritional yeast is three tablespoons per day. When using concentrated substances such as yeast, bee pollen, and ocean algae, it is advisable to take small amounts, such as one tablespoon or less, frequently during the day, rather than one or two large dosages per day.

As a general guideline, I recommend the following:
- Protective amounts: ¼ to 1½ teaspoons, three times a day.

• Therapeutic amounts: 1½ teaspoons to one tablespoon, three times daily.

As with all new foods and supplements, it is a good idea to incorporate nutritional yeast into the diet gradually in order to allow the body to adjust. One should monitor oneself closely to see what, if any, symptoms the new food causes. Equally important, symptoms due to a new food need to be distinguished from symptoms that appear by coincidence. A new, normally healthful food should be given a long enough time period for an accurate trial.

Consumption of an excessive nutritional yeast dose may elicit a temporary sensation of heat and itching, called the niacin heat flush, which subsides within about twenty minutes. This heat flush is a natural feedback mechanism that tells users that they are taking in too high a level of niacin. This reaction produces no known harmful side effects.

Tablets are an expensive form of nutritional yeast, but may be the most convenient or acceptable alternative for some people. It takes from twenty-four to sixty-five tablets, depending on the weight of each tablet, to equal one tablespoon of powdered or flaked nutritional yeast, so the tablets may have to be eaten by the handful. Nutritional yeast is commonly found at most natural foods stores.

Some people drink yeast mixed only with water, while others prefer to mix it with fruit juices such as apple, orange, grapefruit, grape, or pineapple. Still others use tomato juice, vegetable juice, or soup. Experiment to see what works best for you. You can also try it in a "smoothie" made with fresh or dried fruit, or in a natural shake. The flavor of vegetable soups is often improved by adding yeast. For years, commercial soup processors have used yeast for this purpose, and now yeast is used to enhance the flavor in low-sodium products. Many people enjoy adding it to sauces and gravies, to baked foods, and to other cooked foods. Yeast can also be kept in a shaker on the dining table for sprinkling on salads, on popcorn along with natural soy sauce, or on other foods. The yeast imparts a cheesy or nutty flavor.

Nutrition writer Beatrice Trum Hunter says, "Yeast is economical, with no waste. It has a long shelf life and does not require refrigeration. Store it in a tightly closed container that excludes light. Keep it in a cool, dry place."

For most people, primary-grown yeast proves useful as a concentrated food that helps produce optimal health and energy. It is low in fats, calories, and sodium, while being an inexpensive source of protein and other nutrients.

GARLIC

Garlic smells like garlic because of an oil it contains called allicin. The allicin in garlic in turn contains sulfur, which is known to be a natural antibiotic agent. Onions also contain sulfur in the amino acids cysteine and methionine. Cysteine is a well-documented radioprotectant and antioxidant (see Chapter 7). It binds with and deactivates both radioactive isotopes (especially cobalt-60) and toxic heavy metals like cadmium, lead, and mercury. The sulfur in cysteine helps the kidneys and liver detoxify the body. Mature dry onions contain 265 mg. of sulfur per 3.5 oz. average serving.

Garlic has been documented to reduce high blood pressure and blood cholesterol levels, prevent blood clots, reduce fatty deposits that clog arteries, increase the body's uptake of the B vitamins, and stimulate the pituitary gland, according to Lloyd Harris's *The Book of Garlic* (Panjandrum Press, 1974). Garlic contains at least two natural antibiotics that act against some fifteen species of harmful bacteria. It also contains the anti-carcinogenic mineral germanium, which stimulates circulation of oxygen in the body.

Garlic, wild ginseng, and onions may have many as-yet-undiscovered properties for healing. According to N. Tretchikoff, noted Russian herbalist, and Alma Hutchens, co-authors of *Indian Herbology of North America* (Merco, 1973), wild garlic, wild onions, and wild ginseng have been found to contain a substance that both prevents the assimilation of radioactive isotopes and helps to draw them out of the body. In the Soviet Union, scientists have labeled this substance Vitamin X, because its complete function is still not fully understood.[52]

For those who don't like either the taste or smell of garlic, it can still be used in cooking. You can diminish its odor and aftertaste by the way you prepare it. Peel the bulbs whole without breaking or slicing the inner skin. Or cook them whole as cooks do in southern France, for use as a more mild-flavored vegetable. Roasted whole in the juice of other foods as they are cooking, the garlic bulbs lose most of their strong flavor. They leave a somewhat sweet taste in the mouth and do not affect the breath. You can further protect your breath from odor after eating garlic by chewing some parsley or other chlorophyll-rich greens, or some fennel or anise seeds.

Natural foods stores have many garlic preparations for those who prefer not to use the bulb in food. One popular, highly potent Japanese garlic product in which the strong taste and odor have been removed is Kyolic. Some people find that garlic capsules or perles of garlic leave no odor on the breath.

CHLOROPHYLL

Foods rich in chlorophyll have long been used as natural medicines to treat a wide range of diseases. A number of scientific studies conducted over twenty years ago found that chlorophyll-rich foods can decrease radiation toxicity. In 1950, Lourau and Lartigue reported that green cabbage increased the resistance of guinea pigs to radiation.[53] Further research by Duplan with green cabbage in 1953 confirmed Lourau's findings.[54] In 1959 and 1961, the chief of the U.S. Army Nutrition Branch in Chicago found that broccoli, green cabbage, and alfalfa reduced the effects of radiation on guinea pigs by 50 percent.[55, 56]

There are many excellent sources of chlorophyll, such as leafy greens, celery, parsley, the sprouts of any grain or bean, the young shoots of any edible grass, and sunflower greens. Spirulina and chlorella are two microalgae that are rich in chlorophyll and often are recommended by natural healers to prevent or treat various health problems. Chlorophyll is similar in structure to hemoglobin, and chlorophyll obtained from whole foods in its raw or lightly cooked form is considered by many health therapists to be one of nature's finest tonics.

OILS

There is some preliminary evidence that common food oils offer some protection against radiation. While conducting research at the University of California, Dr. James Ashikawa found that mice will survive normally lethal doses of x-rays if they are given common edible unprocessed vegetable oils—especially olive or peanut oils, according to an article entitled "Oils Used to Fight Radiation in Mice" in the May 11, 1960 issue of *The New York Times*.

Six days after that article appeared, Professor Humberto Aviles of Mexico wrote to *The New York Times* and advised that those who work or live near sources of radiation, such as atomic laboratories or nuclear power plants, eat or rub vegetable oils onto the skin for greater protection. In a subsequent series of experiments professors Julian Ibanez and Adolfo Castellanos of the Cajal Institute in Madrid observed that olive oil taken internally fully protected rats against progressive doses of x-rays ranging from 300 to 2,400 roentgens.[57]

In another set of studies by Ibanez and Castellanos, various proportions of olive oil, ranging from zero to 30 percent, were added to the diets of six groups of mice comprised of fifteen males and fifteen females each.

These six groups, plus a single control group that did not receive the olive oil, were irradiated by x-rays for fourteen weeks. After the fourteen-week period, the researchers found that the six groups of mice receiving the olive oil were offered some protection against the damage known to be caused by such irradiation. Mice that did not receive olive oil suffered from the expected radiation damage to the liver, kidneys, lungs, skin, and hair.

The olive oil provided optimal protection when it comprised about 15 percent of the total calories of the diet. This is similar to the quantities of fat and oil used in traditional diets around the world. Fifteen percent of a typical 2,100 calorie diet amounts to 315 calories of fats, which is equivalent to about 2 ½ tablespoons of oil, and is consistent with recommendations from many progressive nutrition experts, such as the late Nathan Pritikin. Diets in which fat comprises approximately 15 percent of the total calories have been shown to protect against heart disease, cancer, adult-onset diabetes, and other serious illnesses.

Fish liver oils have also received some attention. They are a good source of organic iodine and vitamin A, two substances which are known radioprotectants. Dr. Gladys W. Royal discovered that mice exposed to large doses of radioactivity (enough to usually prove fatal within five days) lived from three to six days longer if they were fed cod liver oil as compared with mice which had not eaten the oil.[58] Research in India verifies that fresh peanut oil also has a beneficial effect in preventing and treating radiation injury in mice.[59]

Unrefined vegetable oils are commonly available from most natural foods stores. Cold- or virgin-pressed olive oil contains more chlorophyll and is more nutritious than most other vegetable oils. Olive oil and sesame oil are more resistant to breaking down from heat while cooking, and also have a longer shelf life due to their greater resistance to oxidizing and becoming rancid.

CHAPTER 5

Fighting Radiation & Chemical Toxins with Vitamins & Minerals

Choosing a diet rich in foods that help counteract radiation and environmental pollutants is preferable to relying solely on a variety of vitamin and mineral supplements for protection. In whole foods, natural protective elements occur in an organic and complementary relationship to one another. Whole natural foods may even contain as-yet-undetected elements which enhance protection. It is known that certain vitamin and mineral supplements can significantly protect against radiation and chemical pollutants, but I recommend that these be taken as supplements to a whole foods diet, not as substitutes for one. At the end of the section on each vitamin or mineral, you will find a list of the foods containing the largest amount of that particular nutrient. Also, Appendix One contains a detailed table that describes optimal nutrient combining and lists some of the factors that cause nutrient deficiencies.

Supplements are often used in large (mega) amounts. They can create significant changes in the body and produce definite therapeutic results. They can also be overused or overly relied upon because of their relative convenience. Some supplements, such as vitamins A and D, can cause toxic symptoms if taken in excessive dosages. For this reason, complete information regarding appropriate dosage and possible toxicity is included.

Exposure to radiation or chemical pollutants is destructive to vitamins A, C, E, K, several B vitamins, and essential fatty acids.[1,2] Vitamin C is destroyed almost immediately, although it can be replaced. The destruction of other nutrients can be prevented with natural therapies such as the foods, herbs, vitamins, minerals, and antioxidants discussed in this book.

We are just beginning to witness the results of research into natural therapies that involve the consumption of vitamins, mineral, and other supplements. Hopefully, soon we will see more research into foods, herbs, and other components of holistic health that are not as easily marketed but may be just as important to our overall health as supplements are.

VITAMIN A

Vitamin A is an important nutrient because of its role in strengthening the body's protective mechanisms and helping to build optimal strength. Vitamin A, and especially beta-carotene, helps protect against the adverse effects of radiation, drugs, and chemical pollutants.

Beta-carotene is a precursor of vitamin A, meaning that it is converted into vitamin A by the body. Sometimes referred to as pro-vitamin A, beta-carotene is a yellowish compound found in most yellow, orange, and dark green vegetables. Carrots (from which carotene derives its name), broccoli, collard greens, kale, and other leafy green vegetables are rich sources of carotene.

The other form of vitamin A is derived from animal sources and is sometimes called preformed vitamin A because the animal has already metabolized the carotene from its food into vitamin A. One of the richest sources of preformed vitamin A is fish-liver oil.

Both preformed vitamin A and beta-carotene improve the growth, reparability, elasticity, strength, and resistance of internal and external body tissues. Like bee propolis, these nutrients maintain and tonify the epithelial cells that form the outer protective layer of the skin and internal mucous membranes.

A deficiency of vitamin A or beta-carotene can harm the structure and function of these protective tissues and thus render them vulnerable to diseases. Optimal amounts of vitamin A or beta-carotene can prevent normal cells from mutating into cancerous ones after exposure to a carcinogen, such as a radioisotope or chemical pollutant.

These nutrients also improve resistance and immune response by protecting and strengthening the thymus gland. Vitamin A and beta-carotene help the thymus to produce more T cells, which fight invading organisms and cancer like foot soldiers engaged in hand-to-hand combat. These nutrients also increase the effectiveness of the cells that produce antibodies.

Other protective functions of vitamin A and beta-carotene include aiding the production of adrenal cortex and steroid hormones, helping the synthesis of protein and the nucleic acid RNA, and serving as antioxidant scavengers of free radicals.

It is now well established that vitamin A, and perhaps to a greater extent beta-carotene, have powerful anti-cancer properties and may even play a role in cancer therapy. Between 1928 and 1981 over three hundred studies were published in professional journals documenting the effectiveness of these nutrients against a wide range of carcinogens, including airborne pollutants such as those from cigarette smoke, radioactive fallout, and chemical toxins.

Perhaps the most influential of these studies was reported in the prestigious British medical journal, *Lancet*, by a group of respected American research physicians in 1981.[3] A nineteen-year study of 1,954 middle-aged men conclusively demonstrated that those who consumed low levels of beta-carotene each day suffered a much higher rate of cancer than those who consumed regular amounts of the nutrient. The researchers noted that a below-average intake of beta-carotene preceded the development of cancer, not that the cancer caused the low levels of beta-carotene or vitamin A. The principal sources of carotene were green leafy vegetables, carrots, and broccoli. The protective qualities of beta-carotene were so great that even men who smoked cigarettes and ate regular quantities of carotene-rich foods showed a much lower incidence of cancer than those who did not smoke but abstained from such foods. (Cigarettes, of course, are a powerful carcinogen. As we've seen, however, cigarettes also constitute a sizeable radiation hazard due to their emission of radon and other extremely dangerous radionuclides.)

Interestingly, the study also demonstrated that beta-carotene was far more effective in preventing cancer than vitamin A. This suggests that the vegetable sources of the precursor beta-carotene may be healthier than the animal foods that are rich in vitamin A.

In 1982, the National Research Council of the National Academy of Sciences published *Diet, Nutrition, and Cancer*, a review of the evidence linking diet to cancer. The report showed that some common foods—especially those rich in fat—have a causal link to cancer. It also outlined a diet that could prevent cancer. Among the foods that demonstrated the greatest promise in preventing cancer were those rich in beta-carotene.

As for the specific problem of radiation, vitamin A and beta-carotene have consistently demonstrated radioprotective characteristics. For instance, ever since radiation therapy came into use, patients have experienced burns, lesions, and other skin problems as a result of the process. In 1968, Polish researchers found that applications of vitamin A to the skin of those who had undergone radiotherapy produced improved resistance to skin diseases.[4] In 1974, researchers from India found that vitamin A, when taken internally by humans, hastened recovery from radiation.[5]

In 1984, Dr. Eli Seifter and a team of researchers from the Albert Einstein College of Medicine's department of surgery reported in the *Journal of the National Cancer Institute* that vitamin A and beta-carotene counteracted both partial- and total-body gamma irradiation.[6] Mice were subjected to 450 to 750 rads of total-body gamma radiation from cesium-137 irradiators. Cesium-137, along with iodine-131, were the two most prevalent radioisotopes released during the accident at Chernobyl. Beginning directly after exposure, the mice received vitamin A or beta-carotene supplements. These supplements were "previously found to decrease radiation disease in mice subjected to partial-body x-irradiation," the scientists reported. The study showed that both vitamin A and beta-carotene increased the number and survival time of mice that lived when compared to control animals not fed these nutrients. The treated animals also showed less weight loss, thymus atrophy, adrenal malfunction, and deficiency of lymphocytes in the blood.

Interestingly, a two-day delay before giving the animals the supplements did not greatly change the supplements' effectiveness. However, when the delay was extended to six days, the protective qualities "decreased almost completely," according to the researchers. The longer a radioisotope inhabits the body, the greater damage it does. Therefore, the more a treatment is delayed, the greater the risk of harm from radiation exposure. Significantly, the scientists also found beta-carotene to be a more effective form of therapy than preformed vitamin A.

That same year, Dr. S. M. Levenson and associates, also from the department of surgery, Albert Einstein College of Medicine, tested rats exposed to 175 to 850 rads of whole body radiation.[7] They found that vitamin A or beta-carotene improved the healing of wounds; reduced weight loss, thymic and splenic atrophy, and adrenal enlargement; and prevented gastro-ulceration and an abnormal decrease in red and white blood cell formation.

The National Research Council has set the RDA for vitamin A or beta-carotene at 1,500 International Units (IU) for infants, 3,000 IU for children one to eleven years old, and 5,000 IU for adults.

These RDAs should be increased during any kind of pronounced physical or emotional stress, including exposure to radioactive or chemical toxins. For daily preventive or protective purposes, 10,000 to 20,000 IU of vitamin A, preferably in the form of beta-carotene, are recommended for adults. This amount can easily be derived from the optimal diet discussed in Chapter 8. For therapeutic purposes, 25,000 to 35,000 IU are recommended for adults. During emergencies or crisis situations, intensive exposure may warrant as much as 40,000 to 100,000 IU of beta-carotene, but should be taken for *no more than three to four weeks*. Infants should not consume such high amounts. These amounts can still be supplied in part by a whole foods diet—one-half cup of sliced carrots contains 8,140 IU of beta-carotene; one-half cup of spinach contains 7,290 IU of beta-carotene; and one five-inch sweet potato contains 9,230 IU of beta-carotene.

As for animal sources of vitamin A, one-half pound of calf's liver contains approximately 74,000 IU of preformed vitamin A, and one tablespoon of cod liver oil supplies 11,900 IU of preformed vitamin A. Because the liver stores concentrated amounts of environmental pollutants, many health authorities now discourage the regular use of beef and poultry liver unless high quality is assured, such as liver from organically raised animals, or, better yet, from defatted and dessicated liver supplements that are available at natural foods stores.

Following is a list of some of the foods highest in beta-carotene.

Food Source	IU of Beta-Carotene per 100 grams (3.5 oz.) edible portion
Hot red pepper, dry	77,000
Dandelion greens	14,000
Carrots	11,000
Apricots, dried	10,000
Sea vegetables	140-11,000
Kale leaves	9,300
Collard greens	9,300
Boiled greens	8,800
Watercress	9,300
Sweet potato	8,800
Parsley	8,500
Most other dark leafy greens	4,000-9,000
Apricots, fresh	2,700
Broccoli	2,500
Pumpkin	1,600
Peach	1,330
Ocean Fish	1,000-2,000 (preformed vitamin A)
Cod Liver Oil	11,000 per 1 tablespoon (14 gm.) (preformed vitamin A)

There have been no reported cases of beta-carotene toxicity, whereas toxicity cases have been reported for infants receiving a daily dose of 18,500 IU or more of preformed vitamin A for one to three months. If there is no existing vitamin A deficiency, then daily, ongoing doses of 50,000 IU of preformed vitamin A may be toxic to some people. Vitamin C plus bioflavonoids can help prevent or decrease vitamin A toxicity.

There are many factors that can limit or decrease vitamin A or beta-carotene absorption, including excessive consumption of alcohol or caffeine; excessive intake of iron supplements (especially synthetic iron); the use of cortisone and other drugs; the ingestion of mineral oil (as in some salad dressings); the appearance of gastrointestinal or liver disorders, or infections; the consumption of nitrates, antacids, or processed oils that lack antioxidants; and the advent of cold weather, which diminishes transport and metabolism of both carotene and vitamin A. Diabetics have difficulty metabolizing beta-carotene.

Both vitamin A and beta-carotene are absorbed more readily when optimal amounts of B-complex, vitamins C, D, and E, and zinc are present in the diet.

VITAMIN B COMPLEX

When the first vitamins were identified in the early years of this century, "vitamin B" was thought to be a water-soluble compound that was present in rice polishings and that could prevent the disease beri-beri. Further research showed that this compound was actually a number of substances, and there have now been over two dozen B vitamins identified. As Rudolph Ballantine, M.D., notes in his book *Diet and Nutrition* (Himalayan International Institute, 1978), "The term 'B complex' continues to be useful, however, since to a great extent these substances are found together in nature. Those foods which are rich in one member of the B vitamin complex are very likely to be rich in several of the others." The B complex includes B_1 (thiamine), B_2 (riboflavin), B_3 (niacin), B_6 (pyridoxine), B_{12}, folic acid, pantothenic acid, and some others such as biotin, inositol, choline, PABA, B_{13} (orotic acid), B_{15} (pangamic acid), and B_{17} (laetrile) that are in varying stages of acceptance by the U.S. nutritional establishment.

B-vitamin-rich foods and supplements provide numerous benefits. They help the body to replenish its energy, to metabolize protein and fats, and to regulate the nervous system and brain. They aid in the maintenance of muscle tone, especially in the gastrointestinal tract. They help to prevent fatigue and premature aging, to produce antibodies for the immune system, and to keep red blood cell count normal. They are key factors in the health of skin, hair, teeth, eyes, and mouth. They help regulate many important organs and glands such as the liver, kidneys, adrenals, and pituitary. In addition, they are involved in the production of DNA and RNA, which are important protectors against toxins.

The B vitamins also play a key role in protecting against radiation and pollutants. For instance, vitamins B_6, B_{12}, folic acid, and pantothenic acid have been found to be effective in promoting the resistance of rats to sub-lethal radiation, and in increasing their rate of survival. Experiments in Germany have shown that these nutrients produce a renewed formation of red blood cells and blood platelets which are essential to clotting.[8]

Two more studies showed that B_6, B_{12}, folic acid, and pantothenic acid were effective not only in stimulating the repair of red blood cells[9] but also in doubling laboratory animals' survival time after exposure to normally lethal doses of radiation.[10]

In a Soviet study, pantothenic acid was fed to 1,181 male rats twenty-four days before and thirty days after irradiation.[11] The percentage of rats surviving was increased compared to controls, as was the average length of survival time of those that eventually died. This study also showed that pantothenic acid increased white blood cells, especially when it was administered in low doses.

This latter finding is especially significant if it is applied to humans, since the body's ability to manufacture white blood cells determines whether an illness or pathogen can be overcome. When the body is threatened by a harmful foreign agent, an increase in the white blood cell count, such as that stimulated by pantothenic acid, is necessary for proper immune response. Moreover, the destruction of white blood cells by radiation can last for extended periods of time. Any food substance that could be used to promote white blood cell count would therefore be important in the prevention and treatment of radiation exposure.

Vitamin B_{12} and folic acid when ingested together stimulate repair and replacement of both mature and immature red blood cells in rats exposed to x-irradiation of doses ranging from 600 to 1200 roentgens, according to the findings of researchers A. Morezek and W. Schmidt.[12] Their research also showed that these same vitamins reduced the destruction of red and white blood cells and blood platelets, thus protecting the animals after they were exposed to normally lethal doses of x-rays.

Supplements that normalize red and white blood cell count will have a markedly positive benefit upon human health. This is because the primary function of red blood cells is to deliver oxygen to tissue and to carry away carbon dioxide. The primary function of white blood cells is to act as scavengers of harmful substances, thereby helping the immune system to resist infection.

In a series of German studies on laboratory animals, vitamin B12 was shown to be able to significantly increase survival rates of animals receiving doses of normally lethal radiation.[13] A greater percentage of mice survived when they were administered normal vitamin requirements of B12. Larger doses of B12 were not necessarily the most effective, although large dosage supplementation was better than no extra supplementation. Weight losses that were indicative of ill health were observed in both the treated and the control groups within five days after radiation exposure. The loss was much less severe in the animals treated with vitamin B12 than in the untreated control animals. After the initial weight loss, the average weight of the animals treated with B12 increased more than even the average weight of the control animals that were able to survive for thirty days or more.

Soviet scientists in another study gave the B vitamin inositol to several groups of rats both before and after irradiation.[14] These animals were compared to a control group that was not given the B vitamin, but suffered the same doses of radiation. Thirty percent of the control group survived the radiation, while 67 to 84 percent of the groups given inositol survived. In this experiment, inositol diminished the initial post-irradiation decrease of white blood cells, and it also markedly accelerated the leukocytes' return to normal value.

According to P. V. Atkin, human patients suffering loss of appetite, nausea, and a general feeling of sickness after exposure to radiation therapy experience a pronounced reduction of symptoms when given specific B vitamin supplementation.[15] And according to information offered by Paavo Airola in *How to Get Well* (Health Plus Publishers, 1974), B vitamins offer more than just radiation protection. They help counteract common pollutants, including carbon monoxide, lead, mercury, DDT, nitrates, nitrites, and many toxic drugs.

Other studies have combined vitamin C with B vitamins. In one study 296 human cancer patients were exposed to radiation.[16] Vitamin C was added to the control diet. The result was reduced radiation toxicity. When the whole vitamin B complex was added to the diet along with vitamin C, the new diet was the most effective in reducing digestive problems, nervous disorders, and other side effects resulting from radiation.

In another experiment, thirty dogs were fed various diets.[17] One of the diets contained the vitamin B complex, vitamin C, and vitamin P (bioflavonoids). Vitamins were begun one month before and continued for one to two months after the dogs had been subjected to whole-body irradiation. According to study author Dr. S. R. Perepelkin, "Addition to the diet of vitamins C, P, and the B group of vitamins at the normal requirement amounts and minimum therapeutic doses caused gastric secretory functions to tend to become normal. Mortality of the irradiated dogs was delayed in those treated with normal requirements of the vitamins."

Perepelkin's research showed that when the vitamins were administered in large doses, some of the usual radiation side effects were aggravated. Also, the most acute effects of irradiation were observed in dogs who received milk and eggs in their diet.

These findings point to the need for balanced amounts of nutrients in the diet and the possibility of adverse effects on the immune system when megadoses are administered for an extended period of time. Also, as we will see later on, high-fat foods, including dairy products and eggs, can have an adverse effect on the body's ability to eliminate toxins, especially when they are consumed regularly.

Dried nutritional yeast is the richest natural source of B vitamins as well as being a strong protector against toxins. Other excellent vegetarian sources of B vitamins include whole grains or whole grain cereals, especially wheat, oats, and rice; wheat germ; wheat or rice bran; wild rice; soybeans; peanuts and other legumes; bee pollen; seeds, especially sesame seeds and sunflower seeds; nuts; certain herbs, especially comfrey roots and leaves; vegetables, especially pumpkin, beets, potatoes, and leafy greens; fermented vegetables; sea vegetables; avocados; raisins and dates; and unrefined molasses.

Animal sources of B vitamins include liver (preferably from organic sources or from defatted and desiccated liver supplements), fish, eggs, kidney and heart meats, the white meat of poultry, red muscle meat, and milk products including yogurt and aged cheese. People with allergy, sinus, or hayfever problems, or those who have a tendency to excess mucus build-up, are best advised to limit the amount of milk, other dairy products, and eggs they consume. Regular consumption of milk, other dairy products, eggs, and red meat tend to elevate fat and cholesterol levels.

Human intestinal bacteria also produce B vitamins. Since fermented foods help create healthy intestinal flora, they can stimulate the body to produce some of its own B vitamins. Sulfa drugs and other antibiotics may destroy these valuable bacteria. Fermented foods such as miso, tempeh, tamari, natural soy sauce, raw sauerkraut, fermented vegetables and fruit (chutneys), yogurt kefir, fermented grain drinks such as amasake, and others are available at most natural foods stores and some supermarkets.

Recent studies done on strict vegetarian populations (such as those that eat little or no animal, dairy, or seafood) indicate that the risk of developing a B_{12} deficiency, especially in infants and young children, may be greater than originally thought. If you follow a strict vegan or macrobiotic vegetarian diet, taking vitamin B12 within a whole B-complex supplement may prove beneficial. Otherwise, the addition of small amounts of ocean fish, poultry, dairy products, or meat in your diet could prevent potentially serious problems related to a vitamin B12 deficiency in years to come.

For people who wish to take supplements of B vitamins, whole B complex vitamins are available in low- and high-potency dosages. They work best when vitamins B1, B2, and B6 are present in equal amounts ranging from 50 mg. to 100 mg. per day for adults. B vitamins are water-soluble, so any excess amount is excreted each day. The B vitamin supplements should be taken only with or after a meal, not on an empty stomach—otherwise temporary nausea may develop in a small percentage of people.

It is important to remember that all the B vitamins should be taken together. Large doses of any one of the isolated B complex vitamins may result in high urinary losses of other B vitamins and lead to deficiencies.

Generally, no known toxicity is associated with taking B vitamins. However, some reports indicate the possibility of developing symptoms such as tremors, edema, nervousness, rapid heartbeat, allergies, and neurological disturbances when doses are taken in great excess. Natural forms of the B vitamins are preferable to the synthetic forms because the natural forms have all the B factors, including any which are not yet known. They are also more easily assimilated than the synthetic forms.

B vitamins are lost or destroyed through consumption of refined carbohydrates, sugar, alcohol, coffee, birth control pills or estrogen replacement pills, sulfa drugs, sleeping pills, exposure to stress or external toxins, and excess perspiration.

VITAMIN C AND BIOFLAVONOIDS

The National Research Council of the National Academy of Sciences now recognizes that vitamin C does play a role in the prevention of cancer. Numerous research studies indicate that Vitamin C both improves our immune system response and effectively counteracts radiation and chemical toxins.

Bioflavonoids are water-soluble substances, such as rutin, quercetin, and hesperidin, that often occur in fruits and vegetables as synergistic or complementary companions to vitamin C. Dr. Fred R. Klenner, a pioneer researcher of vitamin C, observed that guinea pigs given megadoses of vitamin C and bioflavonoids were able to survive doses of radiation that were twice the known lethal dose, according to Linda Clark's *Get Well Naturally* (Arco, 1968).

Vitamin C decreases hemorrhaging and cell degeneration in white rats after exposure to plutonium radiation.[18] In this and other experiments, the irradiated rats that were fed vitamin C lived longer, a greater proportion survived, and the usual clinical radiation symptoms were markedly reduced.[19]

Other studies of irradiated animals given vitamin C indicate such varied benefits as greater weight increase and faster recovery after exposure, quicker return to normal gastric function, and accelerated normalization of kidney function.[20-23]

In a study that has implications for the radioprotection of infants in utero, the survival time of irradiated hamster ovary cells was increased by a factor of seven when high concentrations of vitamin C were supplied.[24]

Vitamin C and bioflavonoids (sometimes referred to as vitamin P) often occur together in fruits and vegetables. In a 1949 study conducted by the Atomic Energy Commission, researchers tested five bioflavonoids and found that they reduced the mortality rate in x-rayed dogs by 49 to 60 percent.[25] When ascorbic acid (vitamin C) was used alone, it reduced the mortality rate by 50 percent. When vitamin C and the bioflavonoids were used in combination, the mortality rate was further reduced to only 10 percent (90 percent lived).

Dogs that were subjected to radiation experienced a normalization of gastric functions after the addition to their diets of vitamin C, bioflavonoids, and the B-complex vitamins at the minimum therapeutic dosages.[26]

In studies comparing two groups of irradiated rats, one of which was given bioflavonoids, only 10 percent of the control group survived, while the bioflavonoids group experienced an 80 percent survival rate.[27, 28] It is known that bioflavonoids help strengthen and protect the vessel walls of the circulatory system—especially the capillaries—thereby reducing possible hemorrhaging caused by radiation or toxic chemicals.

Medical researchers James A. Scott, M.D., and Gerald M. Kolodny, M.D., measured the effects of irradiation on normal mice cells given varying amounts of vitamin C and compared them to irradiated mice cells not given vitamin C.[29] According to Scott, then assistant radiologist at Massachusetts General Hospital, Boston, and an instructor at Harvard Medical School, "Our experiment showed that vitamin C can prevent damage from radiation... it somehow keeps the radiation from killing the cells."

Their experiment indicates that the equivalent dosage for humans exposed to intensive radiation would be approximately 10 grams per day—a megadose. Several other authorities on vitamin C therapy concur with this dosage during intensive exposure. Scott concludes that "if vitamins are necessary for human life in small quantities, maybe some people need more, especially in those situations which stress our bodies—such as exposure to radiation and other environmental pollutants. I take 500 mg. per day to be on the safe side."

Anemia, or red blood cell deficiency, is a common symptom after exposure to radiation or environmental pollutants. Vitamin C plays an important role in the absorption of iron, which is necessary for the formation of red blood cells and thus the prevention of anemia. Iron is an "acid-bound" mineral, which means it is more efficiently assimilated when the pH of the stomach is more acidic. Normally, the stomach produces its own hydrochloric acid, which, among its other functions, assists in the assimilation of acid-bound minerals.

Unfortunately, because of improper diet and other factors, many people produce less than optimal amounts of stomach acids, especially as they get older. Hence, acid-bound minerals such as iron are inadequately assimilated.

Vitamin C does not necessarily improve the digestive process. Rather, it helps create a favorable acidic pH in the stomach in order to facilitate absorption of these acid-bound minerals. Many iron-rich foods naturally contain some vitamin C. In order to increase iron assimilation, it is often beneficial for people to take vitamin C and iron-rich foods or supplements together.

When comparing iron sources, one should keep in mind that there are two kinds of iron: naturally occurring ferrous iron (also available in supplement form) and synthetically produced ferric iron. Because the body reduces most iron to ferrous iron before absorption, it is utilized more efficiently than the ferric iron sources (this is true whether the ferrous comes from food or supplement sources). Vitamin C also helps reduce ferric iron to its more easily utilized ferrous form.

Vitamin C is an antioxidant, similar to vitamins A and E, selenium, and S.O.D. (See Chapter 3 for an explanation of antioxidants and their function in protecting against radiation and chemical pollutants.) Because vitamin C is a water-soluble antioxidant, it may help to protect the fat-soluble vitamins A and E, and unsaturated fatty acids.

Vitamin C, together with the bioflavonoids, helps protect against most common pollutants, including lead, mercury, DDT, cadmium, nitrates, nitrites, aluminum, chlorine, cigarette smoke, copper, fluoride, carbon monoxide, arsenic, benzene, pesticides, chromium, PCBs, dioxin, THC, polynuclear aromatic hydrocarbons, and the toxic side effects of many drugs. Vitamin C and bioflavonoids protect against the side effects of many chemical drugs, ranging from antibiotics and aspirin to painkillers and Valium. Massive doses of vitamin C and bioflavonoids have been successfully used in programs to treat drug addiction, including from such drugs as heroin, cocaine, barbiturates, methadone, and marijuana.

Dr. Edward J. Calabrese, associate professor of environmental health at the University of Massachusetts and the author of *Nutrition and Environmental Health* (Wiley, 1980), has stated, "It is now widely accepted that vitamin C markedly affects the toxicity and/or carcinogenicity of greater than fifty pollutants, many of which are ubiquitous in the air, water, and food environments. Vitamin C can actually prevent the formation of nitrosamines in your stomach."

Nitrosamines are cancer-causing agents that can form in the stomach when one eats foods treated with sodium nitrite. Nitrites and nitrates are present in food preservatives, flavorings, and coloring agents, all of which are added to many processed and smoked meats and fish. According to Dr. Steven R. Tannenbaum, professor of toxicology and food chemistry at Massachusetts Institute of Technology, healthy people given a total of 2,000 mg. (2 grams) of vitamin C per day are able to block nitrosamine formation.

To act as a natural detoxifying agent, vitamin C needs to be in the stomach at the same time as the nitrite-treated foods. Vitamin C should be taken several times per day in foods or supplements when one is exposed to radiation or environmental pollution.

Vitamin C loses potency when exposed to air, light, heat, or long periods of storage. Foods tend to lose their vitamin C potency during processing.

Vitamin C and the bioflavonoids have numerous functions in the human body, many of which are relevant to counteracting radiation and environmental pollutants. They are necessary for the growth and repair of body tissues, cells, blood vessels, and bones. They promote capillary integrity and proper permeability. Vitamin C and the bioflavonoids help prevent anemia, as well as ruptures in the capillaries and connective tissue. They build a protective barrier against infections, and they are essential for proper functioning of the adrenal and thyroid glands. The adrenals control the body's ability to properly respond to any kind of physical or emotional stress, including stress from exposure to external toxins, and they have a direct influence on the pancreas and blood sugar levels.

In addition, vitamin C and the bioflavonoids fight bacterial infections and reduce the effects of some allergy-producing substances. They protect the following nutrients against oxidation and aid in their assimilation: vitamins A and E, several of the B vitamins, iron, and calcium.

Unlike most animals, humans cannot manufacture their own vitamin

C in the liver. Our ancestors were exposed to fewer toxins than modern people. They also may have had a considerably higher intake of vitamin C from fresh fruits and vegetables, and because they consumed more food due to their vigorous activities. Many nutritionists now recommend ingestion of doses of vitamin C beyond the usual RDA.

There is considerable controversy over what constitutes proper dosages of vitamin C. Suggestions range from amounts meant to prevent disease, including cancer, to amounts recommended for therapeutic purposes.

The National Research Council recommends 45 mg. of vitamin C per day for adults. Dr. Linus Pauling, two-time Nobel Laureate and Professor of Chemistry at the University of California, Stanford, states that the minimal daily intake for adults should be from 2,000 to 10,000 mg., in part because most animals, under normal, minimal stress conditions, make their own ascorbic acid at levels for which an adult human equivalency would be 2,000 to 10,000 mg. daily. More is manufactured during times of stress. There is obviously an enormous gulf between these authorities. One reason for this variation in dosages is that the need for vitamin C increases when there is more stress, higher body weight, increased activity, faster metabolism, more ailments, or increased age.

Symptoms of toxicity are rare with high intakes of vitamin C because it is a water-soluble vitamin, and the body usually discharges daily whatever it cannot use. However, regular daily intake of greater than 5,000 to 10,000 mg. may cause side effects in some persons. Toxicity symptoms can be a slight burning sensation during urination, excess urination, diarrhea, or skin rashes. These same symptoms are not inevitable signs of excess vitamin C intake, though. They can also be symptoms of exposure to radiation, environmental pollutants, drugs, or other toxins. Regardless, when one is taking large doses of supplements and toxicity symptoms appear, dosages usually should be reduced.

Vitamin C is readily available from common foods, especially leafy green vegetables, broccoli, and certain fruits. When taking greater quantities of vitamin C, the following range of doses is suggested:

• **Prevention and Protection**—250 mg. to 2,000 mg. per day. Regular doses of vitamin C may be advisable, since we are daily exposed to radiation and environmental pollutants.

• **Therapeutic doses preceding or following exposure**—2,000 to 10,000 mg. per day. Therapeutic doses can be taken both before exposure, as in the case of scheduled x-rays or radiation treatments, and after intensive exposure.

Rapidly decreasing the dosage level of vitamin C after regular ingestion of high doses could possibly result in symptoms of scurvy. Therefore, reduction of vitamin C should be done gradually so that the body has time to adjust.

An excessive intake of vitamin C can occasionally cause oxalic acid and uric acid kidney stone formation. If more than 750 mg. of vitamin C is taken daily, calcium, magnesium, B6 (within the whole B complex), and sufficient water to prevent kidney stones should also be considered.

Bioflavonoids are completely nontoxic. Usually, only about one-eighth to one-twelfth the amount of bioflavonoids as vitamin C should be consumed. There is no Recommended Daily Allowance for bioflavonoids. When ingested together, vitamin C and bioflavonoids are more helpful than vitamin C taken alone. Bioflavonoids are necessary for the proper absorption and function of vitamin C. Bioflavonoids occur with vitamin C in natural food sources; synthetic vitamin C usually does not contain bioflavonoids. The edible parts of fruits contain ten times the concentration of bioflavonoids as strained juices.

According to John Kirschmann, Director of Nutrition Search, Inc., and author of the comprehensive *Nutrition Almanac*, "The body's ability to absorb vitamin C is reduced by smoking, stress, high fever, prolonged administration of antibiotics or cortisone, inhalation of DDT or fumes of petroleum, and ingestion of aspirin or other painkillers. Sulfa drugs increase urinary excretion of vitamin C by two or three times the normal amount. Baking soda creates an alkaline medium that destroys vitamin C. In addition, drinking excessive amounts of water will deplete the body's vitamin C. Cooking in copper utensils will destroy the vitamin C content of foods."

Foods high in vitamin C and bioflavonoids include acerola cherries, rosehips, sweet or hot peppers, black currants, kale, parsley, collards, spinach, other dark leafy greens, broccoli, wild violet leaves, strawberries, citrus, other fruits, and the inner pulp of citrus and banana peels. Buckwheat is a nutritious grain that contains a good supply of bioflavonoids.

VITAMIN D

Vitamin D is a fat-soluble vitamin which most humans could derive from sunlight. Only a short exposure every day—about thirty minutes—is necessary for most people to meet the RDA, although the sun's action on the skin is diminished by air pollution, clouds, clothing, window glass, dark suntans, and dry skin. Vitamin D is normally found in the fatty tissues of certain foods. Small amounts are present in sprouted seeds, mushrooms, sunflower seeds; fatty fish such as halibut, mackerel, salmon, sardines, herring, cod, and tuna; egg yolks and dairy products; and organ meats. Fish liver oils are a good source of both vitamins A and D.

Preferably, vitamin D should be derived from sunlight and from natural food sources. Synthetic vitamin D, found in fortified milk and in synthetic supplements which contain "irradiated" ergosterol or calciferol, may be slightly toxic for some people.

Italian researchers in 1966 found that vitamin D, in combination with vitamins A and the whole B complex, helps remove radioactive isotopes such as strontium-85 and strontium-90 from the bones and the body.[30] Vitamin D also helps protect against some common pollutants, including lead and cadmium, according to Airola in *How to Get Well*.

Vitamin D, like vitamin A, can be toxic if taken in excessive dosages, especially for infants and children. Some signs of toxicity are unusual thirst, sore eyes, itching skin, urinary urgency, loss of appetite, nausea, vomiting, diarrhea, muscular weakness, dizziness, and fatigue. These symptoms will disappear within a few days when the overdosage is stopped. People with heart or kidney disorders should be especially careful not to overdose with vitamin D.

Vitamin D is best utilized when taken after meals with vitamin A, and when there is ample calcium, choline (a B vitamin found in lecithin), vitamin C, and phosphorus in the diet. Small amounts of unsaturated fatty acids, sometimes called vitamin F, also aid utilization of vitamin D. The body can store sizeable reserves of vitamins A and D, primarily in the liver. Smaller amounts of D are stored in the intestinal tract. Mineral oil, as is sometimes found in salad dressings, destroys the vitamin D which is already stored in the intestinal tract.

Prolonged deficiency of vitamin D may lead to rickets, tooth decay, pyorrhea, poor bone formation and retarded growth in children, osteomalacia (soft bones), osteoporosis, poor metabolism, weight gain, diabetic distress, muscular weakness, lack of vigor, deficient assimilation of minerals, and premature aging.

In 1968, the U.S. Food and Nutrition Board recommended 400 IU of vitamin D daily for both infants and adults for preventive purposes. An adult therapeutic dosage would range from 400 IU per day to 1,000 IU daily. For children, the daily therapeutic range would go from 400 IU to 500 IU. During an emergency, adult daily dosage could go as high as 2,000 IU, *if taken for no longer than one month.*

Vitamin D not only protects against toxins and radiation, it aids in preventing colds when taken with vitamins A, C, E and F. It promotes the assimilation of calcium, phosphorus, magnesium, and other minerals, thus improving toxin protection and producing strong bones and teeth. Vitamin D helps regulate the thyroid and parathyroid glands, thereby maintaining proper calcium levels in the blood. Calcium is a very important protective mineral that will be discussed later in this chapter.

VITAMIN E

Vitamin E is a fat-soluble nutrient. It was originally credited with being the "fertility vitamin" because it was found that rats on a vitamin E-free diet failed to reproduce. This gave it a reputation (perhaps undeservedly) for increasing virility, although in recent years the public has focused more on its merits as an agent in the prevention and treatment of heart disease. Vitamin E acts in the body as an antioxidant to prevent premature and undesirable oxidation of lipids (fats) in blood serum. It provides more available oxygen to the tissues by preventing the formation of toxic peroxides which cause both free radicals to appear and red blood cells to be destroyed. It prevents unsaturated fatty acids, sex hormones, and fat-soluble vitamins from being destroyed in the body by oxygen. Vitamin E increases the life of red blood cells. It oxygenates tissues and markedly reduces the need for oxygen intake.[31] Vitamin E also produces an anti-cancer, radioprotective effect similar to that of other antioxidants, and aids in the improvement of circulation.

Vitamin E in recommended dosages strengthens the immune system. A deficiency of vitamin E leads to low levels of antibodies, T cells, and B cells. Vitamin E deficiency can also cause a decrease in the size and efficiency of the lymphatic organs and vessels. Although vitamin E is necessary for optimal immune response, excessive intake can reduce the efficiency of the immune system.

Given this immune-boosting potential of vitamin E, it is not surprising that studies have shown that vitamin E dramatically increases survival of mice following exposure to normally lethal doses of radiation—including radioactive cobalt and x-rays.[32] In a National Cancer Institute study, lethal doses of x-rays killed all the mice in the control group, whereas the mice that received vitamin E showed few adverse effects.

Another investigation found that the placentas of irradiated pregnant mice given vitamin E showed less radiation injury than those of mice not receiving vitamin E.[33] The investigators concluded from this study that at least parts of the body, including the blood, might be protected from radiation by vitamin E. This study is also significant in that it indicates vitamin

E may help protect the fetus against radiation.

Vitamin E has been observed to have a positive effect on the blood and to improve anemia following exposure to radiation. A group of Jordanian children suffering from anemia, who had been consistently unresponsive to other therapies, showed significant improvement after vitamin E treatment.[34] As we'll see in the discussion of Siberian ginseng in Chapter 6, substances that protect red blood cells often are reliable protectors against radioactive and chemical toxins.

Radiation destroys leukocytes in both tissues and the blood, according to S. L. Robbins in *Pathologic Basis of Disease* (W. B. Saunders, 1974). In Japan, I. Kurokawa and co-workers found that blood given vitamin E maintained a white cell count twice as high as blood not given vitamin E but exposed to the same radiation.[35]

Vitamin E has also been shown to produce internal and external protection in mice irradiated by cesium-137.[36] This could be especially significant because cesium-137 is a common component of fallout, nuclear power plant leaks and routine emissions, and because it has already been used in food irradiation. Mice that were exposed to gamma radiation experienced the usual marked decline of both the red and white blood cells. The fur of the mice was ruffled and ulcerated after weeks of the exposure. They had lost weight, and were lethargic and irritable. In contrast, mice given vitamin E once a week—either two days before or seven days after irradiation—showed no adverse internal or external effects. Researchers Alan Hecht and Karl Mohrmann concluded that "the antioxidant properties of vitamin E are able to protect the body from damage due to ionizing radiation. Both red and white blood cells were protected from the destructive properties of radiation when this vitamin was administered to mice irradiated daily by gamma radiation. While the unprotected group showed skin ulcerations and ruffling of the fur, the external features of the groups protected by the vitamin remained normal."

The type of vitamin E used in this series of experiments was d-alpha-tocopherol. On a body-weight ratio basis, a human dose of about 900 IU per day for an adult weighing 154 pounds can be extrapolated from the dosage of vitamin E given to the mice (2.7 IU per week).

The destruction of vitamin A and fatty acids by x-ray treatments and other radiation therapy can be largely prevented by megadoses of vitamin E.[37] Vitamin E, applied externally, seems to act similarly to the fresh herb aloe in eliminating severe radiation burns, decreasing pain, and reducing scarring.[38-41] The vomiting, diarrhea, headaches, hemorrhaging, and severe anemia that usually accompany irradiation by cobalt or x-ray treatments have been largely prevented by vitamins B, C, and E, provided that large doses are started several days prior to treatment.[42-48]

After radiation therapy, many harmful substances are formed from the destroyed malignant tissues, but the liver's ability to rid the blood of these substances is greatly enhanced by intake of vitamins C and E, and the eight essential amino acids, especially methionine.

Vitamin E also offers protection against many common pollutants in food, water, air, and the environment. These pollutants include carbon monoxide, nitrogen dioxide, chlorine, cigarette smoke, mercury, nitrates and nitrites, ozone, polynuclear aromatic hydrocarbons, and the damaging or toxic side effects of many drugs, including aspirin. Literally hundreds of articles are published every year in medical journals that demonstrate the therapeutic value of vitamin E for treating cancer, immune dysfunctions, hormonal imbalances, heart disease, stroke, asthma, premature aging, and other health problems that can result from exposure to radiation or chemical pollutants.

Vegetable oils are the richest source of vitamin E, particularly wheat germ oil and soybean oil (which is also a good source of lecithin, discussed in Chapter 7). The best vegetable oils are unrefined. These oils are available at most natural foods stores. Other good sources of vitamin E are whole wheat and other whole grains, raw or sprouted seeds, fresh nuts, green leafy vegetables (especially cabbage), and eggs. The germ of whole grains, such as wheat or rice germ, or the germ oil, is an abundant source of vitamin E if it is fresh.

Vitamin E can be taken in supplement form. Capsules remain fresher much longer than bottled vitamin E oil. For preventive purposes, the preferred form of vitamin E is the mixed tocopherols, which is how vitamin E occurs in nature. However, for therapeutic purposes, the advice of Drs. Evan and Wilfred Shute, among the world's foremost authorities on the therapeutic uses of vitamin E, seems most persuasive. They maintain that the isolated d-alpha-tocopherol is the most effective form of vitamin E available.

The reader should be cautious about using synthetic vitamin E, which is marketed as dl-alpha tocopherol or alpha tocopherol acetate. Synthetic vitamin E has an adverse effect on the absorption of iron. Likewise, consumption of synthetic iron has an adverse effect on the absorption of vitamin E. Also, the use of mineral oil, as in some commercially prepared salad dressings, is not recommended because it has been shown that it inhibits absorption of vitamin E.[49]

The approximate therapeutic daily dosage of d-alpha-tocopherol vitamin E is 400-600 IU. Mixed tocopherols are approximately one-half as potent, and therefore twice as much is usually recommended. Consult an experienced health practitioner before using more than 600 IU of d-alpha-tocopherol or 1,200 IU of mixed tocopherols per day. One IU equals 1 mg.

Vitamin E should be used cautiously if one has high blood pressure or rheumatic heart disease. An initial high dose of vitamin E can increase the blood pressure, or produce rapid deterioration, in chronic rheumatic heart disease patients. If one has either of the above health problems, it is best to consult a physician or a knowledgeable health practitioner who will likely begin with small amounts of E, and then gradually increase the dose.

CALCIUM

Calcium is the most abundant mineral in the human body. It is essential for a wide range of vital body functions, including building bones and teeth and insuring normal growth. Calcium helps the functions of the kidneys, which are primary blood cleansing organs. It helps regulate blood pH, electrolyte balance, and nerve transmission--all of which have protective functions. Calcium also protects against strontium-90, calcium-45, and other radioisotopes.[50-54]

By the mechanism of selective uptake, optimal daily intake of calcium blocks, or at least significantly decreases, the absorption of strontium-90, calcium-45, and other radioactive isotopes by the skeletal system. According to one study, the body is four times more likely to form bones from calcium than from strontium.[55] Calcium also helps to eliminate strontium-90 and other radioactive isotopes that may be already lodged in the bones. Research on humans has shown that the greater the amount of calcium, the lower the absorption and retention of strontium-90.[56]

Doctors from the Veterans Administration Hospital in Hines, Illinois, found that calcium, when combined with magnesium, removed from the blood significant amounts of radioactive strontium, which was then excreted from the body.[57, 58]

That calcium can remove radiostrontium from the blood is important for three reasons. One is that research shows that "newly formed bone has about the same strontium-calcium ratio as is in the blood circulating at the time of formation."[59] The second reason is that fetuses and young children who have rapidly growing bones are especially vulnerable to strontium-90. The third reason is that bones have several important functions such as skeletal support, formation of blood cells, and involvement in our immunological response.

Calcium's ability to protect against toxicity of cadmium, lead, aluminum, fluoride, mercury, and other heavy pollutants has also been recognized.[60, 61]

Usually only 20 to 30 percent of ingested calcium is absorbed, depending on the availability of other nutrients with which calcium works synergistically. For example, in order for calcium to be properly utilized by the body, there must be adequate amounts of phosphorus, the ratio being approximately two calcium molecules for every one of phosphorus. If excessive quantities of food with a high-phosphorus to low-calcium ratio are consumed—such as meat, poultry, fish, beans, and grains—without including calcium-rich foods in the diet, a calcium deficiency could occur. For optimal absorption of calcium, the diet must also contain adequate amounts of vitamins A, C, D, E, and F, magnesium, phosphorus, manganese, iron, and protein. There should also be low but adequate amounts of fats. The best way to achieve a balanced calcium intake is to follow the dietary guidelines outlined in Chapter 8, which provide optimal amounts of this and other nutrients in ratios that are beneficial to the body.

Refined foods have lost calcium and many other important nutrients during processing, thus increasing one's chance of suffering from deficiencies. Other common factors that can limit calcium absorption are stress, caffeine, some kidney or adrenal disorders, and food grown in calcium-deficient soil.

The National Research Council recommends that adults consume 800 mg. of calcium a day. The recommended daily amounts of calcium for children and pregnant or lactating women is 1,000 to 1,400 mg. Some health authorities now say that because calcium deficiencies are quite common in the U.S., even these recommended amounts are conservative. With age, calcium absorption is often even further diminished, especially in women, so extra supplementation should be considered. Whenever you supplement your diet with calcium, add half that amount of its complementary mineral magnesium, which is also a good protective mineral.

Too much calcium can be harmful. Prolonged high intake of calcium and vitamin D have been shown to cause hypercalcemia, which is an excessive amount of calcium in the blood. Prolonged elevated blood calcium may produce excessive calcification of the bones and some tissues, including the kidneys.

Some of the foods richest in both calcium and magnesium are green leafy vegetables (including collard, kale, parsley, and mustard greens), sea vegetables, sesame seeds, almonds, and soybeans and soybean products.

One should be cautious of consuming mineral supplements derived from bone meal, which sometimes contains large amounts of strontium. Also, supplements from deep-mined rock such as dolomite contain high quantities of calcium but may contain lead, copper, and other metals, and be difficult to assimilate. Children and pregnant women are especially vulnerable to the toxins that may be in bone meal and dolomite.

The best forms of supplemental calcium are calcium citrate, gluconate, carbonate, lactate, or amino acid chelated calcium. Several companies now produce high-quality calcium-magnesium supplements that are in balanced proportion to each other and come in a single tablet. These supplements are available at most natural foods stores.

If you grow your own food, make sure that your garden has optimal levels of lime (calcium) and magnesium. Unfortunately, these two minerals have been depleted from a substantial percentage of the soil in the U.S. Acid rain, which is now common, is much more efficiently buffered by soil that has balanced amounts of calcium and magnesium. One can speculate that enriching the soil with calcium would help prevent the plants, by the principle of selective uptake, from absorbing several radioactive isotopes and toxic metals. Indeed, preliminary studies indicate that plants grown in calcium-rich soils absorb less radioactive strontium. More research is needed in this area.

MAGNESIUM

Magnesium has been studied less than calcium, but it seems to have similar radioprotective qualities. Both these minerals are in the same family of elements as strontium; that is, they have the same number of valence electrons. Like calcium, magnesium prevents the uptake of strontium-90 and other radioisotopes, probably by the mechanism of selective uptake. It helps to eliminate already absorbed strontium-90 as well.[62]

One study has shown that exposure to gamma radiation can decrease calcium and magnesium levels in the blood.[63] As a result, optimal levels of both minerals in the diet are essential after one is exposed to higher amounts of radiation.

Magnesium has many other protective functions in the body, including helping to counteract aluminum toxicity. It complements or balances calcium's properties. It aids in the utilization of several important nutrients, including calcium and the vitamins B complex, C, and E. It also helps maintain blood pH balance.

Magnesium deficiency can cause a wide range of problems including a loss of calcium and potassium, kidney disease, muscle cramps and seizures, nervous irritability, confusion, depression, premenstrual syndrome, and coronary heart disease.

Calciferol (synthetic vitamin D) can bind with magnesium and carry it out of the body. Commercial milk usually contains relatively high quantities of calciferol, and overconsumption of milk, especially in children, may contribute to a magnesium deficiency. Fluorine also leaches magnesium from the body, while coffee, alcohol, diuretics, and certain other drugs can deplete the body's magnesium levels. One's magnesium requirement is increased when either blood cholesterol or protein consumption are high. Oxalic acid, found in a few vegetables such as spinach, and phytic acid, found in grains and beans, diminish magnesium absorption.

An optimal diet should contain approximately twice as much calcium as magnesium. (See section on calcium.) Some of the foods highest in calcium and magnesium are sea vegetables, sesame seeds, green leafy vegetables, almonds, soybeans and soybean products, and nuts and seeds. Magnesium is an essential element of chlorophyll in green plants.

The adult Recommended Daily Allowance (RDA) for magnesium is 350 mg., with some nutritionists using therapeutic doses of up to 700 mg. per day. Doses above 700 mg. should be taken only under a doctor's supervision. Prolonged, large amounts of supplementary magnesium can be toxic, especially if the calcium intake is low and the phosphorus intake is also high. The kidneys can usually process even large amounts of magnesium, but are nevertheless taxed under prolonged excessive levels of supplementation. In the event of kidney failure, there is a greater risk of magnesium toxicity.

The standard American diet does not provide even the recommended daily intake of magnesium, let alone optimal intake. Optimal magnesium intake not only gives additional protection from toxins, but also aids in the prevention of a wide range of common ailments.

SELENIUM

Selenium is an essential trace element found in small amounts in animal and plant foods. It is best known as an effective antioxidant. Recent research demonstrates that a diet containing optimal amounts of selenium protects against radioactive and environmental pollutants, fortifies the immune system, and significantly decreases the rate of several different forms of cancer in humans.

Selenium has been shown to decrease the mortality rate of rats exposed to irradiation, and to alleviate leukopenia (abnormal decreases of white blood corpuscles).[64, 65] Selenium greatly reduces cancer in animals exposed to cancer-causing agents.

Various studies have also shown that selenium has the ability to reduce by up to tenfold the rate of cancer in laboratory animals which, because of their genetic vulnerability and forced exposure to carcinogens, usually have an 80 to 90 percent incidence of cancer.[66-74] The lifespans were significantly longer for even the small percentage of selenium-fed animals that did develop cancer.

Studies have shown that people who consume regular amounts of selenium in food or supplemental form experience lower rates of several types of cancer, including bladder, breast, colon, lung, ovary, pancreas, and prostate.[75-85]

Selenium fortifies and stimulates the immune system.[86-88] It is an antioxidant that scavenges dangerous free radicals in the body. When selenium is deficient, humans produce lower amounts of antibodies, including immunoglobulins M and G.[89]

Research indicates that the immune-stimulating properties of the antioxidants selenium and vitamin E are much greater when they are supplied simultaneously than when they are given separately.[90]

Selenium also protects against common environmental pollutants such as lead, mercury, cigarette smoke, cadmium, and polynuclear aromatic hydrocarbons.[91-95] Selenium binds with and neutralizes both methyl mercury and inorganic mercury. It protects against all of mercury's toxic effects.

Selenium's ability to protect against the toxic side effects of mercury is significant, since mercury is prevalent in dental fillings, cosmetics, and some pesticides. Selenium confers several health benefits including reduction of tumors and resistance to many diseases.

Diets in the industrialized West are often deficient in this important micronutrient. The amount of selenium in soil and food varies dramatically from one geographical location to another. The selenium content of animal products is likewise dependent upon the selenium content of the diet fed the animals. Thus, all food tables for selenium content represent, at best, only average amounts. Modern agricultural practices, acid rain, and food processing further contribute to decreased amounts of selenium in our diets.

According to *The Antioxidants* by Passwater and Mindell, Asian diets contain about four times more selenium than Western diets, which, they speculate, may be one reason why "the breast cancer rate is substantially lower in Asian women than in women from Western countries."

Usually good sources of selenium include ocean fish, bee pollen, sea vegetables, whole grains, organ meats (preferably organically grown), nutritional yeast, ground sesame seeds, garlic, onions, mushrooms, broccoli, carrots, cabbage, radishes, and other vegetables. Selenium is more abundant in vegetables that have been grown organically.

The National Research Council has set the RDA for selenium at 50 to 200 micrograms per day. Some health authorities recommend 100 to 300 mcg. per day for optimal nutrition and therapeutic purposes. Taking more than 100 to 200 mcg. of selenium per day in supplement form is not recommended unless one is under the supervision of an experienced health practitioner. Toxicity may begin at 1,000 micrograms per day of inorganic selenium and 2,000 to 3,000 micrograms (2 to 3 grams) of organic selenium. A healthy diet, as outlined in Chapter 8, should fulfill most of the daily requirements for selenium with only moderate supplementation recommended. Selenium is most effective when combined with vitamins A and E, and it also increases the effectiveness of vitamin E.

POTASSIUM

Cesium-137, cesium-134, potassium-40, and potassium-42 are radioactive, competitive sister elements of natural potassium, all of which are in the same chemical family. These radionuclides are absorbed by the body when there is a deficiency of natural potassium. They concentrate primarily in the reproductive organs and the muscles.

Cesium-137 is common in nuclear fallout, and can often be detected in our food, soil, and water. The authors of one study described our biosphere as "contaminated with radiocesium."[96] Researchers discovered that after the accident at Chernobyl, iodine-131 and cesium-137 were the most prevalent radionuclides in samples of food from the U.S.S.R., and from Poland, Hungary, and other parts of Eastern Europe.[97] Cesium-137 is also already being used in some countries to irradiate foods as a means of extending their shelf life at the supermarket.

Research by the Food and Nutrition Board of the National Academy of Sciences demonstrates that natural potassium decreases the concentration of radiocesium.[98] Radioactive cesium is approximately 100 times more concentrated in freshwater organisms than in ocean life, where there is a much greater amount of potassium. The board recommended eating ocean fish, and other ocean products, in preference to freshwater fish.

Research done in the 1960s also supports the observation that natural potassium protects against radioactive cesium and potassium.[99, 100] The latter research indicated that a diet containing ample amounts of natural potassium would significantly increase the probability of survival after radiation exposure. This study also concluded that "an apparent site of radiation injury was the potassium-sodium active transport system," often called the sodium-potassium pump. A proper balance of the minerals sodium and potassium is essential for normal function of muscle tissue, proper conduction of nerve impulse, regulation of osmotic pressure, and maintenance of acid-base balance. Sodium and potassium are the primary electrolytes in the body. Disruption of this important mineral balance by radiation may be a contributing cause of the symptom of nerve enervation (weakness or failure of nerve energy) frequently observed after radiation exposure.

Other protective functions of the mineral potassium are detoxification of the kidneys, and prevention of over acidity by keeping a proper acid-alkaline balance in the blood and tissues.

The RDA for potassium has not been formally established, but many health authorities suggest that a minimum of 2,000 to 6,000 mg. be included in the daily diet. The average American diet provides 1,900 to 5,850 mg. per day. Potassium supplementation is usually not necessary if you eat a healthful diet and minimize the factors that limit potassium. Sudden increases in potassium intake to about 18,000 mg. per day can cause cardiac arrest. Potassium supplementation should be monitored during cases of dehydration, adrenal insufficiency, and kidney failure.

The highest amounts of potassium are found in sea vegetables, beans, fruits, vegetables, whole grains, sunflower seeds, ocean fish, lean meat, and mint leaves. Potatoes, especially potato peelings, parsley, and dried bananas contain large amounts of potassium. Sea vegetables contain an excellent ratio of potassium and sodium. Potassium is more effective when taken with vitamin B6 and with food that contains moderate but appropriate amounts of sodium.

Excessive use of salt can decrease the body's supply of potassium. Other factors that can deplete potassium are excessive consumption of sugar, aspirin, corticosteroid drugs, diuretics, or coffee, and excessive sweating, diarrhea, vomiting, and alcohol. Alcohol can cause double trouble because it also depletes the body's magnesium reserve. The body needs magnesium to retain the supply of potassium in its cells.

Research should be conducted to determine whether foods that have been grown in potassium-enriched or composted soil absorb less radioactive cesium or potassium.

ZINC

Radioactive zinc-65 lodges primarily in the bones and reproductive organs. By the principle of selective uptake, a diet that supplies optimal amounts of the mineral zinc blocks the uptake of zinc-65.

In 1976 the experimental compound zinc DTPA, a chelating agent that has been tried in animal experiments, was used to successfully treat Harold McCluskey, "The Atomic Man" of Prosser, Washington. McCluskey had been exposed to a very high dose of americium-241 during an accident at a Hanford nuclear production facility in southeastern Washington state. Americium-241, which is used in most ionizing-type smoke detectors, is an artificially produced element that is fifty times more radioactive than the plutonium-239 it is made from. At the time, officials said McCluskey's exposure represented the largest amount of radioactive material ever taken in by a surviving nuclear plant worker. He was given a fifty-fifty chance of survival, at best, but managed to pull through due at least in part to the special permission given by the Food and Drug Administration for the administration of zinc DTPA.

Natural zinc will also help the body eliminate several toxic heavy metals, including cadmium, aluminum, lead, and excess copper. Elevated copper levels can depress the immunological response. Zinc also helps protect against cigarette smoke and polynuclear aromatic hydrocarbons.

Zinc is an essential trace mineral that has a variety of functions. It is essential to healthy immune functioning since a deficiency of zinc can result in a weakening and even atrophying of the thymus gland. This gland, located behind the breastbone, is integrally involved in producing T cells. A zinc deficiency can thus lead to a decrease in the number of T cells, or to an imbalance between the types of cells—fighter and suppressor cells—in the immune system. (Suppressor cells turn off the immune system after the fighter cells have rid the body of a pathogen.)

The noted health author and lecturer Arnold Fox, M.D., has said, "Too many fighters, and your immune system can go on fighting even after the battle is won. With no opponent in sight, your immune system may turn on your own body. Too many suppressors, and your immune system will lay down its arms too soon. Not enough zinc can also lead to low levels of blood immunoglobulins. That means your immune system will have difficulty in specifically targeting and destroying germs."

A malfunctioning immune system can leave us vulnerable to a wide range of infections and serious diseases—including Acquired Immune Deficiency Syndrome (AIDS).

Among the many other important functions of zinc is its role in aiding healthy metabolism. Zinc is required in the synthesis of nucleic acids, which are important protectors against toxins. Zinc is necessary for the normal absorption and function of vitamins, especially the B complex. The National Research Council recommends a daily intake of 15 mg. of zinc for adults, 30 mg. for pregnant women, and 45 mg. for lactating women.

Although it is a relatively nontoxic element, excessive intake of zinc interferes with copper absorption, which then causes depleted iron assimilation. Thus, excessive intake of zinc may produce a loss of iron and copper. Excessive zinc intake can also diminish the immunological activity of some white blood cells.

Zinc combines well with several other nutrients to fortify the immune system. These nutrients are vitamin A in the form of beta-carotene, vitamins B_6, B_{12}, folic acid, vitamins C and E, and selenium. Zinc supplementation is more effective when combined with extra vitamin A or beta-carotene, vitamin B_6, vitamin E, calcium, phosphorus, and small amounts of copper.

High amounts of cadmium or copper can decrease zinc absorption. Many vitamin supplements contain copper in small amounts. The National Research Council recommends a daily copper intake of 2 mg. for adults. Excessive copper can be leached into our water supplies through copper-lined pipes. It is also contained in some pharmaceutical drugs, including some birth control pills.

The amount of zinc in our food is decreased by food processing procedures, especially the milling of whole grains into refined flour products. Other factors that can decrease zinc absorption are alcohol consumption, the use of diuretics or corticosteroid drugs, and the removal of excess copper through the use of synthetic chelating compounds.

Ingestion of excessive amounts of calcium, or foods rich in phytic acid and fiber (such as grains), can diminish zinc absorption. If one regularly takes large amounts of these normally beneficial and protective supplements and foods, moderate extra zinc supplementation is recommended.

The best sources of a balanced amount of trace elements are natural, unprocessed foods, preferably grown in well composted or naturally enriched soil. Usually reliable sources of zinc include the germ and the bran of whole grains; nuts and seeds, especially sesame, pumpkin, and sunflower seeds; nutritional yeast; seafood, especially oysters; organ meats; eggs; and peanuts, peas, and other legumes. Although the phytic acid in grains and seeds can decrease the availability of zinc, phytic acid's effect can be diminished by fermentation, by baking with baker's yeast, or by initially soaking the grains and seeds in water and then discarding the water.

The following chart is for those who already take, or would like to take, zinc supplements.

ZINC (mg. per day)		
	Preventive or Protective	Optimal, Therapeutic, or Crisis
Adult Men and Women	15	15-50
Pregnant Women	30	30-50
Lactating Women	40	40-50

Although some therapists have used therapeutic doses of up to 600 mg., doses over 50 mg. should be considered only under a doctor's supervision and for a temporary time period.

Like other supplements, zinc can prove beneficial for a wide range of ailments when it is taken in appropriate dosages.

IRON

The mineral iron, found in every living cell of the body, combines with protein and copper to produce hemoglobin, a component of red blood cells. Hemoglobin carries oxygen in the blood to the tissues, for use in chemical reactions such as the creation of energy. Iron is said therefore to help build red blood cells. It also helps the body to withstand stress, improves the immune response, promotes protein metabolism, and strengthens respiratory action among other functions. Iron deficiencies have been cited as a cause of fatigue, pallid complexion, and anemia.

A number of research studies indicate that exposure to radiation significantly decreases levels of iron in the body. The Russian researchers P. D. Gabovich and I. A. Mikhalyuk found that either low- or high-intensity ultraviolet radiation "adversely affects iron and copper utilization, indicating the necessity of increasing the daily intake of both elements under climatic conditions corresponding to low or excess ultraviolet irradiation."[101]

That ultraviolet radiation, frequently due to climatic conditions, increases our need for iron is especially noteworthy because of the recent conclusive evidence that our diminishing protective ozone layer is already causing intensified exposure to ultraviolet radiation from the sun—thus leading the way to substantially more skin cancers and other health problems.

Research done in Czechoslovakia showed that whole body irradiation disturbed absorption of iron, and functions of red blood cells, plasma, and bone marrow.[102] Other researchers found that gamma-irradiation of the whole body or of the abdomen decreased absorption of iron, vitamin B12, and lipids.[103] A connection was observed between disrupted iron and vitamin B12 assimilation and subsequent diminishment of red blood cell formation. A series of Canadian experiments on rabbits irradiated with cesium-137 produced similar results. "Amounts of iron in the intestinal wall, blood, and liver were significantly less in irradiated rabbits than in controls," researchers said.[104]

Radioactive iron and plutonium, the isotopes similar in structure to iron, can be carried by the body to iron storage sites such as liver, bone marrow, ovaries or testes, and lungs, whenever the body is deficient in iron. According to Helen Caldicott, M.D., an authority on nuclear issues and the health effects of radiation, "Plutonium's iron-like properties also permit the element to cross the highly selective placental barrier and reach the developing fetus, possibly causing . . . damage and subsequent gross deformities in the newborn infant." Preliminary research indicates that, by the process of selective uptake, optimal amounts of iron in the body prevent the absorption of radioactive iron and plutonium.

There are several factors that influence the amount of iron absorbed from the diet. In addition to eating iron-rich foods, consuming optimal amounts of vitamin C improves absorption of iron. The degree of natural stomach acidity regulates the solubility and availability of the iron in food and most supplements. See Chapter 9 for an herbal formula that improves iron assimilation and regulates digestion.

In addition to proper levels of vitamin C and gastric hydrochloric acid, other nutrients that aid iron absorption are calcium, cobalt (a trace mineral), copper, several B-vitamins, magnesium, and phosphorus. Excess phosphorus, which is common in the standard American diet, depletes iron. A proper balance of calcium, iron, magnesium, copper, and phosphorus is crucial, and is available by following the optimal diet outlined in Chapter 8.

Other factors that can decrease iron absorption include overconsumption of antacids, aspirin, and caffeine, diarrhea or menstruation, excess oxalic acid or phytic acid from certain greens or grains, pregnancy, synthetic vitamin E, and some food preservatives such as EDTA.

The best food sources of iron are sea vegetables, seeds, nuts, beans, whole grains, leafy green vegetables, and root vegetables. Dried fruit and molasses contain high levels of iron, but the iron often is not as well absorbed as with other foods. For those who eat animal products, liver and other organ meats such as heart (preferably raised organically), and oysters, sardines, and other fish are good sources of iron.

The National Research Council recommends a daily iron intake of 18 mg. for women, 30 to 60 mg. daily if pregnant, 20 mg. or more if lactating,

10 mg. for men, and 10 to 18 mg. for children. The need for iron increases, however, whenever there is a loss of blood such as in menstruation or hemorrhaging, during periods of growth, and during pregnancy and lactation. Iron has been shown to help counteract the side effects, and help prevent absorption, of several common environmental pollutants such as lead and cadmium. After exposure to pollutants, or radiation from medical tests or power plant leaks, or during any of the above iron-depleting situations, extra iron supplementation of approximately 10 to 18 mg. daily should be considered.

A toxic level of iron has been known to occur due to blood transfusion, a rare genetically caused metabolic disorder, consumption of substantial amounts of red wine containing iron, addiction to certain iron tonics, and prolonged intake of large amounts of iron supplements. Older men are more vulnerable to accumulating excessive iron levels. Unfortunately, no research has been done to distinguish any difference in toxicity between inorganic, synthetic iron supplements, and natural organic iron.

BECOMING SUPPLEMENT SAVVY

All of the previous supplements can easily be obtained at health food stores, natural foods stores, and even drugstores and supermarkets. If you purchase a combined multiple vitamin/mineral supplement, note that most companies load up their multiple supplements with vitamins and leave them deficient in minerals. The reason is that minerals take up too much space—to provide the RDA in one pill would necessitate pills too large to swallow. Therefore, many companies make both a multiple vitamin/mineral supplement and a separate set of multiple minerals. Since vitamins and minerals are equally important, I encourage you to buy both, and from a reputable company, in order to ensure that you receive appropriate amounts of each needed nutrient.

Keep in mind that you might wish to buy extra amounts of specific nutrients, such as beta-carotene vitamin A, vitamins C and E, calcium, magnesium, zinc, and iron. Remember too that B vitamins should be taken together as a whole complex. They should be taken only with or after a meal. Vitamin C and the bioflavonoids can be taken after meals, but they are best taken between meals. The other vitamins and minerals are best taken together with or preferably after meals. People who are concerned about their calcium levels, such as pre- and post-menopausal women and many older people, may benefit by taking part of their calcium/magnesium supplements before bed, as most of the calcium that is leached from bodily tissues occurs at night. Vitamin E and selenium are best taken at the same time since selenium preserves vitamin E.

Look for supplements without artificial flavors, colors, and other additives. All of the above supplements are easy to incorporate into even the most hectic lifestyle.

Fighting Radiation & Chemical Toxins with Herbs

"**A**nd God said, Behold, I have given you every herb-bearing seed, which is upon the face of all the earth, and every tree, in which is the fruit of a tree-yielding seed; to you it shall be for meat. And to every beast of the earth, and to every fowl of the air, and to everything that creepeth upon the earth, wherein there is life, I have given every green herb for meat: and it was so. And God saw everything that He had made, and, behold, it was very good. . . ."

GENESIS 1:29 - 31

"*The mandate of the World Health Organization is to provide health for all by the year 2000 through the worldwide promotion of Herbal Medicine and the arts and crafts of the native healer.*"   U.N. WORLD HEALTH ORGANIZATION

Herbal medicine is the oldest form of physical healing chronicled in human history. More people have been effectively treated with herbs than by any other method. Thousands of books and many millions of people credit this practical system as being responsible for the profound healing of severe health problems. Herbs have long been nature's concentrated medicinal agents or pharmaceuticals, and they've earned a distinguished position among healing therapies. Today, more and more people are going back to this ancient and respected form of medicine. Still, few healers suggest that herbology be the only form of medical treatment, any more than synthetic antibiotics should be. There is no single preeminent modality of healing. But for all our exploration in the molecular and chemical world, the fact that herbs haven't been given greater attention by our modern health care system is both unscientific and tragic.

There is now a renaissance of interest in herbal medicine. Herbs contain a wide array of different medicinal substances that therapeutically affect different parts of the body. Indeed, every part of the body, including the blood, lymphatic, and nervous systems, every organ, and all our glands can be treated effectively with herbs. Certain herbs cleanse, strengthen, and protect the immune system, thereby reinforcing the body's innate self-healing mechanisms and helping people to heal themselves of serious diseases such as cancer.

Herbology is a complex yet potent system. Like other healing arts and sciences, medical herbology requires many years of study to be practiced responsibly and reliably. Uninformed herbal self-treatment is not a good idea. Fortunately, we can draw upon a tradition that is thousands of years old, as well as upon the collective experiences of modern herbalists, for the responsible use of plants as medicine. When using herbs in your own life, consult an experienced and knowledgeable herbalist and, as with any highly potent system, follow the directions accurately and respectfully. The herbal remedies, and especially the herbal formulas, provided in this book are effective and safe at the recommended dosages. They are widely used and have been thoroughly tested by the author as well as by other herbalists and many clients over time.

SIBERIAN GINSENG

Eleuthero, or *Eleutherococcus senticosus*, is frequently called Siberian ginseng because it is native to parts of China and Russia. Its medicinal use differs from other types of ginseng, which belong to the family *Araliaceae*, genus *Panax* (such as North American ginseng, which is *Panax quinquefolius*).

Since 1960, more than 1,000 scientific articles have been written about eleuthero, most of which are in Russian, and the Soviet government has encouraged its testing in more than 100 hospitals and clinics in the U.S.S.R. Eleuthero has been most extensively tested by the well-known plant researcher Dr. I. I. Brekhman and his associates at the Institute of Biologically Active Compounds, part of the Far Eastern Center of the Siberian Division of the U.S.S.R. Academy of Science. Brekhman says, "Results have established that a fluid extract of eleuthero possesses a remarkably wide range of therapeutic activity. For example, it protects the body against stress, radiation, and various chemical toxins."

Eleutherococcus senticosus is frequently referred to as an "adaptogen," which means that it produces an adaptive or normalizing effect on the body. An adaptogenic herb increases the body's ability to adapt to internal or external stress and changing environmental conditions—such as toxins that affect our immunity and vitality. The reason it has a "wide range of therapeutic activity" is that eleuthero can significantly improve the general health, strengthen the immune system, and increase the energy level of those who regularly use it. Eleuthero is consumed throughout the Soviet Union for both the prevention and treatment of disease. That it helps humans overcome both mental and physical stress has been well documented. Russian Olympic athletes regularly take an herbal extract of eleuthero and report noticeable improvements in their performance. In addition to athletes, a wide array of Russians, including soldiers, executives, mine and mountain rescuers, and cosmonauts, regularly take eleuthero extract. Results of studies conducted on eleuthero have been so promising that research scientists held an international symposium on this herb in Hamburg, West Germany in 1980.

Soviet researchers have reported that eleuthero extract has radioprotective abilities, and can be used therapeutically in conditions of acute and chronic radiation sicknesses such as hemorrhaging, severe anemia, dizziness, nausea, vomiting, and headaches due to x-rays.[1] It has been shown to lengthen survival time after exposure, as well. After rats were exposed to large doses of from 1,620 to 7,000 roentgens of prolonged irradiation, eleuthero doubled the rats' lifespan and improved the state of blood and other indices. In another experiment within the same research study, eleuthero neutralized radiation damage and increased the survival period of irradiated mice five times longer than a control group.

Dr. T. M. Khatnashvili, chairman of oncology at the Tbilisi Post-Graduate Medical School in the Soviet Union, used eleuthero extract while treating human patients suffering from cancerous tumors of the lips and mouth.[2] Thirty-eight patients received eleuthero one hour before irradiation, while a control group with the same number and severity of cancers did not. Khatnashvili reported, "Eleuthero considerably improved the patients' general state, appetite, and sleep, and it normalized pathological shifts of respiration, pulse, and arterial pressure."

In those patients receiving eleuthero after exposure to radiation, tumors began to soften three to five days sooner, and the wounds healed within four weeks instead of the usual six to nine weeks. Also, during an observation period of two years, only the eleuthero group showed no signs of relapses or metastases (spreading of cancer from its original site).

Experiments conducted by G. Mainanski showed that antibiotics administered alone were unable to prevent or cure radiation sickness.[3] When animals were treated with both antibiotics and eleuthero, a number of barometers of health either improved or rapidly returned to a normal level.

In a study that was conducted by specialists at the Institute of Oncology in the U.S.S.R., forty of eighty patients with breast cancer received eleuthero extract in a dose of 2 ml. daily for fourteen days.[4] The oncologists concluded, "The most favorable results were observed when eleuthero was administered two to four days prior to the beginning of roentgenotherapy or in parallel with the latter. These patients showed almost no usual reactions to x-radiation, such as indisposition, dizziness, nausea, loss of appetite, etc. Their feeling of well-being and their general state remained good for a long time. Even in patients with third-stage cancer (with metastases) whose conditions were grave, an improvement of mood, general state, and appetite could be achieved after taking three or four doses of *Eleutherococcus*. The arterial pressure, pulse, and respiration rates in *Eleutherococcus*-treated patients were much better than in control patients observed in parallel. No side effects were noted in any case."

Gvamichava et al. determined that eleuthero significantly decreased the toxic side effects of anti-cancer chemotherapy and roentgenotherapy, which were being used to treat mammary gland cancer in humans.[5] After dispensing just 28 ml. of the *Eleutherococcus* extract, the researchers noted that the patients' general condition, appetite, and sleep substantially improved. The researchers "emphatically recommended the use of *Eleutherococcus* in the treatment of mammary gland cancer—including the first, second, or third stage cancer development."

The two series of experiments by Studentzova showed that even one single dose of eleuthero extract reduced the toxic effects of highly lethal and medium-lethal dosages of either radiation therapy or anticancer drugs.[6] It substantially improved both red and white blood cell levels. Other research experiments conducted on animals with cancerous tumors demonstrate that eleuthero definitely inhibits metastasis and the growth of new cancers. In two experiments, however, eleuthero did not affect the growth of existing tumors.[7-9]

Researchers Turkevich and Matreichuk found that eleuthero extract normalized endocrine dysfunctions that were caused by administration of carcinogenic drugs commonly used to treat breast tumor.[10]

According to Brekhman, eleuthero "can be very beneficial in increasing the general resistance of the patient. These tests and others demonstrate the unique ability of *Eleutherococcus* to retard the development of metastases and increase the effect of anticancer agents. These effects, added to its ability to provide antitoxic, antioxidizing, tonic, radioprotective, and therapeutic effects in radiation sickness, as well as reduce the toxic side effects of anticancer preparations, emphasize the need for its use in cancer therapy."[11]

Several more studies show that liquid extract of eleuthero can neutralize the ill effects caused by drugs and other substances.[12] Eleuthero increased the blood supply to the brain of animals anesthetized with ether or other substances.[13, 14] Eleuthero produced a return to normal in rabbits administered injections of cobalt nitrate.[15]

Eleuthero extract protected frogs from normally lethal doses of digitalis, which is commonly used for some heart dysfunctions.[16] The same experiments showed that eleuthero extract strengthened the immune system and increased the resistance levels.

Liquid extract of eleuthero counteracted some of the side effects of cortisone treatment, such as adverse changes in the weight of the adrenals. Eleuthero also caused the weight of the thyroid to return to normal after animals were administered other drugs.[17] *Eleutherococcus* fluid extract prevented an abnormal decrease in white blood cells when rabbits were injected with various toxins.[18]

Other research experiments, in addition to some referred to earlier, indicate that eleuthero offers significant protection against various toxic chemicals and helps counteract their effects. For example, when mice were injected with tetraethyl lead, their conditioned reflexes became damaged. Treatment of these mice with eleuthero restored their conditioned reflexes, and extended their lives 33 percent compared to the untreated mice. In another study, administration of a toxic chemical to guinea pigs resulted in paralysis of lower extremities, increasing emaciation, and the eventual death of all the animals except one. By contrast, all the guinea pigs given the same chemical but treated with eleuthero remained alive; they regained their weight and free use of their extremities.

As noted earlier, exposure to radiation or chemical pollutants can cause prolonged, abnormal shifts in white blood cell counts. Eleuthero extract given to people after exposure to chemical pollutants normalizes both moderately low and some chronically and abnormally high levels of white blood cell counts.

Studies in the U.S. have shown that rats exposed to any kind of stress—whether it is radiation, chemical intoxication, exposure to heat or cold, electric shock, surgery, exhaustion, or immobilization—all demonstrate the same effects, including bloated adrenals and lowered immune response. On rats and other animals, eleuthero extract either prevented or delayed the usual pathological changes due to stress.

Numerous other research studies show that liquid extract of *Eleutherococcus* significantly improved human immune response. Over 1,000 Russian factory workers were administered 4 ml. daily of eleuthero while working for a five-month period in bitterly cold Arctic weather.[19] The eleuthero extract produced a 40 percent decrease in days lost from work and a 50 percent reduction in general sicknesses. No ill side effects were reported.

Administration of 5 ml. daily of eleuthero extract to 445 men working in another inclement area of the Soviet Union caused a 50 percent or greater reduction in a wide range of common cold ailments, including tonsillitis, laryngitis, bronchitis, pharyngitis, acute rhinitis, and acute inflammation of mucous membranes.[20] Several of the above ailments were completely prevented during the three months of harshest weather.

Tests were conducted on 1,200 test-car drivers whose work involved daily emotional strain as well as physical stresses produced by extreme changes in temperature, automobile vibrations, and exhaust fumes.[21] For two years, eleuthero was given in the drivers' tea each day for two months every spring and autumn. Eleuthero produced a dramatic reduction in common illnesses, high blood pressure, and number of working days lost due to influenza.

Several more research studies document that *Eleutherococcus* liquid extract substantially strengthens the immune system and stimulates the immune response in both humans and animals. The spleen and thymus are the two organs that directly control the immune response in humans. Administration of eleuthero extract for eight days prevented the usual reduction of the thymus and spleen following cortisone medication.[22-24]

Eleutherococcus senticosus contains several substances (glycosides) that are similar in structure and function to substances in the herb *Panax ginseng* (discussed next). It also contains other unique polysaccharides that have distinct immune-enhancing properties. Eleuthero stimulates macrophages, granulocytes, and other components of white blood cells that act as scavengers. These scavengers surround, ingest, and neutralize foreign harmful toxins, thereby helping the body to resist infections or other immunological disorders.

The Soviet doctors Pichurina and Bronnikov found that eleuthero extract offered rabbits strong protection against infections and other harmful conditions, including exposure to lethal dysentery microbes.[25]

Eleuthero increases the resistance to the bacteria *Listeria monocytogenes*, which causes infections and meningitis in humans and animals.[26, 27] Fluid extract of eleuthero stimulates the production of antibodies and fosters immunity to other viruses in mammals.[28] It helps build immunity to typhoid.[29, 30] Eleuthero extract increases immunity to other bacteria and viruses, and it helps prevent the side effects of several vaccines commonly used.[31] *Eleutherococcus* prevents abnormal changes in white blood cells caused by subcutaneous administration of milk.[32]

After years of research with humans, Soviet scientists concluded that the eleuthero plant extract increases human resistance to a remarkably wide variety of stressors. The herb preparation helped people cope better under the ordinary stress and tension of modern everyday living; protected against typical stress-induced illnesses; produced a calming effect on people who had endured months of pressure and tension; eased the strain of worry and bottled-up anxiety; relieved tensions of business and sports competition; and delivered a protective effect against the stress of surgery, accidents, certain chemical toxins, radiation, and chronic illnesses.

Eleuthero extract prevents harmful changes in human biochemistry due to stress. These changes include stomach bleeding, unbalanced vitamin C content of adrenal glands, disrupted production of adrenalin, excretion of a number of ketosteroids, and other symptoms of stress.

Eleuthero's ability to increase human resistance to various stressors is typical of so-called adaptogenic or harmonizing herbs. Adaptogenic herbs tend to restore both red and white blood cell counts to normal. They normalize both high and low blood pressure, and improve our immune and stress response systems. Adaptogenic herbs also relax or stimulate as needed certain other body functions.

Exposure to radiation or chemical pollutants can result in any of a variety of nervous system disorders. Soviet scientists have discovered that eleuthero extract has a pronounced therapeutic effect on functional nervous disorders, even in chronic patients.[33] Clinical studies of eleuthero extract were carried out on human patients suffering from irritability and excitedness, insomnia, decreased working capabilities, persistent fears, moodiness, depression, loss of vigor, and extreme exhaustion. Administration of eleuthero consistently brought about an improved sense of well-being, more balanced energy, and regular sleep, and it helped stabilize other physical and emotional factors. There were no side effects recorded.

Eleuthero aids in the absorption and retention of some important protective nutrients. When 2 ml. of eleuthero extract was administered alone or in combination with a multivitamin supplement, it increased the absorption in both men and women of vitamins B and B_2.[34] Liquid extract of eleuthero also increased the retention of vitamin C.[35]

At an International Symposium on *Eleutherococcus* and Ginseng, Soviet scientists reported the wide variety of uses of eleuthero extract. According to N. Tretchikoff, a prominent Russian herbalist, the Soviet government has spent well over the equivalent of 5 million dollars researching eleuthero extract.[36] The results were so impressive that an extract of eleuthero was included in the primary drink of their cosmonauts when they orbited the world for a record-setting 100 days. The Soviets considered eleuthero extract to be the most effective substance they could find for protecting their cosmonauts against the effects of stress and environmental changes, and for increasing their stamina, endurance, and general health.

Although eleuthero extract has been observed to yield quick, symptomatic relief, it is best taken as a tonic in repeated daily doses over time. Richard Lucas, author of *Eleuthero: Health Herb of Russia* (R & M Books, 1973), states that Soviet doctors recommend as a general course of treatment that eleuthero extract be used in the following amounts:

"Adult single doses: 20 to 40 drops before meals, repeated two or three times a day to make the total daily dose of 80 drops. Dosage for children, a single dose: one drop per each year of age, repeated twice a day. A treatment course lasts for 25 to 30 days. Repeated courses are given at one- or two-week intervals, if necessary." Eleuthero extract is best taken by adding the liquid extract to room-temperature or slightly warm water.

Eleutherococcus senticosus extract is currently produced by several companies in North America, and can be purchased from many natural foods stores or from herb companies. If you have any difficulty finding eleuthero extract, you can go to your local health food or natural foods store and have them order the extract for you. An informative book about this herb is *Eleutherococcus Senticosus* (Oriental Healing Arts Institute, 1984) by Bruce Halstead, M.D., and Loretta Hood.

Since 1972, when I first began working with eleuthero, I have had countless clients report beneficial results. My clinical experience is that eleuthero is unique—it is an excellent tonic as well as a gentle yet reliable stimulant. Taken regularly, eleuthero produces long-lasting benefits that are not accompanied by the usual consequences of ingesting synthetic stimulants such as amphetamines, including deterioration of general health and eventual reduction of energy and work capacity. Research experiments on humans, and clinical experience, show that eleuthero not only increases energy levels, it improves the quality and efficiency of the effort as well. *Eleutherococcus senticosus* is a primary substance in the immune-boosting Herbal Formula Three described in Chapter 9.

In a summary of his research on eleuthero, Brekhman, who is probably the world's foremost authority on this herb, says, "The preparations from *Eleutherococcus* are nontoxic and harmless even when they are administered recurringly over a long period of time. These preparations improve and increase quality and quantity of physical and mental work (stimulating and tonic effect). The capacity of *Eleutherococcus* to increase the nonspecific resistance of an organism against the harmful influence of a large number of physical, chemical, and biological factors (adaptogenic effect) is very important."

PANAX GINSENG

Panax ginseng, the Asiatic ginseng native to Manchuria, Korea, and Japan, is probably the most revered herb in human history. *Panax ginseng*, or simply "ginseng," is a tonic herb that strengthens the body's immune system against invasive agents, including radiation and chemical toxins. Its medicinal uses are far too numerous to deal with adequately in this short space. To summarize, it regulates the adrenals and balances digestion. There is a vast body of international research that shows that ginseng and its cousin eleuthero have restorative, stimulating, adaptogenic, and healing capacities. Eleuthero and *Panax ginseng* contain several substances (glycosides) that are similar in structure and function, although each herb also contains other unique substances that have distinct properties and functions.

A number of researchers attending the Third International Ginseng Symposium held in Seoul, South Korea, in 1980, reported the effects of *Panax ginseng* extract on mice that had received ordinarily fatal doses of x-rays. Japanese researchers found that one 6.8 mg. injection of the ginseng extract increased survival from 5 percent in the control group (which was not given the ginseng) to 82.5 percent in the mice that received ginseng.[37]

In another series of experiments, doctors found that a single post-irradiation injection of *Panax ginseng* extract sharply increased the thirty-day survival ratio of x-irradiated mice, rats, and guinea pigs.[38] The ginseng injection accelerated the recovery of red and white blood cells, especially the thrombocytes or blood platelets. *Panax ginseng* enhanced the recovery of blood-forming stem cells in bone marrow. The researchers observed that "even though a dose of 1.8 mg. resulted in significant radioprotection, the survival ratio increased even further with increasing doses of the extract."[39] They also noted that "injection of the extract 1 or 2 days before exposure produced a much more efficacious result," which highlights the importance of an optimal, yet easy to use, preventive program such as the one described in Part III of this book.

Hemorrhage was a symptom of humans exposed to atomic radiations in Hiroshima and Nagasaki. Japanese research doctors found that "*Panax ginseng* prevented hemorrhaging tendency after x-irradiation."[40]

Bone marrow death is one result of radiation damage to blood-forming tissues. It occurs ten to twenty days after exposure to high doses of radiation.[41] *Panax ginseng* extract prevents bone marrow death and accelerates normalization of red and white blood cell counts in animal studies.[42] The extract hastens the return to normal weight of the spleen, the organ that is involved in blood formation and that functions as an important part of the immune system. The researchers also found that *Panax ginseng* aided recovery of mice that had lost the function of their spleens and were also suffering from normally lethal radiation-induced bone marrow dysfunction. They observed that recovery of "thrombocyte blood platelets is very important in survival from radiation-induced bone marrow death." Another researcher, K. Hirashima, observed that, "Since recovery of blood-forming stem cells is a fundamental requirement for a radioprotective substance, this result would confirm the efficacy of ginseng extract as a radioprotective substance."[43]

Two other studies confirm that *Panax ginseng* stimulates bone marrow functions and red blood cell formation—both often adversely affected after irradiation.[44, 45] The researchers also reported their investigations of a variety of substances, including vaccines and crude drugs, that were considered possible radioprotectants. They observed that the root of the *Panax ginseng* plant was more easily assimilated and more effective on humans than the synthetic substances tested. The above evidence was supported by results from another study by Yonezawa, in which a single injection of ginseng extract given to mice after irradiation afforded significant radiation protection.[46]

Research scientists have observed that ginseng increases the rate of production of serum albumin and gamma-globulin (antibodies in blood) as well as DNA, RNA, protein, and lipid (fat) synthesis in bone marrow cells.[47] A Soviet study showed that ginseng root extract allowed human subjects to acclimatize more easily to oxygen-deficient air.[48] Lack of oxygen within the body frequently has been cited as a cause of certain kinds of cancers.

According to Ron Teeguarden in *Chinese Tonic Herbs* (Japan Publications, 1985), "Ginseng is beneficial to both men and women and is used commonly by both. It is a Western myth that ginseng should only be used by men." Teeguarden notes that ginseng is an excellent energy tonic for men and women alike.

Oriental medical authorities describe diseases in somewhat different terms than we do in the West. Traditionally, ginseng is rarely used in what the Chinese call yang conditions, or conditions of excess, such as inflammations or irritations, as manifested by fever, burning sensation, or infection. Similarly, ginseng can strengthen a weak prostate but it is contraindicated for an inflamed prostate (a yang condition). In women, ginseng is contraindicated for excessive menstrual flow (another example of a yang condition), yet it remains quite beneficial for both men and women with deficiency diseases, such as lowered resistance, diminished energy, and some hypofunctions related to the reproductive system in both men and women.

Ginseng may be taken raw or cooked. Many people steam ginseng root until it can be easily sliced into sections about the thickness of a penny. It can also be sucked or chewed. The dried root may be ground into a powder and placed in capsules.

Ginseng extracts from China and Korea are available at most natural foods and health food stores. When buying ginseng, try to obtain the best quality you can afford. Like the Chinese herbalists, I rarely use *Panax ginseng* alone. Over the years, I have combined it with different herbs into various medicinal formulas for some of my clients. Refer to the discussion of Herbal Formulas in Chapter 9 for an excellent preparation that utilizes ginseng to build the immune system.

When using ginseng, it is best to take small amounts regularly over a period of time because ginseng functions best as a tonic that progressively strengthens and balances the system. *Panax ginseng* is not an irritating stimulant such as caffeine. Rather, it has been revered for thousands of years throughout the world because its effects, like those of eleuthero, are gentle yet deep and reliable.

ALOE

During the summer of 1967, I was hired to do research at the world's first medical laser laboratory at Children's Hospital in Cincinnati, Ohio. Every day, after completing my own experiments, I would go into the room where the research animals were housed and do what I could to help some of them heal from their laser burns.

After using several preparations, I observed that a fresh aloe vera gel produced the most impressive healing of various skin disorders, including burns, lesions, and cancers. I also had an opportunity to test the gel on myself after an accidental laser burn, and then on a few willing patients at the laboratory. Each time, aloe consistently and quickly produced impressive results.

Many plant lovers know that aloe can speed the healing of cuts, burns, and other skin problems. Extensive research supports these observations and also documents aloe's value as a radioprotectant.

Of the more than two hundred species of *Aloe*, the following species have shown evidence of being radioprotectants: *Aloe barbadensis* (aloe vera), *Aloe arborescens*, *Aloe striatula*, and *Aloe saponaria*.

Since the very earliest use of x-rays, doctors have found that radiation adversely affects skin tissue, sometimes severely. Often, radiation causes extensive scaling and shredding of skin, severe burning, and continuous and intense itching. It may lead to the oozing of a thin, watery liquid known as serous fluid. In 1935, Dr. E. E. Collins, a Maryland physician, and his brother Creston Collins conducted important studies on the effective use of aloe vera for x-ray dermatitis, which is the inflammation and infection of the skin caused by x-rays.[49, 50] Their reports aroused great interest throughout the medical field.

The Collinses treated more than fifty cases of x-ray and radium burns, skin inflammations, and ulcerated skin tissues. They found that after application of fresh aloe vera the within twenty-four hours itching and burning subsided entirely. Aloe vera subsequently led to a complete restoration of sensation, the return of normal pigmentation, an absence of scarring, and, in general, a markedly improved rate of healing. The researchers used the fresh gel-like material inside the leaf, and left each application on for one to two hours. They carefully washed off each application with warm water, using no soap or medication.

According to Dr. Gilbert Reynolds, who studied the use of aloe as a traditional medicine in Africa:

> Accounts have stated that the leaf of aloe vera (*Aloe barbadensis*) is of great use in the treatment of x-ray burns. . . . A leading Johannesburg dermatologist, when informed that aloe vera leaves were not available locally in South Africa, used the leaves of *Aloe arborescens* in the treatment of x-ray burns. Subsequently . . . he stated 'I have now treated three cases of radiodermatitis [x-ray burns] with the leaf of *Aloe arborescens*. This was used since the aloe vera was unobtainable. My cases were given the split leaf, with the juicy pulp exposed as a dressing on the raw area. The first two patients were given it continuously, while the third had a dressing at night only. All healed well, and far more promptly than one could expect from any other form of local treatment. I conclude from these few cases that this is a valuable method of treatment of x-ray burns.'[51]

Two Soviet researchers tested the emulsions of juices from *Aloe arborescens* and *Aloe striatula*, which were applied externally after radiation treatment to 260 human patients suffering from malignant tumors.[52, 53] They found that the emulsions were of equal effectiveness and that both were far more therapeutic than most synthetic preparations in reducing skin reaction due to irradiation. They said that aloe emulsions were "recommended for preventing the development of local reactions in radiation therapy, in the treatment of dry and moist epidermitis [inflammation of the outer layers of the skin] and treating radiation burns of the second and third degrees. . ." Aloe was also found to accelerate the process of tissue repair and normal cell growth, and to be helpful in treating many other dermatological problems.

According to cancer researcher Dr. James Brown, "Aloe vera tends to keep down keratosis formation of horny growth on skin and ulceration; these effects may tend to slow up, and possibly prevent, changes toward malignancy. We have many patients who have obtained marked relief from pain, cracking, and keratosis of such radiation burns. These include cases of physician's hands burned in their own work, and burns from treatment given over the face and elsewhere. . ."[54]

In 1953, Dr. C. C. Lushbaugh and D. B. Hale performed tests on rabbits and other laboratory animals irradiated with strontium-90 and then treated with the fresh whole leaf of aloe vera.[55] These tests were conducted under the auspices of the U. S. Atomic Energy Commission at the Radiation Burn Center, Los Alamos Proving Grounds. They concluded that, "Treatment with aloe vera was found to hasten. . . reparative phases of the lesion so that complete healing of an ulcer caused by 28,000 rems of beta radiation was accomplished within two months of treatment, while the untreated ulcerations were still not completely healed more than four months after irradiation. It was concluded that aloe vera contains substances that are stimulatory both to the delayed development and delayed healing of ulcerative radiodermatitis, and that because of the growing modern importance of this injury, further investigation of the action of aloe vera should be pursued."

Other researchers have also found that juice from the aloe vera leaf gave excellent results in the treatment of humans experiencing reactions to radiation. A series of tests in the 1960s in various hospitals showed aloe ointment to be 50 percent better than three other remedies considered most advantageous for burn treatment.[56]

After reviewing extensive scientific research on aloe, the Food and Drug Administration stated in 1959 that "upon review, the FDA admits that aloe does actually regenerate skin tissue."[57]

It is optimal to use aloe vera in its fresh form directly from the plant. In studies conducted by Dr. Wendell D. Winters of the University of Texas Health Science Center, a fresh extract from aloe vera was found to speed up healing and to spur growth of new cells far more effectively than commercial preparations of the aloe juice.[58]

Exposure to some radioactive isotopes or certain chemical toxins can cause a wide range of inflammations, infections, and internal and external pains. Drs. John P. Heggers and Martin C. Robson believe aloe vera to contain antibacterial, anti-inflammatory, and pain-relieving properties.[59]

Heggers is director of research and laboratories at the University of Chicago Burn Center, and Robson is director of plastic and reconstructive surgery at the Burn Center. Based on their research with guinea pigs, dogs, a monkey, and finally humans, they concluded that, "Aloe vera has three major properties that are most beneficial in thermal injury [burns]: 1. Aloe vera extract contains an aspirin-like compound which, coupled with the high magnesium content, may be capable of relieving pain; 2. The extract, in concentrations of 70 percent or greater, becomes an effective topical bactericidal against infections common to burns; and 3. Aloe vera appears to negate the interrupted blood flow which usually occurs at a burn site, thus stimulating circulation to the wound and improving tissue regeneration."

The results of many other experiments further document that aloe vera is a reliable radioprotectant.[60-67]

The four species of *Aloe* that have been documented as effective radioprotectants have meaty leaves containing ample quantities of leaf gel. Research indicates that there are different degrees of usefulness among the various true aloes. In my clinical experience, I have found aloe vera (*Aloe barbadensis*) to be the most consistently therapeutic variety for either personal or commercial use.

Aloe has become a popular plant and is easily grown in many areas. It can be grown outside in frost-free climates or indoors in a pot. One of the four species of aloe with known radioprotective qualities should be used in order to receive maximum results. The grower does not need to be a botanist to accurately identify an effective variety of aloe. Dr. William C. Coats, a registered pharmacist and the author of *The Silent Healer: A Modern Study of Aloe Vera*, includes in his book some simple identifying characteristics: "First, the rosette configuration is something that will be consistent with all true aloes. Second, the leaves will be of a triangular spear-like shape coming to a point. In the first two modes of identification it is easy to be fooled by false aloes unless you remember that the leaves of aloe vera will have thorny ridges only along the spines. Otherwise they will be smooth and meaty to the touch, an indication that they are pregnant with gel. Many false aloes will not have meaty leaves and will exhibit bumps or wartlike patterns all over the rind. Additionally, the coloring of many false aloes tends to be darker green while the leaves of a mature aloe vera will be consistently pale green to medium green with yellow flecks or smooth yellow-white highlights. . . ."

The American "aloe" is common in the southwestern deserts of North America. This plant, also called agave or century plant, is actually not an aloe nor is it even related to aloe.

Proper use of the aloe vera plant is important—especially when treating more serious problems such as radiation burns. The most common misuse of aloe vera is the application of gel from immature plants. Though it is generally safe and usually effective to use the younger plants for common household burns, the results obtained are frequently inferior. Coats recommends using plants with "three to five years of growth at a height of from one-and-a-half to four feet and an individual leaf thickness of three inches or more at the base. You don't get that from something growing in a small five-inch pot, and you shouldn't expect to."

Coats also warns against the tendency to "pull leaves from the inner part of the rosette; this is the least potent area. Aloe vera should always be harvested from the outer leaves first, working inward. Not only do these possess leaf-gel with the most medicinal potential, they are also the most nearly ripe. . . . The pulp inside a degenerated leaf loses its potency just like those of many other succulent plants. When it does, it can become bitter and rancid. The gel turns yellowish and mustard-like in color and (if taken internally) can cause some nausea."

Dried aloe is occasionally used in laxative formulas, but it should be taken with guidance. Otherwise intense diarrhea, cramping, or constipation could occur. The medicinal action of dried aloe is quite different from that of fresh aloe, which is more soothing when taken internally. Approach dried aloe with caution.

The gel from the fresh leaf of a mature aloe vera plant is extremely beneficial for disorders of the gastrointestinal tract, including gastric or duodenal ulcers, constipation, and even cancers of the gastrointestinal tract. These disorders are sometimes produced by exposure to irritating or toxic radioactive isotopes or chemical contaminants.

Aloe acts similarly to vitamin A by aiding the growth and repair of body tissues. Both help maintain smooth, soft, disease-free skin. Internally, both aloe and vitamin A give strength to cell walls and help protect the mucous membranes, while reducing susceptibility to infection. Both act as antioxidants and combat the effects of radiation and air-borne pollutants.

There are, however, a few cautions regarding the internal use of aloe. Pregnant women should not ingest aloe vera since it acts to contract the smooth muscles, including those of the uterus. Also, diabetics should consult their physician before taking aloe vera, since there is the possibility that it may stimulate the pancreas to produce more insulin.

Aloe vera is not a panacea, nor is it a cure for most medical ailments as some people have promoted it. However, used properly for the disorders it is known to affect, aloe vera is a powerful healer that has been successfully employed for millennia.

CHAPARRAL

Chaparral (*Larrea divaricata*), sometimes referred to as creosote bush, grows in northern Mexico and the southwestern part of the U.S. In traditional folk medicine, chaparral is considered a strong herb and it is still prescribed today for various health problems. One of chaparral's most active ingredients is a potent antioxidant called NDGA, which stands for nordihydroguaiaretic acid. As previously noted, antioxidants have powerful protective qualities against the effects of radiation and chemical pollutants.

Chemists have used the NDGA from chaparral as an antioxidant to prevent oils, butter, lard, and other fats from spoiling and going rancid. The NDGA in chaparral works by preventing the growth of bacteria.[68] According to several researchers, NDGA has potential as an anticancer and antitumor agent.

In 1960, Dr. Jonathan L. Hartwell of the National Cancer Institute cited several cases of cancer cured with chaparral.[69] In 1968 and 1969, surgeons C.R. Smart and H.Y. Hogle headed a team of researchers who studied the effects of chaparral on tumor growth.[70] They concluded that "the NDGA factor has been very useful in correcting malignant melanoma in many cancer patients."

In 1970, Dr. Ronald S. Pardini and his team of researchers studied the effectiveness of NDGA in cancer therapy and stated that "NDGA also inhibits the tumor electron transport system, which denies such growths the electrical energy they require to exist."[71] The antioxidant NDGA in chaparral stopped and reversed the growth of certain tumors. Its healing effect on malignancies may provide a valuable line of defense after exposure to carcinogenic toxins or radiation. Chaparral is an excellent candidate for further research on potentially protective herbs.

Chaparral is one of nature's better antibiotics. It is useful for treating both bacterial and viral infections. In herbal medicine, chaparral is used for its antiseptic and antibiotic properties. It also works as an "alterative" herb. These herbs help stimulate and improve the body's blood purification and detoxification systems, such as the liver, kidneys, lungs, spleen, bowels, and lymph system. Like the tonic herbs ginseng and eleuthero, chaparral and other alterative herbs should be used in a gradual cleansing program over a period of several weeks or more. This gradual detoxification of the blood system will profoundly improve important body systems—such as the immune system. Certainly unhealthful dietary and lifestyle habits must simultaneously be gradually improved in order to deeply detoxify the blood and strengthen the immune system.

Chaparral should be used with caution and preferably with

supervision. Aside from NDGA, it contains gums, resins, protein, partially characterized esters, acids, alcohol, small amounts of a mixture of sterols, sucrose, and minute amounts of volatile oils. The medicinal parts of chaparral are the leaves and stems.

Chaparral should rarely be used alone. It is best taken in small amounts and combined with other antibiotic herbs such as *Echinacea angustifolia* and goldenseal. (See Herbal Formulas, Chapter 9.) It is advisable to work with a competent herbalist when using chaparral.

If you do take chaparral alone, the best forms are herbal tincture and extract, which are available at most health food or natural foods stores. Several companies make chaparral tincture or extract at different strengths. Follow the directions on the bottle.

The second best method of taking chaparral is in tea form. To make a tea, place one tablespoon of leaves and stems in a covered teapot or jar, pour one quart of boiling water over the tea, cover, let stand for one to eight hours, strain, then drink a quarter of the liquid four times a day. Most people find the taste of chaparral quite unpleasant, which should serve as a cautionary sign. Nature frequently imparts a strong or bitter taste to her powerful medicinal herbs, which serves as a guide for users to ingest only small amounts. The stronger the taste, the greater the probability that the herb contains substances, such as alkaloids or glycosides, that produce an intense effect upon the body. Do not drink more than the amount recommended.

Because of chaparral's taste, many people prefer to take it in tablet form, though it is not as strong as in tincture or tea form. Tablets are available in different strengths. When taking chaparral in tablet, it is best to take an extra 300-750 mg. of vitamin C per day to help the body process the concentrated resins and gums in the herb.

I've been working with chaparral for over two decades, and have used it in various herbal formulas for purifying the blood and lymph systems and for improving immune response. Several clients of mine who have taken chaparral in an herbal formula have subsequently healed themselves of leukemia, cancer, or one or more malignant tumors.

BIO-STRATH

Bio-Strath is a Swiss liquid herbal yeast product that is a combination of *Saccharomyces cerevisiae* yeast (see pages 88–92) and carefully selected wild herbs which have been gathered from fifteen different countries.[72] The herbs are analyzed to be sure they have not been chemically sprayed with pesticides or herbicides.

Bio-Strath was developed by Dr. Walter Strathmeyer, a German physician, and produced by a Swiss engineer, Fred Pestalozzi, who claims it cured him of Meniere's disease.

Bio-Strath has been studied since 1954, and animal and human experiments indicate that it protects against radiation and confers several other health benefits. It seems to improve metabolism and assimilation of nutrients in people who have been irradiated. It may also improve immune function and white blood cell count after exposure to radiation.

The production of Bio-Strath requires two months of fermentation, during which time the herbs are slowly and carefully added to the yeast. The substances added are malt extract, unrefined honey, unprocessed orange juice, and the herbs angelica, balm, basil, camomile, cinnamon, caraway, elder, fennel, horseradish, hyssop, lavender, licorice, peppermint, parsley, sage, and thyme.

All of the nutrients in Bio-Strath are of natural origin. It contains no chemical preservatives, colorings, or flavorings. The medicinal properties of the yeast, herbs, and other substances have not been depleted by common commercial cultivation or processing techniques. During production of Bio-Strath, ingredient temperature is not allowed to exceed about 90 degrees F., so that enzymes are not denatured and the yeasts and other nutrients remain in a state readily absorbable by the body.

When analyzed, the Bio-Strath liquid herbal yeast has been found to have a wide array of nutrients. These nutrients include proteins, carbohydrates, lecithin, the B complex, RNA, DNA, ATP, many minerals, and important enzymes. ATP is the molecule which the body utilizes to store energy for cell functions. It is a naturally occurring chemical energy unit. As is the case with some nutritional yeasts, all the nutrients in Bio-Strath are easily assimilated.

In a series of five experiments, Dr. Hedi Fritz-Niggli, who is head of the department of radiobiology at Zurich University, explored the protective and therapeutic effects of Bio-Strath in 348 white mice given single whole-body irradiation exposures of 500, 700, and 800 rads.[73]

After the dose of 500 rads, Bio-Strath (given as a food supplement before and after irradiation) reduced the mortality rate of mice from 27.8 percent to 11.1 percent. The product also reduced weight loss following irradiation. On the other hand, it did not influence the changes due to irradiation in the blood count and in radiation-sensitive organs.

In mice given a single dose of either 700 or 800 rads (lethal doses in about 90 percent of animals), supplementary feeding with Bio-Strath did not result in any reduction in the mortality rate.

Weight loss is a common result of exposure to radiation. Two indicators of the post-irradiation health of mammals are the percent of weight loss and the rate of weight gained back. Fritz-Niggli observed that mice fed Bio-Strath before and after irradiation lost less weight, and gained weight back more rapidly, than control animals not fed Bio-Strath. Recovery was enhanced by the addition of the Bio-Strath.

Another important observation was that mice fed Bio-Strath preceding exposure showed the same rate of growth as control animals, although their caloric intake had been reduced 18 percent. In growing mice, Bio-Strath improved the absorption of food. This observation was supported by two sets of studies done by H. Sporri and one by J. D. Ireson and colleagues during their investigations on rats.[74-76]

And, in another related study on the growth rate of young rats, J. M. Bagshaw and G.B. Leslie found that, "The administration of Bio-Strath as feed supplement resulted in a final weight increase of 16 percent compared with the control group, even though the number of calories ingested during feeding was less. The addition of the supplement was thus shown to effect a superior metabolic utilization of the animal feed in the rats. . . . The growth-promoting activity of the Bio-Strath supplement is therefore associated with a distinct improvement in the food utilization. It is not clear at present which ingredients of the preparation are responsible for this beneficial effect."[77]

Fritz-Niggli concluded from her own and other experiments that, "The benefits of Bio-Strath on the adverse effects of radiation are due to improved food utilization, a factor often adversely affected because of gastrointestinal involvement after irradiation. It is clear from this study that Bio-Strath helps to protect from the radiation which mammals are subjected to daily as a part of modern life. It would also be suggested that Bio-Strath could be used prophylactically in persons being subjected to radiation therapy."[78]

Fritz-Niggli next undertook a series of six experiments to gain information on the effect of Bio-Strath, given as a food supplement, on irradiation-induced fertility disorders in 177 female mice and their 6,352 offspring.[79] Preliminary experiments on control groups had established that the fertility of female mice was reduced after they had received one whole-body exposure to low doses (25 rads) of radiation, before mating and becoming pregnant. Both the number of successful matings and the size of the resulting litters were reduced when the female mice were exposed to radiation previous to mating.

When Bio-Strath was given to animals under the same conditions, it had no statistically significant effect on the decrease in the percentage of successful matings.[80] However, the size of the litters, which had decreased more than 33 percent in the irradiated mice, rose to the same level of the control group after being fed Bio-Strath. Fritz-Niggli concluded that, "Bio-Strath, given as a food supplement to irradiated mice, has beneficial effects on the radiation-induced depression of fertility."[81]

The results of the above series of experiments suggest that exposure of the whole body to very low levels of radiation, even only once, may decrease the ability of human beings to reproduce unless either preventive therapies are used beforehand or remedial measures taken after exposure to counteract the effects of radiation.

Fritz-Niggli and Dr. C. Michel of the Radiobiologic Institute of Zurich University, Switzerland, conducted research on the effects of Bio-Strath on radiation-induced anomalies (abnormal organs or structures). They state that,

> Contrary to views held in the past and still encountered today, radiation damage is not something that happens immediately at the time of irradiation. The biological effects of radiation are complex and often manifest themselves at the end of a long chain of reactions. Even after irradiation, physical, chemical, and biological means can be employed to abort or enhance the process. The possibility of intervention in the nefarious course of reactions is of particular interest. Substances can be found which reduce damage—they are radiation-protection substances that would, e.g., prevent radiation death caused by nuclear weapons or would protect healthy tissue in the radiotherapy of cancer.
>
> It is well-known that radiotherapy is limited in its application by the risk of radiation damage being caused to normal tissue. The possibility of influencing the effects—such as developmental anomalies—caused by small quantities of radiation appears to be particularly important.[82]

Dr. K.W. Brunner, a German oncologist, directed a series of double-blind studies testing the effect of Bio-Strath on 177 human cancer patients given radiotherapy. He concluded that,

> It is evident from the results of these double-blind experiments that Bio-Strath given regularly (3 teaspoonsful per day = 21 ml.) improved, in several respects, the well-being of human cancer

patients undergoing radiotherapy over a period of time. As assessed by the patients themselves, those in the Bio-Strath groups suffered less from side effects such as loss of appetite and fatigue, and their general well-being was altogether better than that of the controls.

Among the measured parameters, the different progress of the weight curve of the individual is worth special mention. In the Bio-Strath group, the bodyweight remained practically constant during radiation treatment and the one-month period of convalescence. In the control group, however, weight had decreased by an average of 3.00 kg. at the end of the period of observation.

Treatment with Bio-Strath also prevented depression of the hemoglobin level associated with irradiation. The thrombocyte (blood platelet) count showed similar changes in the control and Bio-Strath groups. Blood urea, and the activities of the serum enzymes alkaline phosphatase, SGOT, and SGPt (blood-liver-heart enzymes) remained unchanged in both groups during irradiation and convalescence.[83]

Brunner also observed that Bio-Strath improved a person's condition by enhancing assimilation of nutrients.

According to Drs. J. D. Ireson, E. E. Conway, and F. H. Schwarzenbach, Bio-Strath significantly delayed the development of cancer in mice.[84] In another phase of these studies, cancerous tumors were induced in mice prior to treatment with Bio-Strath. Bio-Strath reduced tumor growth in all groups as compared to control animals. The weight of the solid tumors and the incidence of necroses (localized death of tissue) were both reduced. In another group of mice, the additional feeding of Bio-Strath prior to infection with tumor cells caused a reduction in the initial development rate of the tumor. The doctors concluded from the results of these experiments that treatment with the yeast preparation antagonized, opposed, or counteracted the "take" or early growth of the cancer.

It should be pointed out that a similar experiment at a different institute failed to confirm the effect observed by Ireson et al.[85] In this particular experiment, however, in place of Bio-Strath mice were given an artificial preparation that contained corresponding quantities of calories, vitamins, and minerals. These test mice did not show any difference in tumor development from control animals. The same researchers later repeated the experiment, using Bio-Strath yeast tablets as well as the liquid preparation. This time the earlier positive results were reconfirmed. The efficacy of the tablets was comparable to that of the liquid elixir.

A study published in *Swiss Med* reported that Bio-Strath helps to stabilize the white blood cell count in mice with abnormally low white blood cell counts.[86]

Mice given Bio-Strath have been shown to be more resistant to the effects of E. coli bacteria. One study reported that Bio-Strath-fed mice displayed significant protection against a variety of pathogenic organisms and bacterial infections.[87]

When William Crook, M.D., first published his influential book *The Yeast Connection* in 1984, many healers and physicians began to indiscriminately advise against the use of any yeast product. No differentiation was made between "good yeast" (*Saccharomyces cerevisiae*) and "bad yeast" (*Candida albicans*). In the completely revised and updated edition of *The Yeast Connection* (Random House, 1986), Crook states that "not all patients with candida-related health problems need to avoid the yeast-containing foods. To find out if you need to avoid these foods, follow a yeast-free diet for one week, then eat some yeast and see if it bothers you." Crook goes on to say that benefits could be derived from yeasts other than *Candida albicans*.

John Rippon, Ph.D., of the University of Chicago, a past president of the Medical Mycological [the science of fungi] Society of the Americas, states that, "Not all yeasts contribute to yeast-related problems. *Candida albicans* . . . accounts for the vast variety of yeast-related health problems. On the other hand, *Saccharomyces cerevisiae* yeast, the basic ingredient in the herbal yeast food supplement, Bio-Strath, has been used beneficially for thirty-five years in over thirty-five countries. The difference between *Saccharomyces cerevisiae* and *Candida albicans* is immense." Several other internationally respected medical doctors and health authorities have endorsed Bio-Strath.

I have taken a relatively large amount of space to discuss one type of liquid herbal-yeast product compared to the amount of space devoted to the more commonly available dried, primary-grown nutritional yeasts. It is impossible to determine from current research if one is more effective than the others, and I am not claiming any preference. Certainly Bio-Strath seems to improve the absorption and utilization of nutrients from food. It may also prove to further enhance the benefits of a whole foods diet and recommended food supplements and herbs. The reason I have devoted an extensive discussion to Bio-Strath is because of the relatively large amount of scientific research that has been conducted on this liquid herbal-yeast.

BLACK AND GREEN TEA

Tea, both black and green, is currently being explored for its potential radioprotective properties.

Black and green teas are both made from the same herb, *Thea sinensis*, but each are dried and cured differently. They are also different from the hundreds of other herbal teas commonly available. Green teas are cured without fermentation, and are as popular in China and Japan as coffee is in the West. Black tea is fermented during curing, and India and Sri Lanka are its major producers. Both green and black teas contain sizable amounts of caffeine (1 to 5 percent). They also include up to 27 percent tannins, which have astringent and antibacterial properties. Other substances found in teas are the bioflavonoids quercetin and rutin, which we looked at in Chapter 5. Along with these constituents, according to Albert Y. Leung's book *Chinese Herbal Remedies* (Universe Books, 1984), there are relatively large amounts of vitamin C and more than 300 compounds.

Green tea's use in traditional Chinese medicine first was recorded in sixth-century herbal literature. According to Leung, "Down through the centuries, tea has been described in most major herbals as having the ability to clear one's mind and vision, remove phlegm, facilitate urination, quench thirst, aid digestion, and remove poisons from the body." The usual daily internal dose is 3 to 9 grams (0.1 to 0.3 oz.) taken in the form of a tea, decoction, pills, or powders.

Several studies indicate that black tea helps counteract the effects of radioactive strontium in humans. Researchers Mikhail A. Bokuchova and N.I. Skobeleva report that substances called catechins, found in black tea, protect against the damaging effect of strontium-90 in the human body.[88] They found that catechins absorbed the radioactive isotope and removed it from the body before it reached the bone marrow, in a similar fashion to the action of sodium alginate.

Other studies have indicated that the radioprotective effects of tea catechins are associated with their antioxidative property. The radioprotective effects were shown both when black tea was taken before and after irradiation, and are similar to the radioprotective effects of other natural antioxidants such as vitamins C and E, selenium, and superoxide dismutase, or S.O.D. Thus, tea catechins may have both a preventive and therapeutic function in combating the effects of radiation.

One should be cautious with the use of black or green teas because they contain large amounts of caffeine and tannic acid. High levels of tannin may be carcinogenic. Oriental black and green teas stimulate the nervous system and can cause insomnia, nervousness, or digestive disturbances when taken in large quantity (several cups or more). Green teas are more injurious than black. Taken occasionally by healthy individuals they are relatively harmless.

DEVELOPING FURTHER RESEARCH INTO HERBAL MEDICINE

There are numerous herbs from around the world that have reportedly been used effectively by people to treat leukemia and different kinds of cancers and tumors. And there are countless more that have been used for detoxification or strengthening the immune system and specific organs and glands. It must be remembered that for thousands of years nature has provided us with a wide selection of medicinal herbs. Radiation and chemical pollution are so recent that we have not had the time or economic funding to discover all the remedies that nature makes available. The National Cancer Institute, however, has tested many of these plants—with some promising results.

Some scientists, however, are quite critical of the procedure the NCI uses in screening its plants for antitumor activity. Often plants that fail one type of anticancer test are tested no further. This procedure of quickly discarding a plant if one test is unsuccessful can only result in many of these important herbs being overlooked for possible treatment of other cancers. In fact, independent medical researchers have documented the anticancer effectiveness of certain herbs that had previously been discarded by the NCI after being tested for another form of cancer.[89] Furthermore, these same plants should be tested for potential effectiveness against diseases, other than cancer, that are caused by our modern lifestyle.

Most herbs contain several, not just one or two, active substances that work together to create a therapeutic effect. Therefore, herbs are often more potent when used as a whole substance rather than reducing their effectiveness by isolating only one active component. Some pharmacologists, herbalists, and botanists think that plants, because they are usually compatible with the human body, are the best medicines. This field still holds great promise and I encourage more funding for open-minded research into medicinal herbs. I believe we can combine the advantages of scientific research with the wisdom and experience of centuries of herbal medicine.

For further information about herbs and herbal practitioners, see Appendix Six for the names and addresses of herbal associations.

CHAPTER 7

Fighting Radiation & Chemical Toxins with Miscellaneous Substances

Not only are there various common foods, vitamins and minerals, and certain herbs that can combat the effects of radiation and chemical toxins in the body, but there are also some miscellaneous food substances such as lecithin, thymus extract, cysteine, and pectin, and other more mineral-like substances such as some types of charcoal and clay, and a substance that is becoming very popular now, organic germanium, that may prove useful as part of your optimal health program.

LECITHIN

Lecithin is a phosphorus-containing fatty compound found in many human tissues as well as in plant cells. Good food sources include fish, oatmeal, wheat, soybeans, peanuts, and rice. Lecithin plays an important role in the structure of cell membranes in the body, where it helps to emulsify and regulate blood cholesterol and aids in the movement of fats across the walls of cells. Lecithin thus helps prevent the fatty hardening of arteries and protects the liver and kidneys (key organs for detoxification) and heart.

In addition to phosphorus, lecithin contains some of the vitamin B complex, such as the fatty acids choline and inositol. It helps counteract the effects of radioactive and chemical pollutants throughout the body, especially in the brain and the nervous and reproductive systems.[1]

Lecithin is an important constituent of the myelin sheath, a soft, white, fatty material which surrounds the nerves and brain like a protective insulator. Lecithin's effect on the nervous system can help reduce the stresses associated with our modern lifestyle and with exposure to environmental toxins.[2-5]

Lecithin is particularly useful against strontium-90, x-rays, and the many consumer devices that emit radiation. It also helps to protect the genitals against iodine-131, krypton-85, ruthenium-106, zinc-65, barium-140, potassium-42, and cesium-137. It helps protect against the potent alpha particles emitted by plutonium-239, which are known to concentrate in the genitals. Lecithin can also provide some protection from many common environmental contaminants including lead, mercury, aluminum, DDT, nitrates, nitrites, and the toxic side effects of many drugs.

Lecithin is sometimes called phosphatidyl choline because it is a primary source of choline in the diet. Choline is an important B vitamin that emulsifies or breaks down fats in the body. Equally important, choline is needed to produce the neurotransmitter acetylcholine, which transmits impulses from one nerve cell to another or to a muscle cell. By stimulating greater production of acetylcholine, lecithin prevents memory loss, mania, and tardive dyskinesia (facial tremors similar to Parkinson's disease). Deficiencies of choline and lecithin have been linked to senile dementia, Alzheimer's disease, and other neurological disorders. Lecithin is now being studied as a possible means of prevention and treatment of Alzheimer's disease.

Exposure to radiation, chemical pollutants, or ingestion of certain pharmaceuticals (usually those that alter mood) can decrease the body's reserve of acetylcholine. Thus lecithin may prove useful in preventing or treating disorders of the brain, nervous, or muscular systems that result from exposure to radiation or toxic chemicals.

Lecithin acts as an antioxidant and has a similar effect on the body as selenium, superoxide dismutase, and vitamins A, C, and E. All of these natural antioxidants are protective against radiation and chemical pollutants.

Lecithin increases immunity against viral infections, which can be caused by exposure to toxins. It also increases high-density lipoproteins (the so-called "good" cholesterol which can lower blood cholesterol), thus protecting the cardiovascular system.[6]

Good sources of lecithin include bee pollen (up to 15 percent), egg yolk (8 to 10 percent), fish, and soybeans (0.3 to 0.6 percent). It is found in small amounts in most edible plants. For medicinal purposes, most therapists recommend that one derive a therapeutic dose from supplements. Lecithin supplements are produced from soybeans because soybeans are the least expensive commercial source.

Lecithin supplements are available in liquid, granular, or capsule form. The recommended daily dose of liquid or granular lecithin is one to three tablespoons. Good-quality lecithin can have a mild, nut-like flavor that some people find pleasant. Lecithin granules can be eaten directly, sprinkled on a variety of foods, or added to baked goods. For some people, the thick texture of liquid lecithin renders it less palatable than the granules. However, both the liquid and the granules can be added to other foods with little noticeable change in taste or consistency. There are liquid lecithin products available that can be used to lubricate baking pans to produce a non-stick coating. The baked goods will slide out readily, and the pans will clean quickly and easily.

Lecithin is also available in capsule form. The potency, however, of each gelatin capsule is low—usually about 1,200 milligrams of lecithin. Thus, one would have to swallow about ten or eleven capsules to equal the amount of lecithin in one tablespoon of the granules. During times of exposure to radiation or chemical pollutants, this dosage would have to be taken three times per day to be effective.

It is important to store lecithin properly so that it does not become rancid. Liquid lecithin should be refrigerated after the container is opened. The granules and capsules store best in the refrigerator but can also be kept in a cool, dark, dry cabinet. Once opened, all containers of lecithin should be kept tightly closed.

One caution about the use of lecithin, yeast, and two other supplements, rice bran and fresh wheat germ, is that all four of these contain large amounts of the mineral phosphorus, and comparatively little or no calcium, magnesium, and manganese.

Calcium, phosphorus, magnesium, and manganese work together or synergistically and need to be assimilated in a balanced fashion. The consumption of large amounts of phosphorus alone can create a deficiency of the other minerals, especially calcium and magnesium. Conversely, taking large amounts of calcium and magnesium alone—which is done frequently—can create a deficiency of phosphorus and manganese.

Americans are generally more deficient in calcium than in any other mineral. One reason for this is the current overconsumption of meat, eggs, and poultry—foods which are low in calcium compared to phosphorus, and rich in protein. An abundance of protein in the diet leaches calcium from the body. Petrochemical farming plays a role as well. The soil in industrial countries is frequently deficient in calcium due to reliance upon synthetic chemicals as fertilizers rather than enriching the soil with compost and organic fertilizers.

As we've seen, calcium and magnesium have been well documented as protectants against both radiation and chemical pollutants. Therefore, it is very important not to create a calcium/magnesium deficiency. One should always take supplements in a balanced or proper ratio for optimal results.

The approximate optimal ratio of these minerals is calcium to phosphorus to magnesium to manganese in the ratio of 100 to 75 to 50 to 1.

NUCLEIC ACIDS

Nucleic acids are an important group of organic substances found especially in the nuclei of all living cells. Essential to life, two of the most prominent nucleic acids are ribonucleic acid (RNA) and deoxyribonucleic acid (DNA), which are crucial to the transmission of hereditary patterns.

One study has shown that nucleic acids increase the survival rate of mammals exposed to irradiation.[7] In another experiment, injections of yeast nucleic acids after irradiation were used to increase the survival rate of mice.[8] In a Soviet study, when rats were administered a high-molecular DNA after irradiation, their survival rate jumped by 40 percent.[9] Finally, very small amounts of adenosine triphosphate (ATP, a nucleotide found in muscle tissue that is the immediate source of energy for muscular contractions) were found in one study to produce marked radioprotective and therapeutic effects in mice, rats, and dogs.[10]

Bee pollen, nutritional yeast, and certain sea algae such as chlorella contain relatively large percentages of nucleic acids, including both DNA and RNA. Defatted and desiccated liver supplements also contain good amounts of nucleic acids. Onions contain RNA. Nucleic acids or DNA and RNA are now also sold in the form of supplements at some health food stores. There are no established RDAs for nucleic acids. (For more on the substances RNA and DNA, see Chapter 4 on nutritional yeast.)

Although ATP appears promising, further research with this compound is needed before I would recommend it. Both it and nucleic acids are potent substances. They may be quite effective, but until safety and toxicity levels have been determined, it is probably best to rely upon the foods that contain them, rather than consuming the supplements. The advantage of obtaining these nutrients from foods is that both historical use and scientific research has proven them effective and safe in the amounts recommended. And such potent, concentrated foods as bee pollen, nutritional yeast, and chlorella contain a wide spectrum of complementary nutrients.

CYSTEINE

Cysteine is a naturally occurring amino acid that has been shown to protect against radiation and some environmental pollutants. Amino acids are molecules that bind together to form proteins. Like other amino acids, cysteine contains the elements carbon, nitrogen, hydrogen, and oxygen. Unlike most other amino acids, cysteine also contains the mineral sulfur. Cysteine is an antioxidant that can remove and deactivate free radicals. It is found in abundance in a wide variety of vegetables (see table, Sulfur-Rich Foods).

Cysteine has helped counteract several kinds of radiation in animal studies. Japanese researchers in 1972 found that mice fed cysteine survived 600 rads of x-radiation, whereas 70 percent of the control or non-treated animals died within sixteen days after irradiation.[11]

In 1974, Hungarian researchers found that cysteine protected rats from 900 rads of x-rays.[12] In 1980, Indonesian researchers subjected rats to cobalt-60 gamma irradiation at intensities varying from 100 to 1,600 rads for four weeks.[13] The test rats showed a significant drop in blood hemoglobin. However, "Administration of cysteine fifteen minutes before radiation reduced the irradiation effect on the destruction of hemoglobin," the researchers reported.

Two studies from the Netherlands demonstrated that cysteine diminished radiation's effect of breaking up DNA.[14, 15]

Cysteine and methionine are the only amino acids that contain sulfur. Experiments conducted in Germany and Puerto Rico indicate that the sulfur element in cysteine is at least partially responsible for its radioprotective action. Sulfur protects against the harmful effects of free radicals.

Sulfur-containing cysteine protected rat livers from free radicals generated by exposure to x-rays and cobalt-60.[16, 17] In both sets of studies, cysteine was far more effective than methionine.

Sulfur helps cell mitochondria (small structures in human cells that play a role in the conversion of food to energy) resist radiation, and is known to help repair DNA molecules. Just as natural iodine prevents the uptake of iodine-131, sulfur in cysteine blocks the body's absorption of radioactive sulfur-35.

Because it is an antioxidant that can scavenge free radicals, cysteine also helps detoxify environmental pollutants. It can bind with and neutralize the heavy toxic metals such as cadmium, lead, and mercury, which are then excreted in the urine as harmless compounds.[18-24]

The sulfur in cysteine helps both the kidneys and the liver to detoxify the blood.

Cysteine occurs in sulfur-containing vegetables—most of which are in the cabbage family. The following chart lists the amount of sulfur in a variety of common foods.[25]

SULFUR-RICH FOODS			
Food Source	**Milligrams of sulfur per average serving of 100 grams (3.5 oz) edible portion**	**Food Source**	**Milligrams of sulfur per average serving of 100 grams (3.5 oz) edible portion**
Kale	8,600 mg.	Filberts (nuts)	446 mg.
Watercress	5,390 mg.	Carrots	445 mg.
Brussels Sprouts	3,530 mg.	Brazil nuts	433 mg.
Cabbage	1,710 mg.	Lima beans, fresh	310 mg.
Turnips	1,210 mg.	Soybeans, dried	265 mg.
Cauliflower	1,186 mg.	Onions, mature dry	265 mg.
Raspberries	1,150 mg.	Lima beans, dried	260 mg.
Spinach	1,130 mg.	Barley	240 mg.
Kelp	930 mg.	Eggs 130 mg., dried	103 mg.
Radish	715 mg.	Peas, dried	103 mg.
Okra	710 mg.	Beets	103 mg.
Chard	690 mg.	Brown rice	10 mg.
Peas, fresh	600 mg.	Wheat grain	9 mg.

In addition to eggs, other animal sources of cysteine are fish and meat. Of the three, ocean fish tends to be the least toxic, though this depends on the area in which it is caught.

As was mentioned in Chapter 4, many green vegetables, especially those in the cabbage family, have been documented to protect against radiation, chemical pollutants, and the resulting cancers and tumors. In 1984, the American Cancer Society recommended that we eat at least one or two servings per day of green vegetables. This amount would more than satisfy the recommended daily amount of 850 mg. of cysteine for prevention. In case of exposure to intense amounts of toxins, adults can take up to 2,000 milligrams per day for no more than two to three weeks.

Cysteine is available as a supplement from most natural foods stores. Whenever you are taking extra cysteine, I recommend that you take approximately three times as much vitamin C, a high-potency complete B complex, and a small amount of extra B_6—about 10 mg.

Unfortunately, the research done on cysteine so far has been mostly animal studies. This should be taken into consideration when deciding if you want to take cysteine supplements with a preventive diet, especially when there normally would be an abundant supply of the amino acid in food already. That is assuming, however, that your vegetables have not been irradiated. Two studies demonstrated that irradiation of food, even at the lowest levels tested, caused a significant reduction of cysteine.[26, 27] At the lowest levels, irradiation caused a forty percent reduction of cysteine. Irradiation at the higher levels also produced "considerable destruction" of the B vitamins thiamine and pyridoxine.

PECTIN

Pectin is a water-soluble carbohydrate obtained from ripe fruit and certain other foods. Like the sodium alginate in agar and kelp, pectin has been shown to bond or chelate with radioisotopes, especially strontium-90, and reduce their absorption into the skeletal system.[28-30] Synthetic or commercial pectin, however, has been found to be an ineffective chelating agent. Pectin has also been shown to help prevent assimilation of lead and to help eliminate it from the body, and to lower the harmful types of blood cholesterol known as LDL and VLDL.[31, 32]

Pectin-Rich Foods	per 100 grams (3.5 oz) edible portion
Grapefruit+	3.90
Soybean*	3.45
Orange+	2.96
Carrot	2.00
Banana	.94
Beet	.91
Potato	.83
Apple (whole)	.78
Brussels sprout	.78
Strawberry	.75
Bean	.70

Pectin, which seems to be more effective when obtained from whole foods rather than as a supplement,[33] is found most abundantly in sunflower seeds, soybeans, just beneath the skin of apples, grapefruit, and oranges,

+Most of the pectin in oranges and grapefruit is contained in the white flesh just under the skin, and thus rarely becomes part of the absorbed nutrients.

*While soybeans have a high pectin content, there is no pectin in the soybean product tofu.

and in several types of berries (see table, Pectin-Rich Foods). Organically grown seeds and fruits are better sources of pectin than nonorganic foods because chemical pesticides, fertilizers, and other toxins accumulate primarily in the outer layers of the food and in the embryo (seed, germ, or nut) of whole foods.

PAPAIN

Papain is an organic compound obtainable from papayas. One of the most powerful enzymes known, it breaks down proteins very effectively. In one study, 50 percent of the rats administered papain survived a normally lethal dose of radiation.[34] Papain can now be purchased as a supplement (it is normally sold as a digestive).

THYMUS EXTRACT

In one study, an extract of the thymus organ proved beneficial in treating radiation sickness in mice.[35] Two other studies show that a calf thymus extract stimulates the human body to manufacture T cells, indicating potential benefits to humans for some immunological disorders, including AIDS.[36, 37] The thymus is located behind the breastbone in humans. Little is currently known about the functions of the thymus organ except that it is vital in the development of the immune response in newborns and in the production of T cells. Its removal has been associated with an increased susceptibility to acute infections and chronic immunological diseases at a later time. A thymus extract is currently available from some professional health therapists and natural foods stores.

CHARCOAL

Charcoal's ability to absorb toxins has led to its widespread use in commercial air and water filters. German researchers found that charcoal air filters removed more than 70 percent of radioactive iodine from the air.[38] Today, specially prepared charcoal for internal medicinal use can be obtained in powder, capsule, or tablet form from natural foods stores or most pharmacies, or it can be made at home. And a number of studies have shown that such medicinal charcoal also has the ability to absorb and neutralize radioactive substances and some toxic materials. The magazine

Clinical Toxicology has cited charcoal as the single most valuable agent available for treating poisonings.[39]

French researchers, for instance, report that 10 grams (about 1 tablespoon) of charcoal can absorb about three to seven grams of materials, making it necessary to give at least twice the amount of charcoal as the suspected weight of the toxin taken in.[40]

Taking finely powdered charcoal has been found to be one-and-a-half times as effective as the tablets. David Cooney notes in his book, *Activated Charcoal* (Marcel Dekker, 1980), that in one study humans who took pulverized charcoal absorbed 27 percent of a test drug, whereas those taking the tablets absorbed 52 percent.

One potential concern among health authorities is whether charcoal would absorb and thus deplete the body not only of harmful toxins but of potentially beneficial nutrients. Studies indicate that this concern is unsubstantiated. In one experiment, two groups of rats were fed an identical diet except that one group was also fed charcoal.[41] It was discovered that the charcoal caused no loss of nutrients or deficiencies.

In a study involving sheep, five percent of the total diet was made up of charcoal; a second group of sheep was not given the charcoal.[42] Blood tests and autopsies showed no significant gross or microscopic difference between the two groups of animals. Charcoal apparently did not affect the blood or urinary levels of calcium, copper, iron, magnesium, inorganic phosphorus, potassium, sodium, zinc, creatinine, uric acid, urea nitrogen, alkaline phosphatase, total protein, or urine pH.

Another area of concern has been that the toxins absorbed by charcoal might be released farther down the gastrointestinal tract and then absorbed by the blood. In a study reported in the *Journal of the American Medical Association*, it was determined that charcoal forms a stable complex with toxic materials and does not dissociate the toxins further down the tract.[43]

A good source of further information on charcoal is the book *Home Remedies: Hydrotherapy, Massage, Charcoal and Other Simple Treatments* (Yuchi Pines Institute, 1981) by Agatha Thrash, M.D., and Calvin Thrash, M.D. They note that capsules of "activated charcoal" are roughly twice as potent as tablets. They say, "The oral dosage is one tablespoon of powder stirred into a glass of water, [or] four capsules of activated charcoal, or eight regular tablets taken in the mid-morning and repeated in the mid-afternoon. Food interferes with its effectiveness. Charcoal probably should not be taken regularly over long periods. . . . We have seen no problems with its intermittent use. . . or with regular use for up to twelve weeks."

A commercial charcoal tablet containing 0.44 gm. total material has approximately 0.33 gm. of charcoal, the remainder of the tablet being starch and other substances used to hold the tablet together. Chewing the tablets well before swallowing will substantially increase their effectiveness.

There are no known contraindications to the internal use of charcoal except that it occasionally irritates the bowel of some sensitive people.

CLAY

Raymond Dextreit, in his popular natural healing book entitled *Our Earth Our Cure* (Swan House Publishing, 1974), claims that specially selected clay will absorb excess radioactivity in the body. He states, "Today, when everyone is forcibly submitted to many artificially provoked radioactive aggressions, such as dust in the atmosphere from bomb testing, everything increasing this danger should be avoided. Experiments made with the Geiger counter have demonstrated that dry clay absorbs a very important part of this surrounding radioactivity."

Unfortunately, there is no scientific evidence to support this claim for clay's radioprotective abilities. Clay is worth mentioning, however, because, in addition to Dextreit's claims, I have personally witnessed clay's medicinal effect on a broad range of health problems. I know of many other therapists who have had similar experiences.

Medicinal clay can be taken internally in small amounts or applied externally as an absorbing poultice. It can now be found at most natural foods stores.

Clay is available in a number of different colors depending upon the therapeutic or cosmetic purposes. For absorbing radiation, green clay deserves to be tested first as it seems the most medicinally active. Most importantly, I recommend that readers try to learn more about clay before using it, since care should be taken as to proper use and dosage. I have noticed that clay can produce too stimulating an effect when ingested in large amounts.

ORGANIC GERMANIUM

Organic germanium, or Ge-132, is a health-giving substance of particular promise. Its known capacities as an oxygen catalyst, antimutagen, antioxidant, anticancer agent, and chelating substance indicate that it should be studied for its radioprotective potential in the years to come.

Organic germanium is a synthetic substance composed of the trace element germanium along with carbon, hydrogen, and oxygen. The chemical element germanium along with carbon, hydrogen, and oxygen. The chemical term "organic" in its name refers to the presence of carbon in this compound. Ge-132 was first synthesized by the Japanese researcher Dr. Kazuhiko Asai and his collaborators in 1967. Since that time, it has been extensively studied as a versatile preventive and therapeutic agent.

Ge-132 has been shown to provide protection against toxicity from the heavy metals mercury and cadmium by chelating with them, against some types of ionizing radiation, and against poisoning by PCBs (highly toxic polychlorinated biphenyls).[44-47] Over six million Japanese take Ge-132 supplements every day.

Asai first took an interest in the element germanium, atomic number 32 on the periodic table, in 1950, when he found it in coal deposits while working as a mining engineer in Japan. After reading Russian reports of its anticancer activity, he began to research it himself.

The Russians had analyzed a wide range of plants for their mineral content and had discovered that Oriental medicinal plants were particularly rich in germanium. Asai repeated this analysis and determined the germanium content of the following medicinal plants (reckoned by parts per million, or ppm):

SOURCES OF ORGANIC GERMANIUM	
Shelf fungus (*Trametes cinnabarina Fr.*, a traditional Russian cancer cure)	800-2,000 ppm.
Garlic	754 ppm.
Ginseng (*Panax ginseng*)	320 ppm.
Sushi (*Angelica pubescens Maxim.*)	262 ppm.
Waternut (*Trapa japonica Flerov*)	239 ppm.
Comfrey	152 ppm.
Boxthorn seed (*Lycium Chinese mill*)	124 ppm.
Wisteria knob (gall—*Wisteria floribunda*)	108 ppm.
Aloe	77 ppm.
Chlorella (a type of unicellular green algae)	76 ppm.
Pearl barley	50 ppm.

Twenty years of Japanese laboratory testing and medical case studies on Ge-132 have established it as virtually nontoxic (unlike Ge, or the compound germanium dioxide, which is sometimes sold as a supplement but which could be fatal if taken in excessive doses).[48] Ge-132 is water-soluble, leaving almost no trace in the body twenty to thirty hours after

A catalyst to oxygen assimilation in the body, Ge especially resembles its close relative silicon. They are in the same family of the periodic table (group IVA), and are both effective semiconductors, or electron-transferring materials. Like silicon, Ge-132 tends to form into lattice-like crystals. Through its semiconducting properties it enhances oxygen supply to body cells for increased energy production.

In the textbook *The Pathologic Basis of Disease* (Saunders, 1984), used by a majority of American medical schools, authors S. L. Robbins and Ramzi S. Cotran state, "Hypoxia [oxygen deficiency] is probably the most common cause of cell injury and may also be the ultimate mechanism of damage initiated by a variety of physical, biological, and chemical agents." According to Asai in *The Miracle Cure: Organic Germanium* (Japan Publications, 1980), "My organic germanium compound has proved effective against all sorts of diseases, including cancers of the lung, bladder, larynx, and breast, neurosis, diabetes, hypertension, cardiac insufficiency, inflammation of maxillary sinus, neuralgia, leukemia, softening of the brain, myoma of the uterus, and hepatic cirrhosis. If a line that runs through the many cases of cure taken as isolated points should be found and an hypothesis known to be true to be set up, I should say that all diseases are attributable to deficiency of oxygen. The dangers of an oxygen deficiency in the human body cannot be overemphasized. . . . Germanium greatly enriches oxygen in the living body."

In addition to being an oxygen catalyst, Ge-132 has documented value as an analgesic, an immunostimulant, an antioxidant, a chelatant, and a normalizer of many physiological functions.[49-54] It is also a promising radioprotectant.

According to a study by one of Asai's associates, "Radioactive rays release electrons that destroy cells and blood corpuscles. . . . Germanium floating near the blood corpuscles skillfully catches those released electrons and lets them move around its own nucleus."[55] In this way it prevents the penetration and destruction of blood corpuscles and cells.

In another study, *E. coli* bacteria were exposed to gamma rays from cesium-137 at a dose rate that induced cell mutations.[56] When Ge-132 dissolved in distilled water was introduced into the *E. coli*, mutagenesis of exposed cells was "remarkably reduced" without affecting cellular growth or survival. The authors of this study attribute the antimutagenic effect of Ge-132 to its ability to "improve the fidelity" of DNA replication.

Organic germanium helps to normalize calcium metabolism, possibly through affecting hormone production. Calcium is an essential mineral to the body and a key protectant. In a study of human patients, Ge-132 restored proper sodium, potassium, chloride, and calcium levels in the blood, while returning the balance of pH and red and white blood cell counts to within their normal ranges.[57]

Ge-132 protects cysteine, an amino acid with known protective value, against oxidation.[58] Antioxidant properties of Ge-132 may help it guard cellular electron transfer against the adverse leakage of single electrons to molecular oxygen. Such leakage can generate toxic oxidizing free radicals.[59]

Asai's early research indicated that Ge-132 helps to heal burns without scarring, which should make it a promising candidate for work with radiation burn victims.

Ge-132 is also an immunostimulant which regulates immunity by stimulating production of the antiviral substance interferon.[60] It also increases production of several types of white blood cells, including lymphocytes, macrophages, and B cells.[61] These properties have been found to contribute to its anticancer and antitumor activity,[62] and they contribute to its potential as a protectant.

Recommended dosage levels of Ge-132 for daily preventive use have yet to be established in this country. Twenty-five mg. to 100 mg. per day is the supplementation often used in Japan and is the amount suggested by most U.S. manufacturers. Whether one chooses to use supplements or not, it makes sense to include foods like garlic, pearled barley, and watercress (another plant rich in natural germanium) in one's diet.

More research needs to be done on the possible uses of organic germanium as a protectant, particularly with human subjects. Dosage amounts of Ge-132 have yet to be established for treatment after exposure to various kinds of radiation and toxins. In general, therapeutic doses for specific medical problems are higher than the ones given above as preventive guidelines.

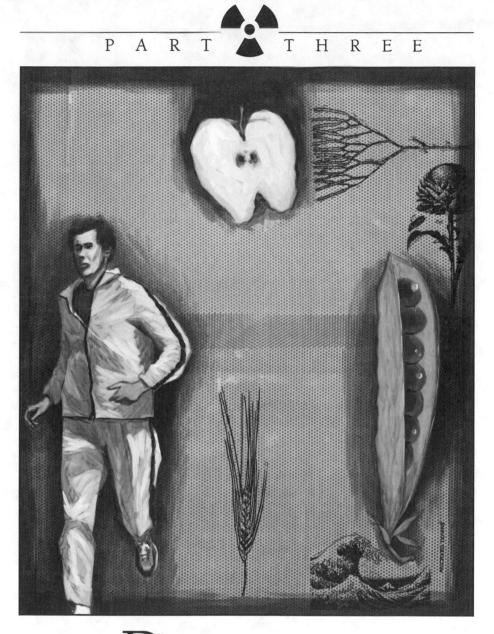

Developing The Optimal Lifestyle For Our Nuclear/chemical Age

CHAPTER 8

Eating for Optimal Health & Longevity

For the past decade scientists and medical doctors have been urging Americans, through the media, to change their diet. One can hardly turn on the television set or pick up a newspaper or magazine without encountering some product that is being advertised for its low fat and cholesterol content. We see an endless parade of presentations on the benefits of pure, natural foods. The reason for this landslide of advice is that scientific evidence is now overwhelming: the typical American diet is laden with toxins and other harmful substances while deficient in vital nutrients.

Our common supermarket foods with their long lists of ingredients are loaded with toxins such as radioisotopes, chemicals, and drugs; they are full of fat and cholesterol and contain excesses of refined grain, sugar, and salt. This diet is now known to cause a variety of degenerative diseases including heart disease, cancers, adult-onset diabetes, gout and other forms of arthritis, liver and kidney diseases, immune disorders, and behavior problems.

Unfortunately, this may be just the tip of the iceberg. Long before the human body manifests symptoms of disease, or succumbs to one or more illnesses, there is a long period of degeneration, in which the organism struggles against the insults of a poisonous and nutritionally deficient diet. The struggle requires energy; the body fights to keep itself alive against an endless barrage of toxins. At the same time, it is deprived of adequate amounts of vitamins, minerals, complex carbohydrates, and fiber. The battle cannot be won. Slow deterioration takes its toll: fatigue, lack of mental clarity, and a weakened immune system are the warning bells along the way to more serious health problems. Eventually, constant pollution from our diets must overcome the body's inherent reserves of strength. The scales are tipped and "suddenly" there is angina (chest pain caused by insufficient oxygen to the heart), heart attack, cancer, immune disorder, liver or kidney disease, a behavior problem, or other serious illness.

Scientific evidence has made this pattern painfully obvious. After much debate and controversy, the medical and scientific communities have finally conceded the point and begun to recommend dietary changes. In 1977 the Senate Select Committee on Nutrition and Human Needs published *Dietary Goals for the United States*. That document urged Americans to reduce their intake of fat, cholesterol, refined grains and other processed foods, sugar, and salt, and to increase their consumption of whole grains, fresh vegetables, fish, and fruit. *Dietary Goals* maintained that six of the ten leading causes of death in the U.S., including cancer, heart disease, and diabetes, were caused by the standard American diet and the toxins in that diet. Two years later, the Surgeon General published the *Surgeon General's Report on Health Promotion and Disease Prevention*, which made the same recommendations as *Dietary Goals*. The next major study, *Diet, Nutrition, and Cancer*, was published in 1982 by the National Research Council of the National Academy of Sciences. The NRC reiterated the basic advice offered by *Dietary Goals* and the Surgeon General, and demonstrated as well that a diet too high in fat had a "causal" relationship to the common cancers, such as those of the breast, prostate, and colon. Fat, as well as being harmful to the body in excessive quantities, contains many toxins.

The diet recommended by all three of those publications was essentially the same. It was based on a predominance of whole grains, fresh vegetables and fruits, beans, and low-fat fish. The reports urged Americans to reduce their intake of processed foods, red meat, dairy products, eggs, and foods laden with sugar and salt. Little did those health authorities realize that the diet they were recommending to prevent degenerative disease was also the diet that would protect against the effects of radiation and chemical pollution.

I have already presented scientific evidence that supports the consumption of certain foods, herbs, and supplements in the prevention and treatment of toxicity sicknesses. But what is equally important is that those foods be part of a regular whole foods diet, a diet that is low in toxins, fat, cholesterol, sugar, refined grains, and synthetic additives. By reducing destructive or disease-promoting substances and increasing foods that contribute to health, we allow our bodies to become stronger and better able to cope with the pollutants in our environment, including radiation and chemical toxins.

OPTIMAL DIET CHARTS

Preventive/Protective Diet

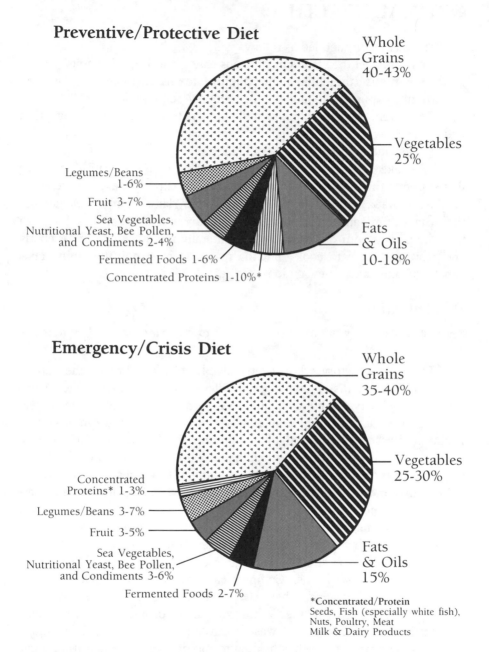

Whole
Grains
40-43%

Vegetables
25%

Legumes/Beans
1-6%

Fruit 3-7%

Sea Vegetables,
Nutritional Yeast, Bee Pollen,
and Condiments 2-4%

Fermented Foods 1-6%

Concentrated Proteins 1-10%*

Fats
& Oils
10-18%

Emergency/Crisis Diet

Whole
Grains
35-40%

Vegetables
25-30%

Concentrated
Proteins* 1-3%

Legumes/Beans 3-7%

Fruit 3-5%

Sea Vegetables,
Nutritional Yeast, Bee Pollen,
and Condiments 3-6%

Fermented Foods 2-7%

Fats
& Oils
15%

*Concentrated/Protein
Seeds, Fish (especially white fish),
Nuts, Poultry, Meat
Milk & Dairy Products

Soups can be made from any healthy combination of some or most of the above food groups, excluding fruits.

THE DIET FOR
OPTIMAL HEALTH

The diet recommended as follows will:
- counteract the effects of previous eating and lifestyle habits
- minimize the current absorption of toxins and detoxify the body after routine exposures to radiation or chemical pollutants
- prevent the absorption of toxins in the future and protect against a wide array of serious diseases
- generate optimal health and vitality.

Let's take a closer look at the diet, at some of the scientific evidence that supports this program, and at what you can expect to experience when you incorporate natural whole foods into your daily regimen. Remember that it takes time and effort to learn to prepare and enjoy new foods. We must be patient with ourselves. We are literally re-educating our tastebuds and relearning how to cook. But the rewards are strong immunity, rejuvenated vitality, and a new outlook on life.

Whole Grains
• *40 percent of daily intake of calories* • *2 to 3 servings of whole grains per day*

Throughout history, whole grains have been referred to as "the staff of life." Whole grains—brown rice, millet, wheat, barley, oats, corn, buckwheat, and rye—are highly nutritious, containing many of the protective nutrients such as the B complex vitamins, vitamin E, phosphorus, magnesium, potassium, zinc, iron, and selenium. Buckwheat and millet have been specifically documented as helping to counteract radiation. These two also contain more protein than the other grains. Buckwheat, millet, and rice are the three most digestible grains, easily tolerated even by those with allergies to wheat and rye.

Whole grains are energy foods. They are a rich source of complex carbohydrates, which provide long-lasting, even-keel energy that endures for hours, rather than the short bursts of nervous energy provided by refined sugars and processed grains. Complex carbohydrates are efficiently metabolized by the body and then cleanly converted into energy without buildup of unnecessary toxins. Whole grains also provide fiber, which aids in digestion and elimination of waste from the intestinal tract. Fiber shortens intestinal transit time, thus helping to rapidly eliminate harmful toxins, including carcinogens, that otherwise might accumulate there.

Whole grains, in addition to providing vitamins, minerals,

carbohydrates, and fiber, also supply small amounts of protein. They are exceedingly low in toxin-laden fat. Because grains are high in bulk-producing fiber and low in fat and calories, they are an ideal food to eat when weight-loss is necessary.

Diets rich in whole grains provide an abundance of the amino acid tryptophan, which scientists at the Massachusetts Institute of Technology have found increases brain levels of the neurotransmitter serotonin. Serotonin increases one's sense of well-being, reduces tension and stress, and improves sleep.

Refined grains, especially white flour and sugar, on the other hand, leach minerals from the tissues, bones, and teeth. The body converts sugar to triglycerides, a kind of fatty acid that accumulates in the bloodstream as blood cholesterol and contributes to heart disease, diabetes, and a weakened immune system. Refined grains and sugars are referred to as "empty calories" because they provide carbohydrate, or fuel, without the necessary vitamins and minerals for healthy metabolism. These refined, or simple, carbohydrates set metabolism in motion but cannot provide the many vitamins and minerals necessary for the body to carry on the multitude of chemical reactions that are the basis of life.

Drs. H. C. Trowell and D. P. Burkitt, editors of *Western Diseases: Their Emergence and Prevention* (Harvard University Press, 1981), were among the pioneer researchers who found that native African peoples, among others, were relatively free of intestinal disease, including cancer of the colon, primarily because of the high fiber content of their diet.

Refined grains, of course, provide no fiber, which makes them difficult to digest. They are also commonly laced with synthetic additives, including artificial flavors, colors, and preservatives. A number of studies have shown that many additives, like other toxins, cause behavioral problems, especially in children. Some additives may be carcinogenic.

In short, whole grains encourage health on all levels while refined grains and sugar debilitate the body and rob it of needed nutrients.

Vegetables

• *25 percent of daily intake* • *2 to 3 servings per day, at least one serving of chlorophyll-rich vegetables*

The vegetable kingdom, with its leafy greens, roots, and tubers, provides an incredibly rich variety of tastes, textures, and colors. Vegetables are the earth's treasure-chest of nutrients, especially vitamins and minerals. Collards, parsley, mustard greens, and kale are rich sources of calcium. One cup of cooked collard greens contains about 320 mg. of calcium; a cup of cooked mustard greens, about 284 mg.; and kale, about 306 mg. A cup of milk, by comparison, provides 270 mg. of calcium, as well as about 40 percent of its calories in toxin-rich fat. Vegetables are uniformly low in fat and contain no cholesterol. Most vegetables are rich in fiber and are easy to digest.

Vegetables provide an abundance of all the necessary vitamins and minerals, including beta-carotene (Vitamin A) and zinc. Vitamins and minerals enhance immune function and are essential to warding off the effects of radiation and chemical pollutants.

In addition to being rich sources of vitamins and minerals, green vegetables, including broccoli, Brussels sprouts, and leafy greens, are rich in chlorophyll, which counteracts radioactive and chemical toxins.

Organic vegetables are far superior to those produced using chemical agricultural methods. Many pesticides, herbicides, and fertilizers are derived from petrochemical sources and have recently been reported by the Food and Drug Administration as possible cancer-causers.

As already noted, many vegetables contain protective and therapeutic qualities. Among those vegetables are parsley, cabbage, broccoli, alfalfa sprouts, mustard greens, collard greens, kale, watercress, carrots, squash, pumpkin, potatoes, sweet potatoes, beets, dark leaf lettuce, other dark leafy greens, onions, and garlic.

Beans and Legumes

• *2 to 7 percent of the daily diet* • *approximately 1 serving per day of beans, tofu, tempeh, or some other bean dish*

Beans and legumes include aduki (also called azuki), black-eyed peas, black soybeans, chickpeas, kidney, lima, lentils, navy beans, pinto beans, soybeans, split peas, and others. They provide protein, fiber, vitamins, minerals, and carbohydrates. All beans are rich in nutrition, but I especially recommend azuki, black soybeans, pintos, black beans, kidney beans, lentils, and chickpeas. In addition to being wonderful sources of nutrition, beans are rich and delicious and can be satisfying and easy to digest when prepared with care. Tofu, tempeh, and natto are highly nutritious, naturally processed soybean-based foods. Beans are rich in amino acids, which are the "building blocks" of proteins, and are the main source of protein for much of the world's population. Meat, chicken, eggs, cheese and other dairy products are the main protein foods in the West, but these are high in toxins, cholesterol, and many synthetic additives including antibiotics and hormones.

Tofu, also known as soybean curd, is high in protein, low in fat, and contains lecithin. It is found at most natural foods stores and in many supermarkets. Tempeh and natto are fermented soybean products. They are available at most natural foods stores, and through macrobiotic mail-order outlets. Tofu and natto can be eaten raw, while tempeh is usually cooked. (In general it is best not to boil a fermented product, since boiling may kill the "friendly" bacteria the food provides.) Tofu and tempeh can be boiled, broiled, fried, or sautéed in 20 minutes or less.

Sea Vegetables

• *2 to 5 percent of the daily diet* • *3 ounces daily*

The common edible sea vegetables are kelp, arame, alaria, dulse, hijiki, Irish moss, kombu, laver, nori, Pacific sea palm, and wakame. They represent a variety of pleasant flavors. Like the sea itself, sea vegetables are bursting with minerals, trace elements, and vitamins. For example, one hundred grams, less than four ounces, of hijiki contains 1,400 mg. of calcium, 56 mg. of phosphorus, 29 mg. of iron, and 150 International Units of vitamin A. Virtually all sea vegetables contain an abundance of the trace elements, including zinc and magnesium. Sea vegetables are easily prepared and are widely available in natural foods stores.

Sodium can be harmful to the kidneys and circulation, especially for people who suffer from heart disease, so most sea vegetables should be soaked before cooking. Soaking, and discarding the soaking water, will reduce the sodium content considerably and make them safe for anyone to eat. There are several good natural foods cookbooks that contain cooking directions and many tasty recipes using sea vegetables.

You do not have to eat great quantities of sea vegetables in order to enjoy their benefits. Because they are so concentrated, a few ounces daily will be sufficient to obtain an abundance of nutrition from them.

Fruit

• *5 percent or less of diet* • *use as a sweetener for desserts or as a snack when desired*

The best guideline for fruit is to try to eat that which is grown locally and in season. This is not always possible, given the realities of modern agriculture and transportation. If you cannot obtain good-quality locally grown fruit, try to choose fruit that is in season in your area. In other words, try to eat fruit that is or could be grown locally. One obviously needs to be flexible with this guideline as well as with others mentioned here.

Try to use the whole fruit, which is richer in fiber and nutrients than just the juice. Whole fruit does not raise blood sugar levels to the extent that juice does with its abundance of too rapidly absorbed fructose. Fruit and fruit juices make wonderful sweeteners in whole grain desserts. Such desserts provide far more nutrition than highly refined ones, and are satisfying without containing excess sugar.

Certain fruits have specific therapeutic capacities. These include apples, for their potassium and pectin content; peaches and apricots for their beta-carotene; bananas for potassium and pectin; and berries for iron, potassium, and pectin. Most commercial citrus fruits are usually picked before they are ripe and thus have high quantities of acid, which leaches minerals. Organic citrus, preferably locally grown, is better-tasting and contains fewer toxins than the trucked-in variety.

Concentrated Proteins

• *1 to 10 percent of the daily diet* • *primarily seeds, nuts, and low-fat animal foods such as fish* • *3 ounces or less per serving of animal foods such as fish*

Appropriate amounts of protein have proven beneficial to the immune system and help to counteract toxins. Again the key is appropriate quantities—either excessive or deficient amounts can cause adverse effects. The optimal diet has been designed to provide the correct amounts of protein and other nutrients. Beans and grains combine well to form high-quality, easily assimilated, complete proteins. Unlike beans and grains, excessive animal proteins or excessive amounts of other concentrated proteins are likely to create subtoxic metabolic waste products.

Ocean fish are the most nutritious form of animal food. They usually contain more vitamins, minerals, polyunsaturated fatty acids, and other nutrients than fresh-water fish. Because they and their environment, the ocean, are so nutrient-dense, they generally contain lower levels of radioactive isotopes and chemical pollutants. The next best animal source of protein is chemical-free poultry, which is available at many natural foods stores and some supermarkets. Animal foods often provide high quantities of important nutrients, especially protein and iron. Many, however, such as red meats, dairy products, eggs, and the skin of poultry, contain high amounts of toxin-laden fat and cholesterol. Ground beef has half or more of its total calories in fat; when it is cooked in oil or lard, as it often is, the fat content goes up. A sirloin steak may contain 75 percent of its calories in fat; a porterhouse steak, 82 percent. A "lean" leg of lamb has about 60 percent of its calories in fat. Spareribs provide 80 percent of their calories as fat; bacon, 82 percent. The white meat of chicken, with the skin, has 50 percent of its calories in fat, but without the skin it is only 23 percent fat.

Most fish, on the other hand, provide very low amounts of fat—as little as 20 percent or less.

Nuts and nut butters can be high in fat. Up to three-quarters of peanut butter's total calories are derived from fat; roasted peanuts, 70 percent; walnuts, 79 percent; sunflower seeds, 71 percent fat. When eating nuts, choose the low-fat varieties and eat them in small quantities. If you regularly eat seeds and nuts, consider soaking them for two to eight hours prior to eating to reduce their high levels of phytic acid, which binds with calcium and other minerals and diminishes their absorption.

Seeds, such as sunflower, pumpkin, and sesame, should be stored in a cool, dark, dry place or in a frost-free refrigerator. Unhulled seeds have a longer shelf life than hulled. Hulled seeds have lost their protective coating and have a relatively higher fat ratio, both of which makes them more vulnerable to rancidity from oxidation.

Fermented Foods

• *Miso soup three to four times weekly* • *Pickles, sauerkraut, tempeh, and natto three to four times per week* • *Shoyu and tamari soy sauce that contain no artificial ingredients*

Miso, a fermented soy product, is rich in B vitamins and friendly bacteria that aid in digestion and the healthy functioning of the intestinal tract. Fermented foods should be part of everyone's diet, and miso is perhaps the best fermented food available. At first, use the milder misos such as barley miso, that have been aged for three to 12 months. The stronger ones, such as hatcho, can be used when one has grown accustomed to miso's flavor. Include wakame and other sea vegetables in your miso soups as a way to add sea vegetables to your diet and enrich their nutritional content. Other vegetables such as onions and carrots are equally delicious in miso soup. Miso can also be used in sauces, in salad dressings, and as a base for stews and bean soups.

Shoyu and tamari are also excellent and savory fermented foods. They contain moderately high levels of sodium, about 17 percent. They should be conservatively added during or at the end of cooking to enhance the flavor of your dishes, rather than used at the table. Like other fermented foods, shoyu and tamari can help strengthen the colon. They are available at natural foods stores and from macrobiotic mail-order outlets.

Total Fats and Oils

• *10 to 17 percent of total calories* • *100 milligrams of cholesterol daily*

Fifteen percent, for instance, of a typical daily diet of 2,100 calories, represents about 2½ tablespoons of vegetable oil. Keep in mind, however, that this figure of 15 percent of calories from fat includes fats used in cooked and prepared foods.

Fat is probably one of the most dangerous constituents in the standard American diet. The typical American consumes as much as 40 to 45 percent of his or her total calories in fat. It is important to remember that fats, especially animal fats, are loaded with radioactive and chemical toxins—far more so than any other type of food. The more fats you regularly include in your diet the more toxins you will absorb, especially when you consume fats from foods higher up on the food chain such as animal sources. Moreover, because toxins easily lodge in fat cells, the more fat you store in your body the more your body will absorb and store those toxins.

Equally important, excess fats or cholesterol have been well documented to have adverse effects on several immune functions and on the protective activity of white blood cells. Also, when a high-fat food is consumed, tiny microns of fat, called chylomicra, invade the bloodstream and raise the fat or lipid content of the blood. This is typically referred to as blood cholesterol. Blood cholesterol causes red blood cells to become sticky around their edges and to adhere to one another. They clump together like a roll of coins, a condition called "the rouleaux effect."

Red blood cells carry oxygen and iron to all the body tissues. The red blood cell is about 7.5 microns in diameter; capillaries, the tiny blood vessels that provide blood to tissues throughout the body, are about 3.5 to 4 microns wide. In order to pass through these tiny vessels, red blood cells must bend or fold, which they do with ease as long as they are not bunched together. Bunched together, they form a bottleneck at the entrance to the capillary, thus preventing blood and oxygen from getting to tissues throughout the body. The tissues begin to suffocate from lack of oxygen; if the condition persists, the tissues will die.

Studies have shown that cow's milk can cause clumping of red blood cells. When high-fat meals are consumed consistently, circulation is reduced throughout the system, and blood cholesterol increases dramatically. Soon, cholesterol balls attach themselves to the walls of vessels and arteries in the condition called atherosclerosis. Atherosclerosis builds within an artery and begins to cut off the flow of blood by reducing the passageway within the artery, causing blood pressure to increase, much like pinching a hose increases water pressure. Eventually, the atherosclerosis, or cholesterol plaque, reduces the amount of blood and oxygen getting to the heart. The heart begins to suffocate from lack of oxygen. It labors heavily to pump blood, while suffocating.

At this point a condition known as coronary insufficiency sets in and the person can begin to suffer from angina pectoris, the characteristic pain in the chest due to heart disease. Eventually the artery can close off entirely; the heart suffocates and a part of the tissue in the heart muscle dies. The result: heart attack.

In a landmark study done in 1987, Dr. David Blankenhorn and his associates at the University of Southern California demonstrated that atherosclerosis could be reversed by lowering blood cholesterol.[1] Blankenhorn showed that by increasing niacin intake and thereby reducing blood cholesterol, the body can actually eliminate, or discharge, the cholesterol plaque that builds up within the walls of the artery. This can be achieved by reducing blood cholesterol to below 160 milligrams, which can be accomplished by following the optimal diet.

A high-fat diet also has been shown to be a primary cause of some common cancers, including cancers of the colon, prostate, and breast. Fat increases bile acids within the body. These bile acids degrade carcinogens and bacteria already present in the intestinal tract, causing the carcinogens to become more active and thus enhancing their cancer-causing capacities. Fat also plays havoc on the hormonal system, raising prolactin and estrogen levels in women and thus giving rise to breast cancer.

As was mentioned in Chapter 3, polyunsaturated fatty acids, as derived from most vegetable oils and fish, are necessary for human health. Taken in moderation, they actually improve immune response. Similarly, certain deep-water ocean fish and their oils benefit the immune system as well as the liver, kidneys, and heart. Balanced amounts of polyunsaturated fatty acids, fish, and fish oils are the key, since both deficiencies and excesses may be harmful to health.

By following the diet described here, you will have no trouble regulating fat and cholesterol. This regulation is essential for health and to minimize ingestion of dangerous toxins.

Condiments

Nutritional yeast, bee pollen, and powdered sea vegetables can be sprinkled on your food at the table. You can choose some of your favorite organic dried herbs and spices, such as basil, oregano, thyme, cumin, and others, mix them together, add some powdered sea vegetables and sprinkle this on your food as a low-sodium, high-nutrient salt substitute. You can also buy a powdered herb seasoning mix from a natural foods store, or buy or make *gomasio*, roasted sesame seeds ground together with sea salt. You can also grind sea salt with whole or powdered sea vegetables.

ADAPTING THE OPTIMAL DIET TO YOU

The diet presented here is an ideal, or optimal, diet. It is similar to some traditional diets practiced around the world and is akin to increasingly popular Western diets such as macrobiotics, the Pritikin diet, and those that grew out of the government studies mentioned earlier.

Realistically, many people who are currently eating a standard American diet are not prepared to quickly change old habits and customs by totally adopting this new diet. It is important to remember that diet is highly personal and individual. I offer guidelines, not unbreakable rules. Personal tastes, cultural heritage, and one's physical strengths and weaknesses all play a role in food choices. I want to emphasize that the foods listed are not intended to be the only foods in your regular diet, but I hope that they will be amply included. Feel free to pick and choose as you wish and to make additions or subtractions. Also, feel free to consult with your doctor or health practitioner to modify and individualize these guidelines to your own specific needs.

Dietary transitions should be made at a pace that is appropriate for you. Rather than focusing on minimizing or eliminating unhealthy foods, I strongly suggest that you focus on increasing healthy foods and on other practices in your optimal health program. Keep your emphasis on the positive and your mind will gradually become less attached to unhealthy, self-destructive habit patterns. Rather than feeling dependent on or craving something that is harmful, your body and emotions will increasingly desire that which makes you feel better over a long period of time. Backsliding is okay if it is occasional and temporary. Worry, guilt, anxiety, and stress hurt the immune system, the adrenals, and metabolism, so don't worry if you occasionally eat questionable foods. You will process the toxins and metabolize them much better if you eat a small amount, allow yourself to enjoy the food, be happy and confident, and, after fulfilling your desire, let it go.

There is plenty of flexibility in these guidelines, and one can use them creatively to incorporate healthful substitutions for foods currently enjoyed. Ethnic and traditional dishes can easily be incorporated into the optimal health program. Pasta made from whole grains can substitute for refined noodles; whole grain breads for white-flour commercial kinds; tofu, tempeh, beans, and fish can become the new protein sources, rather than hamburgers and sausage; high-quality beans and whole grain tortillas in place of beans with lard and refined tortillas; and fresh vegetables rather than canned or frozen. Be creative, and use some of the many excellent natural foods cookbooks available.

Regardless of your current diet, you will find that most of the dietary suggestions can be easily adapted to your lifestyle and can help you to achieve a state of optimal health and resistance to disease. The unique feature of these dietary recommendations is their universal adaptability to the diet of peoples and cultures around the world.

After exposure to intense radiation or chemical pollutants, a high-quality whole foods, mostly vegetarian, diet is the most healthful. Try to minimize or avoid animal foods such as dairy products, eggs, poultry, and red meats, which often contain large quantities of fats and toxins. These foods at the upper end of the food chain tend to concentrate radioactive and chemical contaminants from the environment. Foods at the lower end of the food chain, the plant foods, contain more vitamins, minerals, and other substances known for their ability to increase health and counteract the effects of contaminants.

Sea vegetables are at the very bottom of the food chain and are a very potent protective food. Fruits, vegetables, grains, legumes, seeds, bee pollen, nutritional yeast, and sprouts all contain excellent ratios of vitamins, minerals, chlorophyll, protein, fats, and carbohydrates. As a further consideration, when a person eats lower on the food chain, there is less ecological impact and more energy is conserved.

Digestion begins by chewing food well enough to thoroughly mix it with the digestive enzymes in the mouth. The age-old axiom, "Drink your food and chew your drinks," is still one of the wisest statements ever made about eating. Research now indicates that thorough chewing can also help our immunological response to toxins in our food.

WASHING AWAY TOXINS

Before we take a look at some recipes and the use of supplements for optimal health, I should note that radioactive fallout, whether from routine emissions and leaks from nuclear plants, bomb tests by governments that have not signed the atmospheric test ban treaty, or from industrial or medical sources, is more likely to lodge on edible plants above ground, and on rough-textured or layered plants, than on smooth-skinned and unlayered plants. Careful washing will help to dislodge appreciable amounts of surface fallout from fruits and vegetables. Some people recommend using a dilute apple cider vinegar solution or an extremely dilute bleach solution (approximately one-half teaspoon bleach per gallon of water). After washing the vegetables, rinse them with pure water.

In a German experiment, various methods were tested for removal of surface radioactive contaminants, including radioactive strontium and cesium-137, from vegetables and fruits.[2] The findings are worth quoting at length:

> The methods considered included chemical procedures, such as washing with water or decontamination solutions, and physical methods such as rubbing, brushing, peeling, or covering with a plastic layer and then removing this layer. With contaminated potatoes, hand- or machine-peeling and peeling with lye removed 100 percent of the surface strontium-85 and cesium-137. Washing and brushing removed 70 to 98 percent of these radioisotopes. Soaking in water removed only 15 to 20 percent of the contamination from carrots. Cooking removed 41 to 58 percent while scraping and washing removed 98 percent of the radioisotopes. Washing and brushing removed 60 to 65 percent of the radioisotopes from cucumbers, a plastic sheet removed 15 to 25 percent, and peeling removed 100 percent. Spinach and leeks were difficult to clean by these methods. Washing and brushing of apples removed 65 to 80 percent of the contamination, a plastic sheet removed 20 to 45 percent, and peeling removed 100 percent.

Obviously it is worth using some combination of the above methods as a first line of defense against radioactive and chemical toxins.

RECIPES FOR THE OPTIMAL DIET

The purpose of this book is to document the effectiveness of natural substances that can protect us from the effects of radiation and chemical pollution, not to offer yet another cookbook. Therefore, the number of recipes were kept to a minimum. By including some recipes, however, I am encouraging you to begin to use the foods we've been discussing. In developing these recipes, I've tried to emphasize using a variety of the suggested foods and substances, as well as provide natural foods dishes that look and taste appetizing. I also wanted to help you develop an attitude of experimentation and variation in your cooking. With a little practice, many cooks can use their favorite cookbooks and by making a few strategic substitutions greatly increase the healthfulness of the dishes. There are many good natural foods cookbooks, and I encourage you to go to your natural foods store, food co-op, bookstore, or library to obtain a few of these books. Also, people who have developed good recipes for natural foods are often happy to share—so feel free to ask friends, acquaintances, or chefs for recommendations.

In the following recipes, those foods in italics are the most effective in counteracting toxins.

Salads, Spreads, and Soups

BEET SLAW
MAKES APPROX. 4 CUPS

1 cup unpeeled beets, grated
1 cup grated carrots
1 cup shredded cabbage
½ cup chopped celery
½ cup sunflower seeds
½ teaspoon caraway seed
½ teaspoon dill seed
½ cup chopped onion
Optional: *raisins, apples,* walnuts, *yogurt (preferably soy or goat),* coconut

Mix all ingredients well and sprinkle with *powdered sea vegetable.* Serve with *sprouts, chopped parsley,* or on *leaf lettuce.* Dress with *Slaw Dressing* (below).

SLAW DRESSING

½ cup unrefined vegetable oil
⅓ cup fresh lemon juice
1-2 teaspoons rice syrup or honey (optional)
½ teaspoon bee pollen
½ teaspoon powdered sea vegetable
1 clove garlic, chopped

Shake or blend well.

MOLDED VEGETABLE SALAD

Agar-agar is sometimes referred to as kanten. It is a safe, nontoxic, natural sea vegetable substance that can be used as a gelatin or thickening agent for such diverse foods as gravies and yogurt; non-dairy ice cream, sherbet, and cashew "cheese"; pies and tarts; and vegetable aspics. Gelatins made with agar will set either at room temperature or in the refrigerator.

> *2 teaspoons agar flakes*
> 1¼ cups boiling water
> *2 tablespoons fresh lemon juice*
> 2 tablespoons rice syrup or honey
> *1 teaspoon tamari*
> *1 cup finely chopped cabbage*
> *½ cup chopped celery*
> *½ cup shredded carrots*
> *¼ of a green bell pepper, finely chopped*
> **Optional:** *½ cup beets*

Bring water to a simmer, add agar, and dissolve thoroughly. Remove from the heat and add lemon, honey, and tamari. Immediately stir in the vegetables and pour into a mold. Refrigerate to set.

QUICK HOMEMADE SAUERKRAUT

> wide-mouth canning jars and lids (quart-size)
> *green cabbage*
> sea salt
> boiling water
> **Optional:** mixed pickling spices, caraway seeds, celery
>   seeds, a few juniper berries, peppercorns, *fresh garlic cloves,*
>   dill, *onion,* mild or hot finger (pickling) peppers, diced carrots,
>   whole baby beets

Sterilize jars and lids. Chop green cabbage. If you don't use the dark green outer leaves, save them for soup stock as they are abundant in chlorophyll, minerals, and vitamins (especially vitamin E). Pack the cabbage into the jars. Add 1 teaspoon salt per jar and any optional ingredients. Add boiling water to cover. Seal tightly and shake. Store at room temperature in a dark, dry place. If spices were added, shake jar at least once a day the first week. After the first four days, make sure the lid is sealed as tightly as possible. After six weeks the sauerkraut will be ready. No need to remove scum as in traditional recipes using a crock. Serve at room temperature or chill.

VERY QUICK SAUERKRAUT

Use same ingredients as above. However, instead of chopping the green cabbage, juice it. Then mix the pulp and juice together in the sterilized jars. Add salt, optional ingredients, and enough boiling water to cover. Seal tightly. Shake. Sauerkraut will be ready in 3 days. Again, there is no need to remove the scum.

BASIC SALAD DRESSING
MAKES APPROX. ½-1 CUP

½ cup unrefined vegetable oil
2-3 tablespoons lemon juice
½ teaspoon powdered sea vegetables
Optional ingredients:
¼ cup raw or toasted sesame seeds or sunflower seeds, ground
½ cup chopped parsley
1 clove garlic
½ peeled orange, sectioned, seeds removed
2 teaspoons chopped green pepper
herbs or spices such as ¼ teaspoon marjoram or dill seed, or
⅛ teaspoon celery seed, cumin, or paprika
dash black pepper

Shake all ingredients together in a jar or, if using seeds, parsley, or orange, blend until nearly smooth.

Seeds can be toasted by heating in a dry skillet, preferably cast iron. Shake the skillet gently over moderate heat until the seeds begin to dance (sesame) or turn golden (sunflower). Remove seeds from skillet immediately. If not using a blender, grind them, while warm, in a seed grinder, flour mill, or mortar and pestle.

PROTECTANT SALAD DRESSING

½ cup unrefined vegetable oil (preferably olive, sunflower, or
sesame)
¼ cup liquid lecithin
1 tablespoon bee pollen
½ - ¾ cup fresh lemon juice
1 cup chopped fresh parsley
1 ripe avocado
1-4 tablespoons ground sesame seeds or tahini (optional)

2 *tablespoons miso or powdered sea vegetable*
2 teaspoons sweet basil
Optional ingredients: *1 tablespoon nutritional yeast*, 1 teaspoon
   dill, ¼ - ½ cup honey, 1 tablespoon poppy seeds (poppy
   seeds and honey go well together). Water can be added to
   adjust consistency.

Blend all ingredients well.

HERB VINEGAR

1 part red wine
1 part apple cider vinegar
2-3 garlic cloves, peeled and cut
Optional: tarragon, peppercorns, thyme seeds, oregano, sweet
   basil, dill, or cumin

Combine the red wine and cider vinegar. Add the garlic along with a small
branch of tarragon (or some dried tarragon—be careful, as a little goes a
long way), a few peppercorns, and a pinch of your favorite herbs.

Pour into a bottle (preferably a dark-colored one) and stop tightly with
a cork. Shake vigorously a few times. Store at room temperature in a dark,
dry place. If possible, shake once in a while. After two weeks, you will
have an exquisitely flavored herbal wine vinegar. Use it in salad dressing,
in vinaigrette sauce, or as is, sprinkled over salad with a little unrefined
vegetable oil.

GARBANZO-MISO SPREAD
MAKES ABOUT 4¼ CUPS

4 cups cooked garbanzos (chick peas), mashed or puréed
4 tablespoons tahini or sesame butter
3 tablespoons miso
½ cup dried parsley (or 1 cup chopped fresh parsley)
2 tablespoons extra virgin olive oil
½ teaspoon garlic powder
½ teaspoon basil
juice of 1 lemon

Blend well. Great on sandwiches, crackers, and rice cakes. Serves well as a
dip.

TAHINI-MISO SPREAD
MAKES 1 ¼ CUPS

1 cup tahini or sesame butter
¼ - ⅓ cup miso
lemon juice to taste

Mix together to form a smooth, rich spread. Serve on sandwiches, crackers, celery, or as a vegetable dip.

GOLDEN YEAST GRAVY

2 tablespoons unrefined vegetable oil or butter
½ onion, finely chopped
1 clove garlic, minced
½ cup sliced mushrooms (optional)
½ cup primary-grown nutritional yeast
¼ cup whole grain flour
1½ cups liquid (soymilk, water, or soup stock)
1 tablespoon miso
1 tablespoon bee pollen

Sauté onion, garlic, and mushrooms in oil or butter. Add yeast and flour and sauté a minute longer. Add liquid and stir until mixture thickens. Dissolve miso in ½ cup of water. Remove gravy from heat and add miso and bee pollen.

Seasonings such as dry mustard, pepper, cumin, oregano, or *parsley* may be added.

MISO SPAGHETTI SAUCE

2 tablespoons unrefined vegetable oil
2 small onions, thinly sliced
1 clove garlic, crushed
10 mushrooms, thinly sliced
5 tomatoes, diced
3 green peppers, diced
½ carrot, grated or thinly sliced
2 cups water or soup stock
1 tablespoon primary-grown nutritional yeast
2 bay leaves
4½ tablespoons red, barley, or hatcho miso

1 *tablespoon lecithin*
dash black pepper
dash oregano and/or basil
sunflower and sesame seeds (optional)
alfalfa sprouts, yogurt, or grated Parmesan cheese, for garnish

Heat a heavy pot and coat with oil. Add onions and garlic and sauté until they begin to turn translucent (about 3 minutes). Add the next four ingredients and sauté for 4 more minutes. Add water, yeast, and bay leaves, and bring to a boil. Simmer, uncovered, for 10 minutes. Mix in miso, lecithin, pepper, and herbs and seeds if desired. Simmer, stirring often, for 1 hour. Remove bay leaves. For best flavor, allow to stand for 6 to 8 hours before serving. Reheat and serve over *buckwheat noodles* or spaghetti. Garnish with sprouts, yogurt, or grated cheese.

(Special thanks to William Shurtleff and Akiko Aoyagi, from whose *The Book of Miso* (Ballantine Books, 1976) this recipe was adapted.)

SOUPERNATURAL BEET BORSCHT
SERVES 4

4 cups water or *potato broth*
2 *cups chopped beets*
½ *cup chopped carrot*
1 *cup chopped onion (preferably wild)*
½ *cup chopped potato*
2 *cloves garlic, minced (preferably wild)*
1 *cup finely shredded cabbage*
juice of 1 lemon
2 teaspoons raw honey
1-2 *teaspoons powdered sea vegetable, vegetable salt, or tamari*
½ *cup yogurt (preferably soy or goat)*
1 thinly sliced or chopped cucumber
¼ *cup chopped parsley*

Simmer beets, carrot, onion, potato, and garlic in water or broth for 15-30 minutes. Add cabbage, lemon, honey, and sea vegetable, salt, or tamari. Simmer for another 15 minutes. Serve in bowls, adding a tablespoon of yogurt to each bowl, and garnish with cucumber and parsley.

Optional ingredients: *bell pepper,* chives, dill, paprika, black pepper, mushrooms, 1 tablespoon wine vinegar, 1 tablespoon *lecithin* or butter, *bee pollen, sunflower seeds.*

Optional garnishes: radishes, *dill pickle,* or sliced hard-boiled egg.

Beet Borscht is a wonderful hearty soup either hot or cold. It is especially satisfying with a whole grain bread such as rye or pumpernickel.

SEA VEGETABLE SOUP
SERVES 8

1 cup sea vegetable (dulse, kelp, wakame, etc.)
2 quarts soup stock or water
3 tablespoons unrefined vegetable oil
1 large onion, chopped
1 carrot, chopped
1½ cups chopped broccoli
2 cloves garlic
¼ cup chopped green onion or chives
4 teaspoons primary-grown nutritional yeast
1 teaspoon thyme
1 teaspoon marjoram
dash of cayenne, black pepper, or ginger
2-3 tablespoons miso
Optional ingredients: mushrooms, *potatoes*, barley

Soak sea vegetable for 10 minutes. Add to stock and simmer. Sauté onion, carrot, broccoli, garlic, and green onion in oil for 5 minutes, or until onions are partially translucent. Add vegetables to stock. Add yeast, herbs, and spices. Simmer for 30 minutes. Turn off heat. Remove ½ cup of liquid and dissolve miso in it. Return to soup and heat, but do not boil, for 3 minutes. Adjust seasonings to taste.

Grains and Vegetables

GLAZED BEETS AND CARROTS
SERVES 4-6

4 cups chopped beets and carrots (onions or potatos may be substi-
  tuted for all or part)
1 cup soup stock
1-2 teaspoons tamari
1 cup orange juice
¼ cup lemon juice
¼ cup raw, unfiltered honey, or rice syrup
3½ tablespoons arrowroot powder

2 teaspoons bee pollen
4 sprigs fresh parsley, finely chopped
⅛ - ¼ cup unrefined oil or butter

Boil (or steam) the vegetables with the soup stock. Drain and save the stock. Transfer vegetables to a casserole dish. In another bowl or in a blender, combine the stock with the rest of the ingredients. Mix well. Place in a pot and cook over a low flame until the glaze thickens. Spread on vegetables and reheat in the oven before serving. Garnish with parsley.

Many people think onions are appropriate only in small amounts, complementing salads, hamburgers, or stir-fried vegetables. Onions can also be prepared, however, as a separate dish. In this way one can take full advantage of their protectant properties.

ROASTED ONIONS
SERVES 4

4 large golden Spanish onions
unrefined vegetable oil
garlic cloves (optional)
parsley
alfalfa sprouts
butter
lemon wedges

Wash onions. Trim bottoms, but do not peel. Place onions in an oiled, ovenproof dish. Brush onions with oil, then roast at moderate heat (350 degrees F.) until tender, approximately 1½ hours. A few unpeeled garlic cloves may be added during the final 15 minutes. Serve with parsley and alfalfa sprouts, butter, and lemon wedges. The onions may also be topped with *Golden Yeast Gravy* (recipe on page 187).

BRAISED ONIONS
SERVES 4

4 equally sized onions, about 2 inches high
2 tablespoons unrefined vegetable oil
soup stock (approximately ¼ cup)
herbs such as sage, rosemary, savory, and oregano
chopped parsley
alfalfa sprouts
powdered kelp or dulse

Peel onions. Combine oil and soup stock in a pan to a depth of ¼ inch. Stand onions in pan and sprinkle with your favorite herbs. Cover with a tight-fitting lid and gently simmer for 40 minutes or until tender. Serve on a bed of parsley, sprouts, or any green vegetable. Sprinkle with powdered kelp or dulse. *Golden Yeast Gravy* (page 187) can be served on the side.

Variation: Place sliced tomatoes under the onions while braising.

STUFFED ONIONS
SERVES 4-6

6 medium-sized onions
1 cup cooked buckwheat, millet, or brown rice
½ cup sunflower seed meal
1½ teaspoons miso or 1 tablespoon tamari
½ cup chopped mushrooms
½ cup chopped parsley or cabbage
¼ cup chopped celery
½ teaspoon favorite herb
soup stock or *yeast gravy*

Skin onions and parboil for about 10 minutes. Drain well. Slice the tops off and scoop out the inside, leaving a ¾-inch shell. Chop the removed pulp and combine with the cooked grains, sunflower meal, miso, and mushrooms, and the fresh vegetables and herb. Moisten with soup stock or yeast gravy. Pack onion shell with the filling, and place in roasting pan with enough soup stock to prevent sticking. Bake at 375 degrees F..for 30 minutes. If shells are too soft or thin, bake in well-greased muffin tins.

Variations: Substitute *sauerkraut* and ¼ teaspoon caraway or celery seeds for the vegetables in the filling. Or serve "au gratin": Cover the cooked, stuffed vegetables with a light but thorough coating of bread crumbs, grated cheese, butter or *oil*, and finely ground nuts, then brown until golden.

BUCKWHEAT-STUFFED CABBAGE ROLLS
SERVES 4-5

1 head green cabbage
1 medium onion, chopped
1 clove garlic, minced
¼ lb. mushrooms, sliced
2 tablespoons whole or chopped sunflower seeds (optional)

2 tablespoons unrefined vegetable oil
2 cups cooked buckwheat groats
2 tablespoons chopped fresh parsley
½ teaspoon each rosemary and thyme
1 tablespoon miso
1 tablespoon primary-grown nutritional yeast (optional)
1 egg (optional) or *1 tablespoon lecithin granules*
warm water, vegetable stock, or tomato juice
Optional garnishes include: *chopped fresh parsley, plain yogurt, sunflower seeds*

Carefully peel off 10-12 large cabbage leaves. Steam 3 to 4 at a time in a vegetable steamer until tender, about 3 minutes. Drain and set aside. Sauté onion, garlic, mushrooms, and sunflower seeds in oil until onions are clear and mushrooms are tender. Combine with buckwheat groats, parsley, herbs, miso, and dried yeast, if desired, and mix well. One beaten egg, or a tablespoon of lecithin granules, may be added to bind the mixture. Place 2-3 heaping tablespoons of filling near the base of each cabbage leaf and roll up, tucking in the sides as you go. Two smaller leaves will work if you run out of large leaves, and a small leaf can be used to patch a leaf with holes. Place rolls seam-side down in a baking dish. Add liquid to half cover rolls. Cover dish tightly and bake 45-60 minutes at 350 degrees F. Plain yogurt may be stirred gently into the liquid around the cabbage rolls after removing from oven, or a dollop of yogurt may be spooned onto each serving with a sprinkle of sunflower seeds and chopped parsley.

VEGETABLE GRAIN LOAF
SERVES 4-6

4 cups cooked grain (brown rice, millet, barley, buckwheat, or mixture)
1½ cups cooked lentils
2 tablespoons peanut butter, *sesame butter*, or *tahini*
2 eggs, beaten
2 tablespoons primary-grown nutritional yeast
2 tablespoons miso
1 onion
1 cup chopped celery
½ green pepper
dash celery salt
½ teaspoon thyme

½ teaspoon basil

Mix all ingredients well. Bake in loaf pan for 35-40 minutes. Great with mushroom gravy on top.

Variations: Add *½ cup grated carrot*, 6 oz. tomato paste, *a grated potato*, or *½ cup sunflower seeds*.

SAUTEED BUCKWHEAT NOODLES
SERVES 4

½ cake tofu, cubed
3 tablespoons unrefined vegetable oil
2 cups cabbage or Chinese cabbage, chopped
½ onion, sliced
1 clove garlic, chopped
2 bell peppers, chopped
½ cup sliced mushrooms (optional)
¼ cup sunflower seeds
7 oz. buckwheat noodles, cooked
¼ cup miso
alfalfa sprouts
fresh parsley, chopped
sesame seeds, ground
yogurt (optional)

In a large skillet, sauté tofu in 1 tablespoon oil and ½ tablespoon water. Transfer cooked tofu to a separate container. Sauté cabbage, onion, garlic, peppers, mushrooms, and sunflower seeds in 2 tablespoons oil and 1 table-spoon water until the onions and garlic become clear. Stir in cooked noo-dles and tofu. When noodles are hot, remove the mixture from the heat and stir in miso. Excellent served over a bed of alfalfa sprouts and gar-nished with fresh parsley and ground sesame seeds. If you like, top with a dollop of yogurt.

NORI MAKI SUSHI
SERVES 4

This dish is really not as hard to make as it seems, and it enjoys consistent popularity.

1 cup brown rice, uncooked (buckwheat or ⅔ cup millet may be substituted)
2 cups water

2 tablespoons apple cider vinegar
2 tablespoons honey or rice syrup
5 slices tofu (about ½ lb.)
1 tablespoon apple cider vinegar
1 tablespoon honey or rice syrup
1 cucumber or zucchini
5 spring or green onions
5 umeboshi plums (optional)
10 sheets nori

Cook rice or other grain in water with vinegar and honey until liquid is absorbed and grains are soft. Cool. Press tofu to remove excess liquid (about 15 minutes) and place in a frying pan. Add vinegar and honey and simmer until the liquid is absorbed. Cut tofu into long slices. Cut cucumber and onions into thin, long slices. Toast nori in oven (watch closely—it burns quickly) or by passing back and forth quickly over a flame.

A bamboo sushi mat (which can be found at Oriental shops) works best for rolling the ingredients up into the sheets of nori. Place a sheet of nori on the mat. Spread rice over the lower ¾ of the sheet, about inch thick. Place strips of cucumber, tofu, and onion and dabs of umeboshi plum in a line in the bottom ¼ of the sheet. Roll up. Seal with a little water and let stand for 5 minutes. Slice each roll into 6-8 pieces. Arrange on a platter.

Nori rolls can be served as a main course or as an appetizer. They keep well and are excellent for traveling or as part of a box lunch for work.

TOFU SANDWICH
MAKES 1 SANDWICH

2 slices toasted whole grain bread
slices of tofu, steamed or lightly pan-fried
soy mayonnaise or mustard on one slice of bread
miso on the other slice
sprouts
primary-grown nutritional yeast
slice of avocado
nori or dulse that has been presoaked in water

BUCKWHEAT BREAKFAST

1 cup buckwheat
1 tablespoon unrefined vegetable oil
1 carrot, sliced
¼ cup sunflower seeds
¼ cup roasted sunflower seeds
1 banana, sliced
1 apple, sliced
1 pear, sliced
seeds from ½-1 cardamom or more
dash of cinnamon
1 tablespoon miso
½ cup apple juice

Dry-roast buckwheat. Heat oil. Add groats and next 8 ingredients, and sauté for 10 minutes. Dissolve miso in apple juice and add to skillet. Sauté for an additional minute. Top with *applesauce*, *yogurt*, or ricotta cheese.

BREAKFAST CEREAL

juice or water
⅔ cup rolled oats
¾ cup sunflower seeds
dried fruit as desired
2 tablespoons bee pollen
1½ teaspoons primary-grown nutritional yeast
1½ teaspoons lecithin granules
apples, berries, or other fruit (optional)
liquid: *apple juice or cider*, any other fruit juice, milk, soymilk,
kefir milk, yogurt, clabbered milk

Add juice or water to oats, sunflower seeds, and dried fruit, and let soak overnight. If using water, drain off any excess in the morning. In the morning add bee pollen, nutritional yeast, and lecithin granules. Add juice, cider, soymilk, milk, or yogurt to desired consistency, and stir. (If you add juice to the cereal the night before, you may want to add juice instead of a milk product the next day. Milk when combined with juice can curdle.) Feel free to add other ingredients.

MILLET BREAKFAST

4 cups water
1 tablespoon unrefined vegetable oil
1 cup millet
½ cup dried apricots
½ cup chopped apple
2 teaspoons cinnamon
½ teaspoon nutmeg
1 teaspoon bee pollen
1 teaspoon lecithin

Bring the water to a boil in a pot with a tight-fitting lid. Add oil, millet, apricots, apple, and spices. Gently boil for 45 minutes. Turn off heat. Add bee pollen and lecithin.

You could also add any of the following optional ingredients after the heat is turned off: *1½ teaspoons miso, 1 teaspoon powdered sea vegetable*, 2 tablespoons raw unfiltered honey, *⅓ cup sunflower or ground sesame seeds, ½ cup yogurt, or ½ cup kefir milk.*

BUCKWHEAT PANCAKES
MAKES 6-10

1 cup buckwheat flour
1 cup other whole grain flour
1 teaspoon baking powder
¼ cup carob powder (optional)
2 cups soymilk or water
2 eggs, beaten
1 tablespoon unrefined vegetable oil
1 tablespoon honey
½ cup sunflower seeds

Stir dry ingredients, except for sunflower seeds, together. Add soymilk, eggs, oil, and honey and mix briefly. Add sunflower seeds last. Cook on hot, lightly oiled griddle.

Desserts

FRUIT TOPPING (TZIMMES) FOR PANCAKES, TOAST, POTATO LATKES, OR FOR USE AS A CHUTNEY

1 lb. (3 cups) pitted dried fruits—raisins, apricots, prunes, etc.
water for soaking fruit
2 cups berries (blueberries, raspberries, or halved strawberries)
1 or 2 apples, grated
¼ - ½ cup sunflower seeds
1 slice (or more) lemon or lime
½ teaspoon cinnamon
½ teaspoon allspice
½ teaspoon cloves
2 tablespoons butter
1-3 teaspoons agar

Wash dried fruit and soak in water, covered, for one hour. Drain water and reserve. Combine all ingredients, except for agar, in a pot with ½ cup of the soaking liquid. Bring to a boil, then cook over very low heat for one or two hours, adding more liquid as needed. To thicken, add one to three teaspoons agar dissolved in ¼ cup cooled, reserved liquid; cook an additional 5 minutes and stir. Topping keeps well in the refrigerator for up to one week, or it may be frozen.

FRUIT GELATIN

To make a tasty fruit gelatin, mix one tablespoon of agar flakes with one cup of water. Simmer the mixture for two minutes or until the agar is completely dissolved and let cool slightly. Add two cups fruit juice and some fresh or dried fruit. Optional ingredients such as honey, coconut flakes, seeds, vanilla or almond extract, etc., can also be added. Place the mixture in the refrigerator and it will gel within two hours.

APPLE CRISP

6 cups thinly sliced apples
6 tablespoons honey or rice syrup
2 teaspoons unrefined vegetable oil
4 tablespoons butter
2 tablespoons soymilk

½ cup honey, rice syrup, maply syrup, or Sucanat
2 tablespoons whole grain flour
2½ cups oat flakes
½ cup sunflower seed meal
1 teaspoon cinnamon

Mix the apples, honey, and oil. Spread in a baking dish and set aside. To the butter and soymilk add sweetener, flour, oats, sunflower meal, and cinnamon. Spread over apples. Cover and bake at 350 degrees F. for 20 minutes. Remove, cover, and bake another 15 minutes.

HALVAH
SERVES 12

1 cup sunflower seeds
1 cup sesame seeds
½ cup carob powder
1 tablespoon bee pollen
2 tablespoons sesame oil or butter
½ teaspoon vanilla extract
¼ teaspoon almond extract
½ - ¾ cup honey
Optional: peanut butter, coconut, *pumpkin seeds*

Grind sesame seeds and sunflower seeds in coffee bean grinder, flour mill, blender, or with a mortar and pestle. In a large bowl mix the ground seeds, carob powder, and bee pollen. Heat the oil or butter and add the vanilla and almond extracts. Dribble over the dry mix. Add honey and mix well. The mixture can be eaten as is, or rolled into little balls and refrigerated or frozen. Because honey works as a mild natural preservative and is somewhat antibacterial, halvah keeps at room temperature for several days.

JELLIED APPLE-MISO DESSERT
SERVES 5

5 apples, peeled and cut into quarters
1 cup water
½ cup raisins
1 tablespoon lemon juice
2 tablespoons honey, rice syrup, or maple syrup
2 tablespoons sesame butter or tahini
¼ - ½ teaspoon cinnamon

1 teaspoon agar flakes
1 tablespoon miso
yogurt (optional)

Combine apples and water. Boil, then cover pan and simmer for 10 minutes. Remove apples and place in mold. Add rest of ingredients to the liquid except for miso and yogurt and simmer for an additional 5 minutes. Add the miso, mix well, and pour into the mold. Cool to room temperature, then refrigerate for a couple of hours. If you like, place a dollop of yogurt on top.

SOFT YOGURT ICE CREAM WITH BERRIES

2 teaspoons agar flakes
¼ cup cold water
6 teaspoons nonfat dry milk
¼ cup water
2 cups yogurt
¼ cup raw honey
1 cup fresh or frozen berries
2 teaspoons bee pollen
Optional: vanilla or almond extract, cinnamon, raw carob powder

Stir agar into ¼ cup cold water. Bring mixture to a slow boil, cook for two minutes, and then let cool. In a blender, mix the dry milk and ¼ cup room-temperature water. Then, while the blender is on slow-speed, add these ingredients in the following order: agar and water mixture, yogurt, honey, berries, and bee pollen. Pour ingredients into the central vortex of the blender to insure an even mixture. Freeze to desired consistency. For those who have a non-centrifugal juicer that makes ice cream, try freezing the blended mix in ice cube trays. Then run through the juicer so it comes out with the texture of a soft ice cream.

Drinks

GREEN CHLOROPHYLL DRINK

Use any combination of the following greens, all of which contain chlorophyll: parsley, celery, spinach, collards, turnip greens, chard, leaf or romaine lettuce, kale, endive, watercress, bell peppers, peeled cucumber, green cabbage, alfalfa sprouts, sprouted sunflower seeds, sprouted clover seeds, specially grown edible grasses such as from wheat, rye, barley, or buckwheat.

Wash greens. Blend in a blender with water. Strain well and drink. Or, if you have a juicer, juice your favorite combination.

Optional ingredients: *A small amount of chopped carrot* or *beet* can be added to the blender or juicer.

SIMPLY DELICIOUS HEALTH DRINK

8 oz. Chlorophyll Green Drink or fresh, raw apple juice
1 tablespoon primary-grown nutritional yeast
1 tablespoon lecithin
1½ tablespoons chlorella or spirulina
2-3 teaspoons honey or rice syrup
1 teaspoon bee pollen
1-2 tablespoons carob powder
Optional: nutmeg, cinnamon, or *banana*

Mix ingredients in a blender or with a whisk. Serve hot or cold. I recommend taking *200-300 mg. of calcium* and *100-150 mg. of magnesium* with this drink.

COMPLETE PROTECTANT HEALTH DRINK

1 tablespoon primary-grown nutritional yeast
1 tablespoon lecithin
¼ - 1 tablespoon domestic bee pollen
¼ cup yogurt (if not using yogurt, include *1 tablespoon acidophilus culture*)
⅛ - ¼ cup sunflower seeds or meal
1 cup raw apple juice
1 cup water
Fruit such as a banana or apple, or ¼ cup berries
Optional ingredients:1 teaspoon powdered dulse or kelp (preferably kelp for sodium alginate and iodine and other minerals)
¼ cup carob powder
2 teaspoons cinnamon
1 oz. chlorophyll juice (can be extracted from a juiced, or blended and strained green vegetable such as parsley)
1 teaspoon pure vanilla extract and/or almond extract

1 raw egg yolk
honey or rice syrup, to taste
¼ *teaspoon liquid extract of Siberian ginseng*
⅛ *teaspoon extract or tincture or ¼ teaspoon powdered Panax ginseng (preferably wild or finest quality available)*
1½ *teaspoons calcium lactate or 4 teaspoons calcium gluconate*
½ *teaspoon magnesium oxide*
10,000-25,000 units vitamin A
400 units vitamin D
400 units vitamin E (d-alpha) or 800 I.U. mixed tocopherol

Grind the sunflower seeds in an electric coffee bean or other grinder. Also, sesame seeds can be used but they must be ground first.

Calcium lactate and calcium gluconate taste slightly chalky, and many people dislike the taste of magnesium oxide. Thus, it may be preferable to take these substances in supplement form rather than to include them in this drink.

Combine ingredients and blend in a liquifier, blender, electric mixer, or with an egg beater. This formula should be adjusted to taste. Any ingredient may be decreased or omitted, provided that, during crisis situations or increased exposure to radiation, it is obtained at some other time during the day.

Grind the sunflower seeds in an electric coffee bean or other grinder. Also, sesame seeds (a possible protectant) can be used but they must be ground first.

Women choosing to use Panax ginseng should be aware of a special caution. Ginseng, a "yang" herb, traditionally was taken mostly by men, except in special circumstances. Today, as Westerners are exposed to numerous "yin" substances such as sweets, drugs, pollutants, radiation, and other sources of stress, more and more Western women are using ginseng regularly with excellent results. However, after working with herbs closely for over two decades, I strongly recommend that women consult with a well-trained and experienced herbalist before taking this herb for normal, ongoing use. For crisis situations such as increased exposure to radiation or environmental pollution, ginseng can be used by almost everyone for limited periods of time. It is probably the most revered herb in human history—countless books have been written on its use. Among its many medicinal functions, it regulates the adrenals and balances the digestion.

Many people who find themselves on the go prefer to make their health drink at night, refrigerate it, then drink it the next day for a quick, supernutritious breakfast or snack.

This health drink is quite complete and is intended for the individual who feels in a state of deficient health or who is in a crisis situation such as increased exposure to radiation or pollution. For normal conditions, feel free to simplify it to your desired needs and tastes.

SUPPLEMENTS FOR ADDED SAFETY

The optimal healthful diet and recipes I have described are the basis or centerpiece of preventive protection and partial treatment against radiation and chemical pollutants in our environment. You may, however, want to increase your intake of certain protective and therapeutic nutrients and other supplemental substances.

Listed below are two adult dosage ranges of each vitamin and mineral I have discussed. Unless you are exposed to intensive amounts of radioactive or chemical toxins, begin by taking the preventive or protective dosage levels. In order to correct probable previous deficiencies, a majority of people, including those already eating a healthy diet, would benefit by gradually increasing the dosage levels to the therapeutic amounts. The therapeutic amounts should be taken by most people for at least four to eight weeks—a relatively short period of time in one's life.

After that time, if you are feeling consistently healthy, energetic, and balanced, you may begin to gradually decrease dosage levels back to the protective or preventive levels. The small percentage of readers who have a consistently pure and healthy diet from high-quality foods, and who feel consistently healthy, can try further decreasing their amount of supplements. Frankly, these people are rare. An overwhelming majority of people will greatly benefit by maintaining the preventive or protective levels.

Regardless, whenever you are exposed to higher amounts of toxins, or whenever you feel ill or feel symptoms developing, you should return to the therapeutic dosage levels for a short period of time. The therapeutic amounts should be taken for at least three to seven days after symptoms cease, since absence of symptoms does not necessarily mean that optimal internal health has been achieved.

Many people who have been on this optimal diet, supplement, and total health program for six months or more begin to feel a greater internal sensitivity and a deepening of intuition. You can then begin to trust your own feelings about which foods, herbs, supplements, or other holistic therapies would benefit you. Feel free and encouraged to make modifications in order to individualize your complete holistic health program. Remember, though, that the program presented here has been proven by clinical experience to be the most beneficial for the widest range of people to protect, detoxify, and produce optimal health and vitality in our nuclear and chemical age.

Be sure to read the guidelines for and usages of each vitamin and mineral in Chapter 5 and Appendix One. These sections also describe how vitamins and minerals work together and advise which additional nutrients to take when specific supplements are added to or needed in your diet.

Nutrient	Preventive or Protective Amount	Therapeutic Amount
Vitamin A (preferably (beta-carotene)	10,000 to 20,000 IU	25,000 to 100,000 IU of beta-carotene (to avoid toxic dose)
B Vitamins:		
B1 Thiamine	10 to 50 mg.	50 to 100 mg.
B2 Riboflavin	10 to 50 mg.	50 to 100 mg.
B3 Niacin	50 to 100 mg.	100 to 200 mg.
B5 Pantothenic Acid	10 to 50 mg.	50 to 100 mg.
B6 Pyridoxine	10 to 50 mg.	50 to 100 mg.
B12 Cyanocobalamin	5 to 75 mcg.	75 to 100 mcg.
Biotin	100 to 150 mcg.	150 to 300 mcg.
Folic Acid	0.1 to 0.4 mg.	0.4 to 2.0 mg.
Para-aminobenzoic Acid	10 to 50 mg.	50 to 100 mg. (PABA)
Choline	25 to 50 mg.	50 to 500 mg.
Inositol	25 to 50 mg.	50 to 500 mg.
Vitamin C	250 to 2,000 mg.	2,000 to 10,000 mg.
Vitamin D	400 to 500 IU	500 to 1,000 IU
Vitamin E	50 to 200 IU of d-alpha, or 100-400 of mixed tocopherals	200 to 600 IU of d-alpha or 400-1200 of mixed tocopherals
Calcium	400 to 800 mg.	800 to 1200 mg.
Magnesium	200 to 400 mg.	400 to 600 mg.
Iodine	100 micrograms	150 micrograms
Iron	10 mg.	12 to 18 mg.
Selenium	100 to 200 micrograms	200 to 300 micrograms
Zinc	15 to 35 mg.	35 to 50 mg.

CHAPTER 9

Further Self-Help Guidelines for Fighting Radiation & Chemical Toxins

Ror the past decade, people have been asking me for help in treating health problems resulting from exposure to radiation or environmental pollutants. Some of these people were calling from long distances, which prevented me from working directly with them. As a result, I developed a set of general guidelines not only for essential foods and supplements, but for powerful herbal formulas and for ways to benefit from such activities as exercise, saunas, and detoxifying baths, that could be used by anyone suffering from common toxins.

HERBAL FORMULAS FOR PREVENTION AND THERAPY

Many herbalists prefer to work with herbal formulas rather than individual herbs because of the opportunity to create a balance of herbs that blend well together. Herbal blends or formulas often produce a deeper, broader, and more consistent effect than individual herbs. These herbal formulas can be used in addition to any of the food substances already mentioned. They should not be viewed as substitutes for a good diet but rather as potent, therapeutic complements to the dietary guidelines already outlined.

The herbal formulas below include a general herbal formula for detoxification (Formula One), an herbal antibiotic tincture (Formula Two), an immune system booster (Formula Three), and a digestive regulator (Formula Four). All have been used with great success by many of my clients as well as by other therapists.

The information on these herbal formulas is provided both to offer reliable, safe, and effective self-help procedures and to stimulate further scientific research into herbal medicines.

Formula One: Blood and Lymph Cleanser

Formula One purifies and stimulates the blood and lymph. The herbs in this formula have been cited as helpful against a wide range of problems associated with the blood and/or lymph systems, including radiation, environmental pollutants, venereal disease, herpes, drug detoxification, cysts, tumors, polyps, venereal warts, and some cancers.

Quantity	Herb
2 oz.	purple coneflower (*Echinacea angustifolium* or *purpurea*)
1 oz.	Jamaican sarsaparilla (*Smilax ornata*)
1 oz.	burdock root (*Arctium lappa*)
1 oz.	barberry root or Oregon grape root (*Berberis vulgaris* or *Berberis aquifolium*)
3/5 oz.	red clover blossoms (*Trifolium protense*)
1/2 oz.	violet leaves (*Viola odorata*)
1/2 oz.	dried parsley leaves (*Petroselinum* spp) or 1/3 oz. gravel root (*Eupatorium purpereum*)
1/2 oz.	cleavers (*Gallium aparine*)
2/5 oz.	chaparral (*Larrea divaricata*)
1/2 oz.	Chinese licorice root (*Glycyrrhizae uralensis*)
1/2 oz.	dandelion root (*Taraxacum officinale*)
1/2 oz.	yellow dock root (*Rumex crispus*)

Combine the above herbs in the proportion given. If you wish to make a tincture—which is the most effective and convenient form of the formula, follow the tincture directions given in Formula Two. Adult dosage of a tincture is 30-60 drops, depending on the severity of the problem, four times per day.

If you wish to make a tea or powdered capsules, grind up the herbal combination into a powder using a coffee grinder, flour mill, mortar and pestle, meat grinder, or suribachi (a Japanese grinding bowl available at natural foods stores or Oriental groceries). Once the mixture is powdered, you can make either a tea or portable gelatin capsules.

To make a tea, infuse ½ oz. or one heaping tablespoon of the powder in approximately eight ounces of hot water, let it steep for 20 minutes or more, strain well, then sip about 2 ounces four times daily on an empty stomach. If you would rather take the herbs in dry form take two well-packed "00" capsules or one level teaspoon of the herb powder with warm water four times a day.

Store herbs in a tightly sealed glass jar in a cool, dark, dry place. Herbs are medicines and should be treated with respect and gratitude. An attitude of love and gratitude is especially helpful in healing because any medicine taken with the right frame of mind becomes all the more powerful.

Echinacea angustifolia is considered by many experienced professional herbalists as the king of the blood and lymph purifiers. It is the most effective, yet safe, blood and lymphatic cleanser from North America and one of the most respected in the entire botanical kingdom. It can be taken internally in comparatively large amounts.

Although it is nontoxic, I have observed that echinacea may cause mild dizziness or nausea for a short time in a small percentage of people. Should this happen to you, combine a small amount of Chinese licorice root (discussed in Formula Three) with echinacea, such as in the one-to-four ratio of this formula.

Research conducted in 1969 showed that preparations of echinacea help protect patients receiving x-rays and radiotherapy.[1] Echinacea improved the production of leukocytes by the bone marrow.

In a related function, echinacea is now considered an excellent immune system stimulant and strengthener. In 1950, researchers found that echinacea exhibited mild antibiotic activity against Streptococci and *Staphylococcus aureus*.[2] Further research in 1953 confirmed that echinacea produced antibacterial properties against Streptococci.[3] Studies conducted soon afterward showed that echinacea was significantly more effective than cortisone in both preventing and treating Streptococcus infection.[4]

Other research conducted in 1953 by O. Kuhn at the Zoological Institute of the University of Cologne determined that Echinacin (a purified extract made from the root of echinacea) activated white blood cells and stimulated the regeneration of the cellular connective tissue and the epidermis (the outer layer of skin).[5] Kuhn's investigations also indicated that Echinacin neutralizes a harmful enzyme which is involved in the development of the infection process. Several subsequent studies confirmed this and other infection-fighting properties of echinacea, including its ability to increase the number of white blood cell granulocytes and improve the rate of phagocytosis.[6,11]

In 1972, two researchers from the United States Department of Agriculture found a substance in the essential oils of echinacea root that destroys cancerous cells and/or contains tumor-inhibiting capabilities. The distilled oil inhibits both Walker's carcinosarcoma (cancer arising from underlying tissue such as muscles, organs, or glands) and lymphocytic leukemia. The echinacea oil was inactive in lymphoid leukemia.[12]

In 1978, Germany was again the location for two important sets of research studies on echinacea. The first set of experiments determined that echinacea extract has an interferon-like activity. When cells are exposed to viruses, interferon (one or more proteins which help to protect non-infected cells against viral infections) is produced. Two scientists from the University of Frankfort's Center for Biological Chemistry found that extracts of *Echinacea purpurea* and Echinacin have an interferon-like activity in protecting cells against viral-induced influenza, herpes, and canker sores. Echinacin is used in Germany as an influenza preventive.[13]

Another set of experiments conducted in Germany in 1978 found that echinacea was effective in the treatment of allergies.[14] Echinacea helps prevent inflammation of tissue which can be due to harmful, foreign toxins.

In 1981, scientists at the Institute of Pharmaceutical Biology, University of Munich, tested *Echinacea purpurea* and found that it contains two carbohydrate substances possessing immunostimulating properties. These carbohydrate substances stimulate important T cell activity 20 to 30 percent more than a common, highly potent T cell stimulator.[15,16]

Steven Foster, a widely respected botanist and author of many informative, well-documented articles and books on herbology, states in *Echinacea Exalted* (Ozark Beneficial Plant Project, 1985):

> The immune system-stimulating effects of Echinacea is one of the most important scientific findings to date for this genus. Immunostimulants are compounds that stimulate the immune system in a nonspecific manner. The pharmacological effects of nonspecific immunostimulants fade relatively quickly, thus they have to be administered quite frequently or continuously. An increase in phagocytosis (by macrophages) and granulocytes are important factors in immunostimulation. Immunostimulants could become alternatives or adjuncts to chemotherapy, and may help prevent infections by activating the immune system in persons whose immune response has become impaired. Immunostimulants are potentially useful in some cancers and infectious diseases.

There is currently more research being conducted on *Echinacea purpurea* in Germany. *Echinacea purpurea* is used rather than *Echinacea angustifolium* primarily because *E. purpurea* can be easily cultivated in Germany. No conclusive research has been conducted yet as to which species of echinacea, *E. angustifolium* or *E. purpurea*, is a more potent immunostimulant. To date, *Echinacea angustifolium* has been used more in the U.S. for a wider variety of other health problems. And, with the current rapid increase in immune-related diseases, such as AIDS and Epstein-Barr, echinacea may prove to be an extremely valuable herb because it is a potent T cell stimulator.

In the 1950s, Dr. Jonathan L. Hartwell of the National Cancer Institute (NCI) in Bethesda, Maryland conducted an investigation into literature that described plants useful against cancers and tumors. He reviewed over 1,000 books from around the world and communicated extensively with the NCI and the American Cancer Society. In 1960 he reported some of his findings in an article entitled "Plant Remedies for Cancer" that appeared in *Cancer Chemotherapy Reports.*[17] In his article, Hartwell discussed some of the herbs used in Formula One. He found that in the Southwest, burdock root is combined with yellow dock and sarsaparilla and consumed orally as a tea for cancer in general. Pills made from an extract (a concentrated tea) of dandelion are effectively used for general cancer. Red clover blossoms are made into a tea and widely used for cancer in general and breast cancer specifically. The roots of sarsaparilla are boiled and taken orally as a tea for general cancer. Violet leaves are used throughout the U.S. for general cancer treatment, either in a tea alone or frequently combined with red clover and yellow dock root. Yellow dock root has been used for a wide range of blood/lymph problems and for cancer in general.

Barberry or Oregon grape root is an excellent liver stimulant and tonic. Echinacea, goldenseal, sarsaparilla, and Oregon grape root are reportedly beneficial for minimizing the drastic side effects caused by chemotherapy, according to Dr. John Heinerman in *The Treatment of Cancer with Herbs* (Bi World Publishers, 1984).

Chinese licorice root will be discussed in Formula Three for its capacity to stimulate detoxification and to help blend or harmonize other strong detoxifying herbs.

Formula Two: Antibiotic and Antiviral Tincture

This is an effective and reliable antibiotic and antiviral tincture. Tinctures are concentrated herbal extracts that are preserved with alcohol and can be kept for a long time. They are usually used when herbs have to be

taken over a long period of time—such as tonic or alterative herbs like ginseng, eleuthero, chaparral, and *Echinacea angustifolium*. Tinctures can be
carried around easily and taken in just a little water or under the tongue.
They are particularly useful for herbs that do not taste good. Also, tinctures
are preferred by many herbalists when treating severe infections or other
immunological problems because tinctures can be rapidly absorbed and
their dosages can be easily changed. The manifestation and sequence of
many immunological problems tend to change rapidly, and it is easier to
gauge dosages when using drops.

Quantity	Herb
3 oz.	purple coneflower (*Echinacea angustifolium* or *purpurea*)
1 1/2 oz.	goldenseal root (*Hydrastis canadensis*)
1 oz.	burdock root (*Arctium lappa*)
1/2 oz.	myrrh (*Commiphora myrrha*)
1/3 oz.	chaparral (*Larrea divaricata*)

Combine the herbs with 1½ pints of alcohol such as vodka, brandy,
gin, or rum. Tinctures are usually prepared with an alcohol content ranging
from 30 to 60 percent by using 60 to 120 proof drinking alcohol. Combine herbs and alcohol in a container with a tight stopper or lid. Let mixture stand at room temperature in a dark place for fourteen days, shaking
container two or more times daily. Let the herbs settle and pour off the
tincture. Strain what is left through a filter or a fine cloth such as muslin.
Pour the liquids into a dark glass bottle and cap it tightly. Most people
prefer to fill and carry around a one-ounce amber jar with a dropper-type
lid. These are available at most pharmacies.

The amount of tincture to be taken in a single adult dose varies from
30-60 drops (approximately ½ - 1 teaspoon), depending upon the severity
of the problem, three to six times daily. The tincture can be added to ¼ -
½ cup room-temperature or slightly warm water and drunk; or, better yet,
the drops can be taken under the tongue if the person can tolerate the taste.

The total amount of alcohol ingested is quite small, and for most people does not cause a problem. However, if the use of alcohol even in this
amount must be restricted, the tincture may be made with apple cider vinegar or glycerine. Most herbalists prefer to use alcohol because it extracts
and preserves better. The recommended amount of tincture can be added
to a steaming cup of water and then stirred in order to vaporize the alcohol.

This tincture can also be used externally for its astringent, antiseptic, antibacterial, antiviral, and antifungal properties. Because it helps for a wide array of skin problems and skin infections, this tincture applied externally helps the body resist harmful external agents. It also makes an effective, though unpleasant-tasting, mouthwash for spongy gums, pyorrhea, sore throat, and other ailments requiring an astringent.

In Formula One, I described the powerful antiobiotic, antiviral properties of echinacea.

Goldenseal root has long occupied a preeminent position in herbal tradition, and many claims have been made for it. Although it is not the panacea some have touted it to be, it is an excellent tonic for epithelial tissue all along the digestive/gastrointestinal tract.

Goldenseal contains the strong alkaloids hydrastine and berberine. It was widely used by Native Americans and by the early frontier settlers. In 1860 goldenseal was declared an official drug in the *U.S. Pharmacopoeia*. Currently hydrastine is used in several over-the-counter ophthalmic preparations such as eyewash and eye drops.[18] Besides being a tonic for epithelial tissue throughout the gastrointestinal tract, goldenseal tonifies the liver and kidneys, thus helping these organs better filter and purify the blood. Goldenseal helps these organs eliminate toxic drugs, including heroin, and other dangerous substances from the bloodstream and the body.[19]

Goldenseal is both an antiseptic and another natural antibacterial agent. However, because it is a powerful herb, it should not be overused or abused. Excessive use of goldenseal in larger than recommended amounts, or for a prolonged period of time, will eventually diminish favorable intestinal flora or bacteria which will then decrease production and absorption of important B vitamins.

If you are exposed to toxins and do take goldenseal regularly, it is best to also regularly eat some fermented food, such as miso, to help restore the necessary balance of healthful bacteria in the digestive tract.

Pregnant women who might have a tendency to miscarry should avoid the use of goldenseal unless it is in very small doses (such as in Formula Two). Large doses of goldenseal contract the uterus. Similarly, if you have a tendency towards hypoglycemia, only very small amounts of goldenseal should be used.

Burdock root is a good blood and kidney cleanser, thus producing general healing effects on the whole body. Burdock clears the kidneys of excess wastes and acids, especially uric acid, by increasing the flow of urine. It also helps clear the blood of harmful acids, an important function because studies have shown that an overly acidic bloodstream can both impair kidney function and leave a person far more vulnerable to the harmful effects of radiation and chemical pollutants.[20] Burdock root provides an abundance of iron, which makes it of further value for the blood. One of the medicinal components of burdock root is a volatile oil that both stimulates kidney function and possesses a diaphoretic or sweat-promoting property. When burdock root is taken internally, this volatile oil is eliminated from the sweat glands, carrying toxic wastes out with it. Burdock root is often used when there is an infection or fever due to an invasion of harmful external toxins.

Myrrh is an oil gum-resin. In ancient times, it was one of the primary herbs used in making what was considered a holy ointment. Myrrh was one of two herbs, along with frankincense, said to have been presented at the birth of Jesus. It was also one of two herbs, along with aloe, which Nicodemus brought in mixture form to use for burying Jesus. Today myrrh is used in many countries of the Near and Far East as an astringent tonic and, in a few cases, as an external curing agent for skin cancer.

In 1975, Dr. Guido Majno, a Harvard pathologist, had myrrh clinically tested to accurately determine its bacteria-fighting properties. He states in *The Healing Hand* that laboratory results conclusively demonstrated that bacterium-like *Staphylococcus aureus* simply cannot exist in a typical wound when a fluid solution of myrrh is applied. Myrrh's usefulness for internal and external cancers is now being further investigated in those parts of the world (particularly Egypt and Israel) where it is most commonly used for medicinal purposes.

Myrrh is a strong antiseptic. It destroys putrefaction in the intestines and prevents blood absorption of toxins. From clinical experience, professional herbalists have observed that myrrh combines well with goldenseal. Myrrh contains strong gums and resinous materials. Myrrh should be taken internally only in small amounts and for short periods of time since it contains potent volatile oils that are toxic in large amounts. Small doses of myrrh will help remove toxins from the stomach and intestines.

Formula Three: Immune System Builder

This herbal formula helps improve immune response and could prove to be a useful defense against the initial inflammation and infections that are often experienced after exposure to radiation and environmental pollutants.

Quantity	Herbs
2 oz.	bee propolis
1 oz.	Siberian ginseng (*Eleutherococcus senticosus*)
1 oz.	Chinese astragalus (*Astragalus membranaceus*)
1 oz.	Chinese ginseng (*Panax ginseng*)
1 oz.	ligustrum (*Ligustrum lucidum*)
½ oz.	crab apple tree bark (*Pyrus malus*)
½ oz.	Chinese licorice root (*Glycyrrhizae uralensis*)

Formula Three can be made either as a tea or, preferably, as a tincture. Follow the directions and dosages provided for Formula Two.

I've already discussed bee propolis, Siberian ginseng, and *Panax ginseng*, so we will concentrate here on the other ingredients in Formula Three. As Ron Teeguarden notes in *Chinese Tonic Herbs*:

Extracts of *Astragalus membranaceous* have shown in vitro antibacterial effects as well as hypoglycemic activity in animals.

A recent article published in *Cancer,* a publication of the American Cancer Society, reports that the aqueous extract of *Astragalus membranaceus* restored the immune functions in 90 percent of cancer patients studied. The article states that the cellular immune response is usually impaired in cancer patients, especially in those with advanced disease. Immune response is further compromised by radiation and/or chemotherapy. Astragalus has been found to be a "response modifier" which favorably modulates the subnormal immune apparatus of cancer patients. In studies performed at the National Cancer Institute and five other leading American Cancer Research Institutes over the past eight years, it has been positively shown that astragalus strengthens a cancer patient's immune system. Researchers believed, on the basis of cell studies, that astragalus augments those white blood cells that fight disease and removes some of those that make the body more vulnerable to it. There is clinical evidence that cancer patients given astragalus during chemotherapy or radiation, both of which reduce the body's natural immunity while attacking the cancer, recover significantly faster and live longer. It is evident that nothing in astragalus directly attacks cancers themselves, but instead strengthens the body's own immune system.

The Chinese are currently conducting more extensive research on astragalus as an immune enhancer than on any other immunological herb. Astragalus seems to combine well with another Chinese herb called ligustrum.

Chinese herbalists have long considered ligustrum excellent for strengthening the immune system and improving circulation. It also acts as a cleansing tonic, toning and detoxifying the liver. Modern scientists have found ligustrum to contain extremely powerful immune system stimulants. It has several properties and functions identical to *Astragalus membranaceus*. Medical researchers are doing extensive studies with ligustrum to determine its possible use in the treatment of cancer, AIDS, and other immune system dysfunctions, and for the prevention or treatment of some of the symptoms of old age.

Research performed by the Cancer Institute of the Chinese Academy of Medical Sciences in Beijing lends further support to the concept that extracts of astragalus and ligustrum may indeed act as biological response modifiers due to the presence of one or more extremely potent, naturally occurring immune stimulants.

Chinese medical doctors are using 4,000-year-old herbal prescriptions to strengthen the immune system, effectively fight cancer, and reduce tumors. Two of these herbs, *Astragalus membranaceus* and *Ligustrum lucidum*, are being researched at a major U.S. facility, according to a report in the *Medical Tribune*.[21] Preliminary experiments at the University of Texas M.D. Anderson Hospital and Tumor Institute indicate that the activity of these two Chinese herbs stimulates the white blood cells and thus measurably boosts defenses of the host organism.

Dr. Giora Mavligit, professor of medicine and internist at the Texas research center, and a team of investigators report that astragalus and ligustrum had a profound restorative effect on the immune system of cancer patients. Ninety percent of the cancer patients tested with the astragalus extract exhibited a restored reaction, as did 70 percent of the cancer patients who received ligustrum. Mavligit told the *Tribune*, "We have not seen anything close to this in terms of immune augmentation or restoration. There is definitely a significant increase in in-vitro stimulation of the immune system. . . . Chinese medicine has been in existence for thousands of years. There must be something to it or else they would not be maintaining it." Currently, medicinal herbs still occupy about 75 percent of the regular Chinese materia medica.

Dr. Baldwin Tom, immunologist at the University of Texas Health Science Center in Houston, said in the *Tribune* article, "Used as an adjunct to chemotherapy, Chinese herbs offer a fresh new approach to treating cancer patients. . . . In the next ten years the cancer field and the biological response modifier are going to really explode, and within that explosion will be herbal medicine."

Eastern and Western doctors have begun sharing their knowledge and methods with each other. In 1984, scientists from around the world met at an international symposium entitled, "The Interaction of Traditional Chinese Medicine and Western Medicine." After reviewing research presented at this meeting, Tom reported, "I think you have the best of both worlds if you couple Western ideas and thoughts, in terms of how to monitor physiology, with the Chinese philosophy of looking at the whole person. In the West we look at systems through disease rather than homeostatic systems [a state of equilibrium or balance between different but interdependent elements of an organism]. The West does not respond scientifically to phenomenology."

Crab-apple tree bark has been used to tonify the spleen and regulate immunological responses. It is difficult to find at natural foods stores. The best source is to pick it wild yourself and then dry it. If you cannot find it, just delete it from the formula.

Chinese licorice root is a delicious herb that mixes well with most other herbs and consistently produces an improved state of well-being. I have seen Chinese licorice root's effect on many different people over many years and I appreciate the therapeutic ability of this herb by itself and also its ability to help other strong herbs blend or harmonize with each other.

According to Teeguarden:

Licorice root stands next to ginseng in importance in Chinese herbalism. It is the most widely used of all Chinese herbs. It is known as the "Grandfather of Chinese herbs," as the "Great Adjunct," and as the "Great Detoxifier." It is used as a harmonizing ingredient in a large number of Chinese herbal recipes and is itself an excellent tonic and longevity herb. . . . Chinese licorice root is a very different herb from the Western variety of licorice, *Glycyrrhizae glabra.* The Western variety can cause nervousness, an obviously undesirable side effect. To the contrary, Chinese licorice, *Glycyrrhizae uralensis,* is energizing but calming, and does not have the side effects associated with Western licorice. Be *sure* to use Chinese licorice root. . . .

In pharmaceutical tests, it has been found that glycyrrhizin has a function similar to that of adrenocortical hormones. It is almost identical to the adrenal steroids. Laboratory tests in

China have demonstrated that extracts of *Radix Glycyrrhizae* can help to eliminate or detoxify over 1,200 known toxins. This remarkable capacity as a detoxifying agent is virtually unparalleled in the realm of pharmacology. . . . Recent studies have shown that licorice combined with ginseng is a specific pituitary tonic, improving overall hormonal functioning. Compounds isolated from this herb have been found to have anti-inflammatory, antibacterial, and antitussive activity.

Chinese herbalists consider licorice to be able to help expel poisons and toxins from the body and to cancel any side effects from other herbs used with it. I have noticed that Chinese licorice root also consistently builds or normalizes energy levels for most people, thus making it beneficial for hypoglycemia and some other problems related to the pancreas and adrenals. Frequent large doses of licorice, however, are contraindicated for people with high blood pressure, or for women who have high estrogen levels or who are pregnant and have a history of miscarriage.

Formula Four: Digestive Stabilizer

Digestive disturbances and anemia are common disorders among all mammals after exposure to radiation and chemical toxins. The ability to secrete pepsin and other gastric juices is greatly hampered or lost in rats, for example, after exposure to lethal and sublethal doses of radiation.[22] Under normal conditions, gastric juices produce proper acid pH in the stomach, which assists in the assimilation of iron—thus helping to prevent anemia. The decrease or loss of gastric secretions may contribute to other disorders resulting from radiation or chemical toxins, such as nausea, anemia, and reduced immune response.

Thus, it would be helpful to find a safe, effective remedy to regulate and encourage digestion after exposure to radiation or chemical pollutants. Improved gastric secretions would no doubt provide further protection and perhaps help the body recover more quickly from the debilitating effects of exposure.

Hydrochloric acid (HCL) and pepsin supplements are becoming popular in certain health circles. Certainly, HCL and pepsin offer quick symptomatic relief for insufficient digestive juices. Digestive enzyme supplements, however, leave the user's body less able to produce its own enzymes, thus risking the danger of creating an ongoing dependency. A better choice is herbs that have been used successfully for over 4,000 years to stimulate the body to produce its own digestive juices. For example, gentian root is used in many parts of the world for regulating digestion. It has been used effectively for both hypo- and hyperactive gastric secretion.

I have developed the following herbal formula to effectively regulate the secretion of digestive juices, stimulate the entire digestive system, stimulate the liver, and improve assimilation of iron. In the event of exposure to radiation or chemical toxins and the resultant side effects, such a formula may be helpful in restoring certain digestive functions, particularly the production of gastric juices.

Quantity	Herb
2 parts	gentian root (*Gentiana lutea*)
2 parts	organic lemon peel or organic orange peel
1 part	either cardamom, fennel, or anise seeds; or 1 part (total) any combination of these seeds

Both lemon peel and orange peel are abundant in bioflavonoids and combine well with gentian root. Organically grown citrus is best since sprays and coloring agents lodge in the peel of commercially grown citrus.

Grind herbs into as fine a powder as possible. Take 2 full "00," fifteen-grain capsules or ½ teaspoon of herb powder with warm water before meals. Or, as a bitter tea, take one teaspoon of the mixture per small cup of water and drink before meals.

Many people will prefer to take the above combination in capsule or powder form, since the tea tastes bitter.

THE ROLE OF EXERCISE, SAUNAS, & DE-TOX BATHS

Radioactive fallout and environmental pollutants descend with rain, snow, and wind. They are especially concentrated if it has not rained or snowed in a while, thus allowing the amount of contaminants to build up in the upper atmosphere. Fallout, and other radiation and environmental pollutants, can enter through the lungs and skin, which explains why there is much more sickness reported after a rain or snow following a prolonged dry spell. Let's take a look next at how exercise, sweating, and especially bathing may prove helpful.

Regular exercise has proven beneficial to health, especially if it is aerobic exercise. Among the many benefits of aerobic exercise are that it:

• strengthens the heart and lungs • stimulates every organ and gland • moves the blood and lymph • helps regulate the nerves and muscles • causes the body to temporarily overheat, thus helping both to kill some internal pathogens and to release toxins via perspiration • stimulates bone functions such as blood production • stimulates the immune system • creates a heightened sense of self-confidence and emotional well-being

Regular aerobic activity means working out at a moderate pace for at least 30 minutes or more, usually every other day.

When starting an exercise program, choose a sport that you feel you will enjoy. Preferably, the sport should use your legs—such as brisk walking, easy jogging, bicycling, or swimming. *Start out with a pace and distance that is very easy and enjoyable.* Exercise at a tempo that does not wind you, such that you could still have a normal conversation without panting. Increase your speed and/or distance *gradually* over an extended period of time. Be patient, but remain consistent and committed. Continue to exercise every other day. If you are over forty years of age or if you have had chronic health problems, it is recommended that you have a physical exam by a physician before beginning an exercise program.

Some of the older exercise books tend to lock people into rigid training schedules. People do not progress at the same rate. Therefore, I especially recommend that you individualize your exercise program by training at a certain percentage of your maximum heartbeat. As you gradually get in better shape, increase the intensity or duration of your workout to maintain the desired percentage of your maximum heartbeat. This method allows you to accurately individualize your own training program by working with your own biofeedback system—your heartbeat.

To determine your maximum heartbeat, subtract your age from 220. Most people should begin an exercise program by working out at an intensity that causes the heart to beat at approximately 70 percent of maximum heartbeat. For example, if you are forty years old, your maximum heartbeat is approximately 220 - 40 = 180. You would begin an exercise program by working out at a speed or intensity to cause your heart to beat at approximately 126 beats per minute (180 x 70 percent). As your training capacity gradually improves, you will need to gradually increase the speed or duration of your workout in order to keep your heart beating at the number you calculate as optimal for your level of fitness. Remember, your workouts should be regular, preferably every other day, and optimally they should last for approximately thirty continuous minutes or more.

Remember, exercise and sports should not be literal "work outs" as in "no pain, no gain." You will benefit most over a long period of time if you keep your exercise activities playful. Do everything you can to have fun and enjoy this physical, and emotional, play. Within one to two months you will begin to experience the beginnings of profoundly positive physical and emotional changes.

A traditional worldwide method of using water and heat to detoxify is the sauna, a form of hydrotherapy. A sauna will help cleanse the skin, especially if an appropriate method of brushing the skin is used. It will clean out the seven-to-eight million sweat-secreting and oil-secreting glands found in the skin. (Because of the chemical composition of sweat, the skin is sometimes referred to as the "third kidney" and considered the largest eliminative organ.) Equally important, a good sauna will temporarily and intentionally overheat the entire body, thus stimulating the immune system.

I have occasionally used saunas since 1972 in my clinical practice. The saunas often produced improved results—as determined by both blood tests and interviews of the clients before and after a series of treatments.

In addition to taking a sauna, a "detoxification bath" may possibly be helpful in removing external radiation or pollutants. To take a detox bath, fill a bathtub to a normal bathing depth with water (preferably filtered or purified) as hot as can be comfortably tolerated. First add one pound of baking soda and then add one pound of salt, preferably sun-dried sea salt or salt from a deep mine. Rock salt is not as effective, and ordinary iodized table salt, depleted of other minerals, is ineffective.

This cleansing, drawing bath works best if you keep as much of the body submerged as possible for twenty to fifty minutes. Only one person should use this bath before the tub is drained and cleaned. You will want to take a short shower after completing this bath to wash off the soda, salt, and various pollutants.

The baking soda-salt bath treatment can be quite cleansing and may aid in the removal of radioactive and chemical pollutants on the skin. (The scientific evidence is not as solid as it is for foods, herbs, and vitamins.) Some of my clients have felt tired and drained afterwards. To prevent this feeling and to help revitalize yourself, drink a total of at least two cups of water before, during, and after the bath.

After the bath it may be beneficial to take a nap, pray, meditate, or do a visualization. As a sample visualization, see your body permeated and surrounded by light and a strong, positive, healing energy. Try to see the toxins in and on your body as dark energies that are washed away by the healing water and light.

This bath treatment is said to have powerful effects and therefore is rarely done more than once every two or three days. If you are exposed to a daily source of radiation or external pollutants, you could take a ten-to-twenty-five minute bath treatment each day.

It is obvious that there are many potential natural substances and therapies that may offer substantial protection from radiation and environmental pollutants. Because of widespread interest in natural self-healing, especially in foreign countries, there are numerous other areas being explored. For example, the radioprotective properties of certain mosses, ferns, and fungi are being scientifically explored as a means to restore normal blood values and body weight, preserve fertility, and generally strengthen the protective power of animals receiving irradiation.[23]

Investigation is also being initiated into other areas of naturopathy and holistic health, including professional massage therapy and focusing mental, emotional, or spiritual energies through such techniques as prayer, meditation, and visualization. There have been many claims, yet up to this point the protective and detoxifying potential of these techniques has been evaluated primarily by intuitive methods, although there has been some preliminary scientific research. Especially noteworthy is the work of O. Carl Simonton, M.D., and Stephanie Simonton-Atchley, internationally respected cancer researchers who have conducted pioneering work on how visualizations and positive mental attitudes can combat tumors and improve immune response. My own clinical experience is that several of these approaches can be helpful as adjunct or complementary therapies. These areas should now be researched with an open scientific mind. One should, however, be just as wary of indiscriminate over-enthusiasm as of closed-mindedness. Certainly, both doubters and believers should take a scientific wait-and-see attitude.

TOWARD A HOLISTIC HEALTH PROGRAM

The substances discussed in this book offer humanity substantial protection against radioactive and chemical toxins. It should be noted that all of the testing has been done using only one or two of the substances together, and usually for only a very limited amount of time. I would like to see tests designed that employ a comprehensive protective or therapeutic diet, supplement, and herbal program over an extended period of time. Only then would the combined effectiveness of these substances be determined for both preventive and treatment purposes.

It should be remembered that each individual's metabolic needs may vary slightly, thus probably necessitating slightly different dosages for optimal nutrition and health. Consequently, the dosages listed must be viewed as approximate. I hope that one of the results of this book will be to catalyze further research.

The diet, supplement, and herbal program described herein is based on the best available research and many years of experience in trying to help people who have suffered from the side effects of radiation and chemical pollutants. You certainly need not do everything mentioned in this book to derive the benefits of the program. Indeed, the program is so rich in nutritive, protective, and therapeutic capacities that you need only follow the diet and choose the herbs or supplements you feel are appropriate to your situation. The diet and supplement program given here is designed as the best general optimal health program for the widest range of people. Feel free to modify aspects of either the diet or supplement program in order to satisfy your individual needs. You might choose to add one or more of the other substances I have discussed in order to even more effectively cope with a particular toxin or existing health problem.

A program that goes beyond detoxification, one that aims to produce optimum health and vitality, should be holistic—that is, it should include health-promoting modalities and therapies for the mind, emotions, and spirit as well as for the body. You will benefit by regular, enjoyable exercise, occasional saunas or "detox" baths, and a regular religious or spiritual practice that you feel comfortable with. Scientific research has now repeatedly documented the benefits of positive thought, visualizations, therapeutic massage and bodywork, and other holistic health therapies to help improve the immune system and develop optimum health.

Many books and articles report on the detoxification and rejuvenation benefits of short-term fasts. My clinical experience is that many, though not all, people would benefit by an occasional fast of from one to three days on fruit or vegetable juice, or a mono-food fast. I discourage fasting, however, before or after exposure to intensive amounts of toxins. Because of the amount of toxins already stored in the body, especially those in the fat or adipose tissue that are metabolized and released more rapidly during fasting, longer fasts should be attempted only if one has already experienced shorter fasts with no ill effects. For similar reasons, my clinical experience is that water fasts can be more harmful than beneficial for a significant percentage of people living in an industrial society. Indeed, one research experiment, done on rabbits irradiated by a cesium-137 source, indicated that a water fast caused radioactivity in the blood to decrease, yet it also caused radioactivity in the wall of the intestines and in other tissue to rise.[24]

People who are over forty, women who are pregnant, and anyone who has any kind of health problem may still be helped by saunas, an occasional fast, or especially regular exercise, but they should first consult with a trusted physician or health therapist. The program, with optimal diet, vitamins and minerals, other food supplements, and herbs, is designed for everyone, except for the few exceptions.

In summary, this program is meant to strengthen our bodies, minds, and spirits against a host of insults present in our world. There is no single element in this diet that should be viewed as a magic bullet against disease, radiation, or chemical toxins. Rather, we are dealing with our health from a holistic perspective, recognizing that life encompasses biochemical mechanisms, the power of our minds, and the spiritual will to direct our energies toward a desired goal.

This diet, herb, and supplement program, along with the other self-help therapies, were developed in response to the feeling of impotence that many people have when confronted with problems of such scope and magnitude. There is a great deal we can do to protect ourselves, our families, and our friends from radioactive and chemical toxins. The first step is to adopt the diet and health program described here that will create optimum health combined with reliable protection. As we are establishing our own good health, we can work towards minimizing the threats of toxins in our own lives, and in those of our children, our grandchildren, our friends, and our extended world family.

The specific remedies and the optimum diet presented in this book prevent and counteract the effects of a wide range of common and dangerous toxins, which nutrition author Jeffrey Bland, Ph.D., has called, "the primary cause of chronic degenerative diseases." Yet, even if all radioactive and chemical toxins were miraculously eliminated from this planet tomorrow, their lingering effects would continue to have severe consequences upon our bodies and our planet for generations to come. Therefore, this book was written in order to provide you with reliable, effective, and safe self-help remedies for prevention and treatment. I have sought to offer holistic health solutions in the truest sense of the meaning.

Holistic health care has become popular and widespread. The term "holistic" implies integrating physical, emotional, mental, and spiritual aspects of the individual, plus it considers the larger perspective, the dynamic interplay between the individual and society. The holistic approach does not artificially separate or isolate these two overlapping worlds.

Holistic health care is an integration of the individual with his or her whole self and with the environment—the larger *Self*—thus producing a state of balance wherein our innate capacity for self-healing manifests optimal health and well-being. It is an approach to living a healthy life in balance and harmony with one's internal and external world.

Holistic health care strives to work simultaneously on both the causes of the problems as well as the symptoms. As holistic thinkers, we seek cures for the physical problems of radioactive and chemical toxins, while exploring emotional, intellectual, and spiritual facets of these problems. We need to seek cures for society as well as for individuals.

As herbalist Steven Foster has said, "The best way to deal with the problem of radioactivity is to eliminate the problem at its source. That source is not necessarily only nuclear power plants or uranium mines, but the way of thinking that has produced this, the ultimate monstrosity of an energy-greedy society."

Today the world is faced with global nuclear and ecological problems that threaten our health and our very survival. Our society is increasingly concerned with meeting its gargantuan needs for energy. The nuclear energy industry, as well as other technologies, are being developed despite the incredible risks they present to our health and survival. Many people choose not to think about these and other seemingly overwhelming predicaments. When one first tries to face the enormity of current problems, according to Jonathan Schell in *The Fate of the Earth* (Knopf, 1982), "One might feel sick, whereas when one pushes it out of mind, as apparently one must do most of the time in order to carry on with life, one feels well again. But this feeling of well-being is based on a denial of the most important realities of our time, and therefore is itself a kind of sickness. A society that systematically shuts its eyes to urgent perils to its physical survival and fails to take any steps to save itself cannot be called psychologically well."

Are we really more readily willing to risk global suicide than we are willing to risk changing our minds and habits? If not, we first need to change our tribal consciousness to a species consciousness. We need to replace our "survival of the fittest, fastest, and biggest" attitude with a survival of the planet attitude. It is time we acknowledge and accept our differences, yet realize that ultimately our best defense it to learn to live with more concern for our connectedness.

How, then, can we resolve these problems and create an environment where we can live vital lives with optimal health? It is obviously unrealistic to consider moving millions of people to cleaner environments—isolated islands and ecosystems are available to a fortunate few, perhaps, but not to all. No, our solutions must be societal ones in which our problems are not continually recreated and made worse. Nor is the solution to attempt to immediately eradicate all technologies and industries that cause pollution. To a great extent, our urban societies have grown dependent upon the complex machinery of the twentieth century. Rather, the solution lies in finding a way to integrate some of these technologies and industries with a greater concern for the health and survival of people and our planet.

For instance, innovative solutions to our energy problem may include safer technologies such as solar, geothermal, or hydroelectric alternatives, as well as a greater concern for conservation and recycling. Our best long-term solutions for other political, social, and economic problems should have in common peaceful attitudes and actions, and a more simplified life-style. Eating naturally produced foods, developing appropriate technologies, and "thinking locally, acting globally," are all part of what's being called "right livelihood," the attempt to live in a way that promotes the general quality of life for all people.

As we approach the year 2000, we stand at a precipice, poised to take nothing less than a collective evolutionary leap. Symbolically, like the Israelites during the Biblical Exodus, we must be willing to undergo a simi-lar process in which we use faith and trust to help us drop our chains. We must be willing to let old and destructive habits gently and nonviolently fall away, and evolve new and healthier ones. And, again symbolically, we can travel or evolve towards the "promised land"—not as isolated individuals, but as a group, a community of humankind. In order to let go of our insecurities and bondage, we as individuals, families, societies, and eventu-ally as world citizens, need to be willing to live harmoniously.

According to Willis W. Harman, Ph.D., author and lecturer on the transformation and future of society, "We should not make the mistake of thinking we will find separate solutions to the nuclear dilemma, nor world poverty and hunger, nor pollution, nor urban ills, nor resource crises, nor alienation and loss of meaning in modern society. The solution must be common to all these problems, because they are all interrelated. They will be solved together or not at all."

We must keep in mind that modern technology is not inherently des-tructive. However, we must finally learn to harness and wisely channel that which we have created, rather than letting our devices control our destiny. Human intelligence will seek to survive and prosper physically, emotionally, and spiritually. As concerned individuals and groups, we can learn to use our inventiveness to help us better fit into the natural order of the universe rather than trying to control, and eventually disrupt, our world. We can use our technology for humanitarian concerns. As citizens we can act on our social responsibility. Fortunately, our Constitution encourages us to exer-cise this right. We can do this by lovingly and nonviolently urging and motivating politicians, large multinational corporations, and those who con-trol the bureaucratic power structure to serve the needs of the general popu-lace. We can draw upon our deepest religious/spiritual/social values and become more accountable to the spirit of bettering the world.

Through helping each other to become more conscious of the need for world harmony, we can do more than strengthen our immune systems and counteract toxins, more than end our energy problems, more than even stop the current competition to exploit natural resources. We can use this healing crisis as a time to transform some of our attitudes and actions. We can restore our trust and faith and set the stage for fostering our deepest yearnings and needs—holistic health, well-being, and cooperation on a global level.

Notes

CHAPTER ONE

1. R. C. McMillan and S. A. Horne, Eye Exposure from Thoriated Optical Glass, *Proceedings of the Third International Congress of the Radiation Protection Association*, 1973, Washington D.C., pp. 882-888.

2. Michael Castleman, Are Cigarettes Radioactive?, *Medical Self Care*, Fall 1980, vol. 10, pp. 20-23.

3. Edward Martell, Tobacco Radioactivity and Cancer in Smokers, *American Scientist*, vol. 63, July/August 1975, pp. 404-412.

4. K. W. Taylor, N. L. Patt, and H. E. Johns, Variations in X-Ray Exposures to Patients, *The Journal of the Canadian Association of Radiologists*, 30: 6-11.

CHAPTER TWO

1. J. Blosser, *National Engineer*, October 13, 1981, 16.

2. M. Murozumi et al., *Geochim Cosmochim. Acta*, 1969, 33: 1247.

3. D. M. Settle and C. C. Patterson, *Science*, 1980, 207: 1167.

4. C. C. Patterson, *Arch. Environ. Health*, 1965, 11: 334.

5. E. J. Erickson et al., *N. Engl. J. Med.*, 1979, 300: 946.

6. P. Grandjean et al., *J. Environ. Pathol. Toxical*, 1979, 2: 781.

7. L. Hecker et al., *Arch. Environ. Health*, 1974, 29: 181.

8. S. Piomell et al., *Science*, 1980, 210: 1135-1137.

9. E. Cheraskin and W. M. Ringsdorf, Prevalence of Possible Lead Toxicity as Determined by Hair Analysis, *J. Orthomol. Psych.*, 1979, 8 (2): 82-83.

10. J. Blosser, *op. cit.*

11. *Ibid.*

12. O. David et al., *Lancet*, 1972, 2: 900-903.

13. O. David et al., *Amer. J. Psychiatry*, 1976, 133: 1155-1158.

14. H. L. Needleman, *New England Journal of Medicine*, 1979, 300: 689-695.

15. L. R. Ember, *Chem. Eng. News*, June 23, 1980, pp. 28-35.

16. C. Patterson and D. Settle, *Science*, 1980, 207: 1167-1176.

17. H. G. Petering, *Environ. Health Pers.*, 1978, 25: 141-145.

18. K. Tsuchiya and S. Lwao, *Environ. Health Pers.*, 1978, 25: 119-124.

19. R. Papauiabbiym et al., *J. Orthomol. Psychiatry*, 1978, 7 (2): 94-106.
20. Problem Children: Lead and What to Do About It, *Prevention*, October 1973, p. 87.
21. D. S. Klauder and H. G. Petering, *Environ. Health Pers.*, 1975, 12: 77-80.
22. *Science News*, 1981, 118: 136.
23. H. G. Petering, *op. cit.*
24. Problem Children: Lead and What to Do About It, *op. cit.*
25. K. Tsuchiya and S. Lwao, *op. cit.*
26. D. S. Klauder, *op. cit.*
27. H. G. Petering, *op. cit.*
28. Problem Children: Lead and What to Do About It, *op. cit.*
29. N. Johnson, *Trace Element Metabolism in Man and Animals*, July 1977, Bavaria, Germany.
30. A. Aldanazarov and S. Sabdeova, *Chem. Abstr.*, 1981, 55: 26204g.
31. S. Caccuri and A. Cesaro, *Chem. Abstr.*, 1946, 40: 3532.
32. L. Pecora, *Panminerua Med.*, 1966, 8: 284.
33. G. Acocella, *Chem. Abstr.*, 1967, 60: 15038h.
34. G. Pokotilenko, *Chem Abstr.*, 1964, 60: 15038h.
35. A. Herada, *Jap. J. Nat. Health*, 1955, 24: 143.
36. G. Saita, *Med. Lav.*, 1955, 46: 404.
37. G. Garminati, *Chem. Abstr.*, 1959, 53: 15359b.
38. G. R. Bratton, *Med. World News*, May 25, 1981, p. 3.
39. G. R. Bratton, *op. cit.*
40. R. Papauiabbiym et al., *J. Orthomol. Psychiatry*, 1978, 7 (2): 94-106.
41. J. Blosser, *op. cit*
42. A. Ki. Koshchev et al., *Gig. Tr. Prov. Zabol*, 1970, 14 (1): 52-54.
43. R. Goyer, *Env. Health Pers.*, 1972, 2: 73.
44. A. K. Koshchev, *op. cit.*
45. R. Goyer, *op. cit.*
46. L. Friberg et al., *Cadmium in the Environment*, 1971, CRC Press.
47. M. W. Neathery and W. J. Miller, *J. Dairy Sci.*, 1975, 58 (12): 1767-1781.
48. W. J. Miller et al., *J. Dairy Sci.*, 1968, 51: 1836.
49. M. W. Neathery et al., *J. Dairy Sci.*, 1974, 57: 1177.
50. K. J. Ellis et al., *Science*, July 20, 1979, 205: 323-324.
51. H. A. Schroeder, *J. Chronic Dis.*, 1965, 18: 647.
52. H. A. Schroeder, *J. Amer. Med. Assoc.*, 1964, 1987: 358.
53. R. E. Carroll, *J. Amer. Med. Assoc.*, 1968, 195: 267.
54. G. F. Nordberg, *AMBIO*, 1974, 3 (2): 55-66.
55. M. H. Bhattacharya and B. D. Whelton, *FASEB Meeting*, Anaheim, Calif., (April, 1980).
56. *Science News*, 1980, 117: 262.
57. A. Huag, *Composition and Properties of Alginates*, Report No. 30, Norwegian Seaweed Research Institute (Trondheim), 1964.
58. C. H. Hill et al., *J. Nutr.*, 1963, 80 (3): 227-235.
59. K. Mason et al., *Anat. Rec.*, 1964, 148 (2): 309.
60. G. W. Powell et al., *J. Nutr.*, 1964, 84 (3): 205-214.
61. R. J. Banis et al., *Proc. Soc. Exp. Biol. Med.*, 1969, 130 (3): 802-806.
62. O. J. Lucis et al., *Arch. Environ. Health*, 1969, 19 (3): 334-336.
63. S. Suzuki et al., *Ind. Health*, 1969, 7 (3/4): 155-162.
64. K. Ohkata, *Nichidai Lyaku Zasshi*, 1972, 31 (2): 105-124.
65. P. E. Corneliussen, *Pest. Monitor J.*, 1972, 5: 313.
66. S. Fox, *J. Food Sci.*, 1974, 39 (2): 321-324.
67. T. Maji et al., *Nutr. Rep. Int.*, 1974, 10 (3): 139-149.
68. P. W. Washo et al., *Nutr. Rep. Int.*, 1974, 10 (3): 139-149.
69. W. G. Pond et al., *Proc. Soc. Exp. Biol. Med.*, 1975, 148 (3): 665-668.

70. W. J. Broad, *Science*, 1981, 213: 1341-1344.

71. P. E. Spargo and C. A. Pounds, *Notes and Records Royal Soc. London*, 1979, 34: 11.

72. D. W. Eggleston, Effect of Dental Amalgam and Nickel Alloys on T-Lymphocytes: Preliminary Report, *Journal of Prosthetic Dentistry*, 51 (5): 617-623.

73. Y. Sugiura et al., *J. Amer. Chem. Soc.*, 1976, 98 (8): 2339-2341.

74. G. F. Nordberg, in: *Effects and Dose Response Relationships of Toxic Metals*, 88-91.

75. S. Potter et al., *J. Nutr.*, 1974, 104 (5): 638-647.

76. *Nature*, 1975, 238-239.

77. D. R. Crapper et al., *Science News*, October 1, 1977, 219.

78. Is Aluminum Harmless?, *Nutrition Review*, 1980, 38 (7): 242.

79. D. R. Crapper-McLachan, M. D., University of Toronto, Toronto, Canada, *personal interview*, 1982.

CHAPTER THREE

1. Denham Harman, Role of Free Radicals in Mutation, Cancer, Aging, and the Maintenance of Life, *Radiat. Res*, vol. 16, 1962, pp. 753-764.

2. Sr. Rosalie Bertell, *Health Hazards from Low Level Radiation*, reprinted by Environmental Action Reprint Service.

3. W. R. Beisel, R. Edelman, K. Nauss, and R. M. Suskind, Single Nutrient Effects on Immunologic Functions. *JAMA*, 1981, 245 (1): 53-8.

4. W. R. Beisel, Single Nutrients and Immunity, *Am. J. Clin. Nutr.*, 1982, 35: 417-68.

5. S. Dreizen, Nutrition and the Immune Response: A Review, *Int. J. Vitam. Nutr. Res.*, 1978, 49: 220-28.

6. *Ibid.*

7. M. Jurin and I. F. Tannock, Influence of Vitamin A on Immunological Response, *Immunology*, 1972, 23: 283-7.

8. H. C. Stoerk and T. F. Zucker, Nutritional Effects on the Development and Atrophy of the Thymus, *Proc. Soc. Exp. Biol. Med.*, 1944, 56: 151-3.

9. A. E. Axelrod, B. B. Carter, R. H. McCoy, and R. Geisinger, Circulating Antibodies in Vitamin-deficiency States: I. Pyridoxine, Riboflavin, and Pantothenic Acid Deficiencies, *Proc. Soc. Exp. Biol. Med.*, 1947, 66: 137-40.

10. J. Pruzansky and A. E. Axelrod, Antibody Production to Diphtheria Toxoid in Vitamin Deficiency States, *Proc. Soc. Exp. Biol. Med.*, 1955, 89: 323-5.

11. E. M. Cranton and J. P. Frackelton, Free Radical Pathology in Age-associated Disease: Treatment with EDTA Chelation, Nutrition, and Antioxidants, *J. Holist. Med.*, in press, 1984, 6 (1).

12. W. R. Beisel, R. Edelman, K. Nauss, and R. M. Suskind, *op. cit.*

13. W. R. Beisel, Single Nutrients and Immunity, *op. cit.*.

14. R. E. Hodges, W. B. Bean, and M. A. Ohlson, Factors Affecting Human Antibody Response: V. Combined Deficiencies of Pantothenic and Pyridoxine, *Am. J. Clin. Nutr.*, 1962, 11: 187-199.

15. A. E. Axelrod, Immune Processes in Vitamin Deficiency States, *Am. J. Clin. Nutr.*, 1971, 24: 265-71.

16. R. Edelman, Cell-mediated Immune Response in Protein-calorie Malnutrition: A Review, pp. 47-75. R. M. Suskind, (ed.), *Malnutrition and the Immune Response*, 1977, Ravin Press, New York.

17. W. R. Beisel, Malnutrition and the Immune Response, pp. 1-19, in Neuberger, A. and Jukes, T. A., (eds.), *Biochemistry of Nutrition I*, 1979, University Park Press, Baltimore.

18. A. E. Axelrod, *op. cit*

19. R. Edelman, *op. cit.*

20. S. Dreizen, *op. cit.*

21. R. Edelman, *op. cit.*

22. S. Dreizen, *op. cit.*

23. W. R. Beisel, Malnutrition and the Immune Response, *op. cit*

24. L. Pauling, *Vitamin C and the Common Cold*, W. H. Freeman and Co., 1970.

25. W. Prinz, R. Bortz, B. Bregin, and M. Hersch, The Effect of Ascorbic Acid Supplementation on Some Parameters of the Human Immunological Defense System, *Int. J. Vitam. Nutr. Res.*, 1977, 47: 248-57.

26. S. Vallance, Relationship Between Ascorbic Acid and Serum Proteins of the Immune System, 1977, *Brit. Med. J.*, 2: 437-8.

27. L. A. Boxer, A. M. Watanabe, et al., Correction of Leukocyte Function in Chediak-Higashi Syndrome by Ascorbate, *N. Eng. J. Med.*, 1976, 295: 1041-5.

28. H. B. Demopoulos, Control of Free Radicals in Biological Systems, *Fed. Proc.*, 1973, 32 (8): 1903-8.

29. E. M. Cranton and J. P. Frackelton, *op. cit.*

30. E. Cameron and L. Pauling, *Cancer and Vitamin C*, Linus Pauling Institute of Science and Medicine, Menlo Park, Calif., 1979, p. 238.

31. *Ibid.*

32. F. R. Klenner, Significance of High Daily Intake of Ascorbic Acid in Preventive Medicine, pp. 51-59, in Williams, R. J., and Kalita, D. K., (eds.), *A Physician's Handbook on Orthomolecular Medicine*, Keats Publishing Co., 1977.

33. *Ibid.*

34. P. A. Campbell, H. R. Cooper, R. H. Heinzerling, and R. P. Tengerdy, Vitamin E Enhances in vitro Immune Response by Normal and Nonadherent Spleen Cells, *Proc. Soc. Exp. Biol. Med.*, 1974, 146: 465-9.

35. R. Edelman, *op. cit.*

36. R. H. Heinzerling, C. F. Nockels, C. L. Quarles, and R. P. Tengerdy, Protection of Chicks Against E. coli Infection by Dietary Supplementation with Vitamin E, *Proc. Soc. Exp. Biol. Med.*, 1974, 146: 279-83.

37. R. H. Heinzerling, R. P. Tengerdy, L. L. Wick, and D. C. Leuker, Vitamin E Protects Mice against Diplococcus pneumoniae Type I Infection, *Infect. Immun.*, 1974, 10: 1292-5.

38. R. P. Ellis and M. W. Vorhies, Effect of Supplemental Dietary Vitamin E on the Serologic Response of Swine to an Escherichia Coli Bacterin, *J. Am. Vet. Med. Assoc.*, 1976, 168: 231-2.

39. T. L. Barber, C. F. Nockels, and M. M. Jochim, Vitamin E Enhancement of Venezuelan Equine Encephalomyelitis Antibody Response in Guinea Pigs, *Am. J. Vet. Res.*, 1977, 38: 731-4.

40. D. Harman, M. L. Heidrick, and D. E. Eddy, Free Radical Theory of Aging: Effect of Free-radical-reaction Inhibitors on the Immune Response, *J. Am. Geriatr. Soc.*, 1977, 25: 400-7.

41. L. M. Pelus and H. R. Strausser, Prostaglandins and the Immune Response, *Life Sci.*, 1977, 20: 903-14.

42. S. Ayers, Jr., and R. Mihan, Is Vitamin E Involved in the Autoimmune Mechanism?, *Cutis*, 1978, 21: 321-5.

43. R. O. Likoff, M. M. Mathias, C. F. Nockels, and R. P. Tengerdy, Vitamin E Enhancement of Immunity: Mediated by the Prostaglandins?, *Fed. Proc.*, 1978, 37: 829.

44. L. Machlin, Vitamin E and Prostaglandins (PG), pp. 179-89, in deDuve, C., and Hayaishi, O., (eds.), *Tocopherol, Oxygen, and Biomembranes*, Elsevier/North Holland Biomedical Press, Amsterdam, 1978.

45. R. P. Tengerdy, R. H. Heinzerling, and M. M. Mathias, Effect of Vitamin E on Disease Resistance and Immune Responses, pp. 191-200, in deDuve, C., and Hayaishi, O. (eds.), *Tocopherol, Oxygen, and Biomembranes*, Elsevier/North Holland Biomedical Press, Amsterdam, 1978.

46. C. F. Nockels, Protective Effects of Supplemental Vitamin E Against Infection, *Fed. Proc.*, 1979, 38: 2134-8.

47. L. M. Corwin and J. Shloss, Influence of Vitamin E on the Mitogenic Response of Murine Lymphoid Cells, *J. Nutr.*, 1980, 110: 916-23.

48. J. S. Prasad, Effect of Vitamin E Supplementation on Leukocyte Function, *Am. J. Clin. Nutr.*, 1980, 33: 606-8.

49. H. B. Demopoulos, *op. cit.*

50. E. M. Cranton and J. P. Frackelton, *op. cit.*

51. W. R. Beisel, R. Edelman, K. Nauss, and R. M. Suskind, *op. cit.*

52. W. R. Beisel, Single Nutrients and Immunity, *op. cit.*.

53. H. M. Korchak and J. E. Smolen, The Role of Calcium Movements in Human Neutrophil (PMN) Activation, *Fed. Proc.*, 1981, 40: 753.

54. J. H. Wang and D. M. Waisman, Calmodulin and Its Role in the Second-messenger System, *Curr. Top Cell Reg.*, 1979, 15: 47-107.

55. J. M. Oleske, J. D. Bogden, R. Garcia, A. De La Cruz, R. Cooper, and A. B. Minnefor, Plasma Zinc and Copper in Primary and Secondary Immunodeficiency Disorders, *Biol. Trace El. Res.*, 1983, 5: 189-94.

56. P. M. Newberne, C. E. Hunt, and V. R. Young, The Role of Diet and the Reticuloendothelial System in the Response of Rats to Salmonella typhimurium Infection, *Br. J. Exp. Pathol.*, 1968, 49: 448-57.

57. V. J. Vaughn and E. D. Weinberg, Candida albicans Dimorphism and Virulence: Role of Copper, *Mycopathologia*, 1978, 64: 39-42.

58. T. A. Omole and O. A. Onawunmi, Effect of Copper on Growth and Serum Constituents of Immunized and Non-immunized Rabbits Infected with Trypanosoma brucei, *Ann. Parasitol*, 1979, (Paris), 54: 495-506.

59. C. H. Hill, Influence of Time and Exposure to High Levels of Minerals on the Susceptibility of Chicks to Salmonella gallinarum, *J. Nutr.*, 1980, 110: 433-6.

60. R. L. Gross and P. M. Newberne, Role of Nutrition in Immunologic Function, *Physiol. Rev.*, 1980, 60: 188-302.

61. D. R. Williams, *An Introduction to Bio-inorganic Chemistry*, Charles C. Thomas, Springfield, Ill., 1976, p. 402.

62. E. M. Cranton and J. P. Frackelton, *op. cit.*

63. T. P. Stossel, Quantitative Studies in Phagocytosis, Kinetic Effects of Cations and Heat-labile Opsinin, *J. Cell. Biol.*, 1973, 58: 346-56.

64. J. Fletcher, J. Mather, M. J. Lewis, and G. Whiting, Mouth Lesions in Iron-deficient Anemia: Relationship to Candida albicans in Saliva and to Impairment of Lymphocyte Transformation, *J. Infect. Dis.*, 1975, 131: 44-50.

65. H. Rothenbacher and A. R. Sherman, Target Organ Pathology in Iron-deficient Suckling Rats, *J. Nutr.*, 1980, 110: 1648-54.

66. B. S. Baliga, S. Kuvibidila, S. Tygart, and R. M. Suskind, Effect of Dietary Iron on T-cell Membrane Proteins, *Clin. Res.*, 1981, 29: 622A.

67. A. Jacobs and D. H. M. Joynson, Lymphocyte Function and Iron-Deficiency Anemia, *Lancet*, 1974, 2: 844.

68. C. Bhaskaram and V. Reddy, Cell-mediated Immunity in Iron- and Vitamin-deficient Children, *Br. Med. J.*, 1975, 3: 522.

69. L. G. MacDougall, R. Anderson, G. M. McNab, and J. Katz, The Immune Response in Iron-deficient Children: Impaired Cellular Defense Mechanisms with Altered Humoral Components, *J. Pediatr.*, 1975, 86: 833-43.

70. C. Hersko, A. Karsai, L. Eylon, and G. Izak, The Effect of Chronic Iron Deficiency on Some Biochemical Functions of the Human Hemopoietic Tissue, *Blood*, 1970, 36: 321-9.

71. A. Arbeter, L. Echeverri, D. Franco et al., Nutrition and Infection, *Fed. Proc*, 1971, 30: 1421-8.

72. D. R. Williams, *op. cit.*

73. Nutraletter, Iron and Copper Supplementation: Benefit vs. Risk, *Advanced Medical Nutrition*, 1983, 1 (6): 1-4.

74. E. M. Cranton and J. P. Frackelton, *op. cit.*

75. H. McFarlane, S. Reddy, K. J. Adcock et al., Immunity, Transferrin, and Survival in Kwashiorkor, *Br. Med. J.*, 1970, 4: 286-70.

76. A. E. J. Masawe, J. M. Muindi, and G. B. R. Swai, Infections in Iron-Deficiency and Other Types of Anemia in the Tropics, *Lancet*, 1974, 2: 314-6.

77. M. J. Murray, A. B.Murray, N. J. Murray, and M. B. Murray, Refeeding-malaria and Hyperferraemia, *Lancet*, 1975, 1: 653-4.

78. M. J. Murray and A. B. Murray, Adverse Effect of Iron Repletion on Infection, *Am. J. Clin. Nutr.*, 1978, 31: 700.

79. M. J. Murray, A. B. Murray, M. B. Murray, and C. J. Murray, The Adverse Effect of Iron Repletion on the Course of Certain Infections, *Br. Med. J.*, 1978, 2: 1113-5.

80. M. J. Murray, A. B. Murray, N. J. Murray, and M. B. Murray, Diet and Cerebral Malaria: The Effect of Famine and Refeeding, *Am. J. Clin. Nutr.*, 1978, 31: 57-61.

81. S. J. Klebanoff and W. L. Green, Degradation of Thyroid Hormones by Phagocytosing Human Leukocytes, *J. Clin. Invest.*, 1973, 52: 60-72.

82. D. L. Haggard, H. D. Stowe, G. H. Conner, and D. W. Johnson, Immunological Effects of Experimental Iodine Toxicosis in Young Cattle, *Am. J. Vet. Res.*, 1980, 41: 539-43.

83. H. K. Kashiwa and G. F. Hungerford, Blood Leukocyte Response in Rats Fed a Magnesium-Deficient Diet, *Proc. Soc. Exp. Biol. Med.*, 1958, 99: 441-3.

84. G. F. Hungerford and E. F. Karson, The Eosinophilia of Magnesium Deficiency, *Blood*, 1960, 16: 1642-50.

85. P. Bois, Effect of Magnesium Deficiency on Mast Cells and Urinary Histamine in Rats, *Br. J. Exp. Pathol.*, 1963, 44: 151-5.

86. P. A. McCreary, H. A. Battifora, G. H. Laing, and G. M. Hass, Protective Effect of Magnesium Deficiency in Experimental Allergic Encephalomyelitis in the Rat, *Proc. Soc. Exp. Biol. Med.*, 1966, 121: 1130-3.

87. P. A. McCreary, H. A. Battifora, B. M. Hahneman et al., Leukocytosis, Bone Marrow Hyperplasia and Leukemia in Chronic Magnesium Deficiency in the Rat, *Blood*, 1967, 29: 683-90.

88. H. A. Battifora, P. A. McCreary, B. M. Hahneman et al., Chronic Magnesium Deficiency in the Rat, Studies of Chronic Myelogenous Leukemia, *Arch. Pathol.*, 1968, 86: 610-20.

89. P. McCreary, G. Laing, and G. Hass, Susceptibility of Normal and Magnesium-deficient Rats to Weekly Subtumorigenic Doses of Liver Lymphoma Cells, *Am. J. Pathol.*, 1973, 70: 89a-90a.

90. G. M. Hass, G. H. Laing, P. A. McCreary, and R. M. Galt, Magnesium Deprivation in the Rat Causes Loss of Induced Immunity to Malignant Lymphoma, *Clin. Res.*, 1978, 26: 710A.

91. G. M. Hass, P. A. McCreary, G. H. Laing, and R. M. Galt, Lymphoproliferative and Immunologic Aspects of Magnesium Deficiency, pp. 185-200, in Cantin, M., and Seelig, M., (eds.), *Magnesium in Health and Disease*, Spectrum, Jamaica, New York, 1980.

92. M. Rabinovitch and M. J. DeStefano, Macrophage Spreading in Vitro II., Manganese and Other Metals as Inducers or as Co-factors for Induced Spreading, *Exp. Cell. Res.*, 1973, 79: 423-30.

93. B. E. Sheffy and R. D. Schultz, Influence of Vitamin E and Selenium on Immune Response Mechanisms, *Fed. Proc.*, 1979, 38: 2139-43.

94. R. S. Desowitz and J. W. Barnwell, Effect of Selenium and Dimethyl Dioctadecyl Ammonium Bromide on the Vaccine-induced Immunity of Swiss-Webster Mice Against Malaria (Plasmodium Berghei), *Infect. Immun,*, 1980, 27: 87-9.

95. R. Boyne and J. R. Arthur, Alterations of Neutrophil Function in Selenium-deficient Cattle, *J. Comp. Pathol.*, 1979, 89: 151-8.

96. P. J. Fraker, P. DePasquale-Jardieu, C. M. Zwickl, and R. W. Luecke, Regeneration of T-cell Helper Function in Zinc-deficient Adult Mice, *Proc. Natl. Acad. Sci. USA*, 1978, 75:

5660-4.

97. T. Tanaka, G. Fernandes, C. Tsao et al., Effects of Zinc Deficiency on Lymphoid Tissues and on the Immune Functions of A/Jax Mice, *Fed. Proc.*, 1978, 37: 931.

98. R. W. Luecke and P. J. Fraker, The Effect of Varying Dietary Zinc Levels on Growth and Antibody-mediate Response in Two Strains of Mice, *J. Nutr.*, 1979, 109: 1373-6.

99. P. DePasquale-Jardieu and P. J. Fraker, The Role of Corticosterone in the Loss in Immune Function in the Zinc-deficient A/J Mouse, *J. Nutr.*, 1979, 109: 1847-55.

100. R. K. Chandra, Cell-mediated Immunity in Genetically Obese (C57 BL/67 ob/ob) Mice, *Am. J. Clin. Nutr.*, 1980, 33: 13-6.

101. P. DePasquale-Jardieu and P. J. Fraker, Further Characterization of the Role of Corticosterone in the Loss of Humoral Immunity in Zinc-deficient A/J Mice as Determined by Adrenalectomy, *J. Immunol.*, 1980, 124: 2650-5.

102. Macrophages in Vitro, *Environ. Res.*, 1975, 9: 32-47.

103. J. Patrick, B. E. Golden, and M. H. N. Golden, Leukocyte Sodium Transport and Dietary Zinc in Protein Energy Malnutrition, *Am. J. Clin. Nutr.*, 1980, 33: 617-20.

104. E. S. Lennard, A. B. Bjornson, H. G. Petering, and J. W. Alexander, An Immunologic and Nutritional Evaluation of Burn Neutrophil Function, *J. Surg. Res.*, 1974, 16: 286-98.

105. J. M. Oleske, J. D. Bogden, R. Garcia, A. De La Cruz, R. Cooper, and A. B. Minnefor, *op. cit.*

106. W. R. Beisel, Single Nutrients and Immunity, *Am. J. Clin. Nutr.*, 1982, 35: 417-68.

107. Ibid.

108. R. L. Gross and P. M. Newberne, *op. cit.*

109. D. G. Jose and R. A. Good, Quantitative Effects of Nutritional Essential Amino Acid Deficiency Upon Immune Responses to Tumors in Mice, *J. Exp. Med.*, 1973, 137: 1-9.

110. Cranton and Frackelton, *op. cit.*

111. R. W. Wannemacher, Jr., G. A. McNamee, Jr., R. E. Dinterman, and D. L. Bunner, Effect of Diet and Pneumococcal Infection on Protein Dynamics of Blood Lymphocytes in Cynomolgus Monkeys, pp. 414-6, in Blackburn, G. L., et al., (eds.), *Amino Acids*, John Wright, PSG Inc., Boston, 1983.

112. Beisel, *op. cit.*

113. K. Dewey and F. Nuzum, The Effect of Cholesterol on Phagocytosis, *J. Infect. Dis.*, 1914, 15: 472-82.

114. R. L. Costello, L. W. Hedgecock, and T. R. Hamilton, Alternation of Resistance of the Rat to Tuberculosis When Maintained on an Atherogenic Diet, *J. Exp. Med.*, 1962, 116: 835-46.

115. D. M. Klurfeld, M. J. Allison, E. Gerszten, and H. P. Dalton, Alterations of Host Defenses Paralleling Cholesterol-induced Atherogenesis, II, Immunologic Studies of Rabbits, *J. Med.*, 1979, 10: 49-64.

116. R. H. Fiser, Jr., J. C. Denniston, V. G. McGann et al., Altered Immune Functions in Hypercholesterolemic Monkeys, *Infect. Immun.*, 1973, 8: 105-9.

117. SS-H Chen, Requirement of Cholesterol for Successful Blastogenesis in Mitogen-stimulated Lymphocytes, *Fed. Proc.*, 1978, 37: 377.

118. M. U. Dianzani, M. V. Torrielli, R. A. Canuto et al., The Influence of Enrichment with Cholesterol on the Phagocytic Activity of Rat Macrophages, *J. Pathol.*, 1976, 118: 193-9.

119. H. A. Chapman, Jr., and H. B. Hibbs, Jr., Modulation of Macrophage Tumoricidal Capability by Components of Normal Serum: A Central Role for Lipid, *Science*, 1977, 197: 282-5.

120. N. R. DiLuzio, and W. R. Wooles, Depression of Phagocytic Activity and Immune Response by Methyl Palmitate, *Am. J. Physiol.*, 1964, 206: 939-43.

121. A. Berken and B. Benacerraf, Depression of Reticuloendothelial System Phagocytic Function by Ingested Lipids, *Proc. Soc. Exp. Biol. Med.*, 1968, 128: 793-5.

122. P. M. Newberne, Overnutrition and Resistance of Dogs to Distemper Virus, *Fed. Proc. Fed. Am. Soc. Exp. Biol.*, 1966, 25: 1701.

123. R. K. Chandra and B. Au, Spleen Hemolytic Plague Forming Cell Response and Generation of Cytotoxic Cells in Genetically Obese (C57B1/6J ob/ob) Mice, *Int. Arch. Allergy App. Immunol.*, in press, 1980.

124. H. P. Hawley and G. B. Gordon, The Effects of Long Chain Free Fatty Acids on Human Neutrophil Function and Structure, *Lab. Invest.*, 1976, 34: 216-22.

125. E. N. Wardle, Immunosuppression by Fatty Acids, *Lancet*, 1976, 2: 423.

126. J. Nordenstrom, C. Jarstrand, and A. Wiernik, Decreased Chemotactic and Random Migration of Leukocytes during Intralipid Infusion, *Am. J. Clin. Nutr.*, 1979, 32: 2416-22.

127. A. E. Stuart, G. Biozzi, C. Stiffel et al., The Stimulation and Depression of Reticuloendothelial Phagocytic Function by Simple Lipids, *Br. J. Exp. Pathol.*, 1960, 41: 599-604.

128. J. Mertin, D. Hughes, B. K. Shenton, and J. P. Dickinson, In Vitro Inhibition by Unsaturated Fatty Acids of the PPD and PHA Induced Lymphocyte Response, *Klin Wochenschr*, 1974, 52: 248-50.

129. C. J. Meade, How Arachidonic Acid Depresses Thymic Weight, *Int. Arch. Allergy Appl. Immunol.*, 1979, 59: 432-6.

130. K. L. Erickson, C. J. McNeill, M. E. Gershwin, and J. B. Ossman, Influence of Dietary Fat Concentration and Saturation on Immune Ontogeny in Mice, *J. Nutr.*, 1980, 110: 1555-72.

131. J. W. De Wille, P. J. Fraker, and D. R. Romsos, Effects of Essential Fatty Acid Deficiency, and Various Levels of Dietary Polyunsaturated Fatty Acids, on Humoral Immunity in Mice, *J. Nutr.*, 1979, 109: 1018-27.

132. Erickson et al., *op. cit.*

133. J. Mertin and R. Hunt, Influence of Polyunsaturated Fatty Acids on Survival of Skin Allografts and Tumor Incidence in Mice, *Proc. Natl. Acad. Sci. USA*, 1976, 73: 928-31.

134. L. Krause, M. Williams, and S. A. Broitman, Relationship of Diet High in Lipid and Cholesterol on Immune Function in Rats Given 1, 2, Dimethyl Hydrazin (DMH), *Am. J. Clin. Nutr.*, 1980, 33: 937.

135. J. Mertin and D. Hughes, Specific Inhibitory Action of Polyunsaturated Fatty Acids on Lymphocyte Transformation Induced by PHA and PPD, *Int. Arch. Allergy Appl. Immunol.*, 1975, 48: 203-10.

136. H. Offner and J. Clausen, The Enhancing Effect of Unsaturated Fatty Acids on E Rosette Formation, *Int. Arch. Allergy Appl. Immunol.*, 1978, 56: 376-9.

137. V. Utermohlen, J. Sierra, and R. Smith, Effects of Fatty Acids on Lymphocyte Agglutination in Vitro and in Vivo, *Fed. Proc.*, 1980, 39: 675.

138. R. K. Chandra, *Immunology of Nutritional Disorders*, Year Book Medical Publishers, Inc., Chicago, 1980, p. 100.

139. L. D. Koller, Immunosuppression Produced by Lead, Cadmium, and Mercury, *Am. J. Vet. Res.*, 1973, 34: 1457-8.

140. L. D. Koller, J. H. Exon, and J. G. Roan, Antibody Suppression by Cadmium, *Arch. Environ. Health*, 1975, 30: 598-601.

141. L. D. Koller, J. H. Exon, and J. G. Roan, Humoral Antibody Response in Mice after Single Dose Exposure to Lead or Cadmium, *Proc. Soc. Exp. Biol. Med.*, 1976, 151: 339-42.

142. L. D. Koller and J. A. Brauner, Decreased B-Lymphocyte Response After Exposure to Lead and Cadmium, *Toxicol. Appl. Pharmacol.*, 1977, 42: 621-4.

143. M. D. Waters, D. E. Gardner, C. Aranyi, and D. L. Coffin, Metal Toxicity for Rabbit Alveolar Macrophages in Vitro, *Environ. Res.*, 1975, 9: 32-47.

144. L. D. Loose, J. B. Silkworth, and D. W. Simpson, Influence of Cadmium on the Phagocytic and Microbial Activity of Murine Peritoneal Macrophages, Pulmonary Alveolar Macrophages, and Polymorphonuclear Neutrophils, *Infect. Immun.*, 1978, 22: 378-81.

145. J. A. Cook, E. O. Hoffman, and N. R. DiLuzio, Influence of Lead and Cadmium on the Susceptibility of Rats to Bacterial Challenge, *Proc. Soc. Exp. Biol. Med.*, 1975, 150: 741-7.

146. J. H. Gainer, Effects of Heavy Metals and of Deficiency of Zinc on Mortality Rates in Mice Infected with Encephalomyocarditis Virus, *Am. J. Vet. Res.*, 1977, 38: 869-72.

147. Cook et al., *op. cit.*

148. Gainer, *op. cit.*

149. Koller, *op. cit.*

150. L. D. Koller and S. Kovacic, Decreased Antibody Formation in Mice Exposed to Lead, *Nature*, 1974, 250: 148-50.

151. B. A. Neilan and L. Taddeini, Effect of Lead Exposure on B and T Lymphocytes in Mice, *Clin. Res.*, 1979, 27: 223A.

152. G. Ohi, M. Fukuda, H. Seto, and H. Yagyu, Effect of Methylmercury on Humoral Immune Responses in Mice under Conditions Simulated to Practical Situations, *Bull. Environ. Contamination Toxicol.*, 1976, 15: 175-80.

153. L. D. Koller, Methylmercury: Effect on Oncogenic and Nononcogenic Viruses in Mice, *Am. J. Vet. Res.*, 1975, 36: 1501-4.

154. Gainer, *op. cit.*

CHAPTER FOUR

1. Y. Tanaka, J. Stara et al., Application of Algal Polysaccharides as In Vivo Binders of Metal Pollutants, *Proceedings of the Seventh International Seaweed Symposium, Aug. 8-12, 1971*, John Wiley & Sons, 1971, p. 603.

2. S. C. Skoryna et al., Suppression of Intestinal Absorption of Radiostrontium by Substances Occurring in Phaeophyceae, *Proceedings of the Fifth International Seaweed Symposium, August 25-28, 1965*, Pergamon Press, 1966, pp. 396-397, 399.

3. S. C. Skoryna et al., *Canadian Medical Association Journal*, vol. 91, 1964, p. 285.

4. S. C. Skoryna et al., Suppression of Intestinal Absorption of Radiostrontium by Substances Occurring in Phaeophyceae, *op. cit.*, p. 397.

5. J. F. Stara, Metabolism of Internal Emitters—Repressive Action of Sodium Alginate on Absorption of Radiostrontium in Kittens, *Abstr. Symp. Nuc. Med.*, Omaha, 1965.

6. Y. Tanaka, *op. cit.*, p. 602.

7. S. C. Skoryna and Y. Tanaka, *Proc. Sixth Int. Seaweed Symp.*, (Madrid: Secretaria de la Marina Mercante), p. 737.

8. Y. Tanaka, D. Waldron-Edward, and S. C. Skoryna, *Canadian Medical Association Journal*, vol. 99, 1968, pp. 169-175.

9. Y. Tanaka, S. C. Skoryna, and D. Waldron-Edward, *Canadian Medical Association Journal*, vol. 98, 1968, pp. 1179-82.

10. Z. V. Dubrovina et al., Protective Action of Alginic Acid and Sodium Alginate on the Receipt by the Body of Radioactive Elements Through Gastrointestinal Tract, *Gig. Sanit.*, May 1969, no. 5, pp. 105-107.

11. Y. Tanaka, D. Waldron-Edward, and S. C. Skoryna, *op. cit.*

12. A. Sutton et al., Medical Research Council, Haswell, England, Reduction in the Absorption of Dietary Strontium in Children by an Alginate Derivation, *International Journal of Radiation Biology*, 1971, 19: 79-85.

13. S. C. Skoryna et al., Suppression of Intestinal Absorption of Radiostrontium by Substances Occurring in Phaeophyceae, *op. cit.*, pp. 400-403.

14. K. Nezel, Reduction of the Retention of Radioactive Strontium in Laying Hens, *Archiv. fur Geflugelkunde*, vol. 37, no. 3, 1973, pp. 97-101.

15. D. Waldron-Edward et al., *Nature*, 1965, 205: 1117.

16. S. C. Skoryna, Suppression of Intestinal Absorption of Radiostrontium by Substances Occurring in Phaeophyceae, *op. cit.*

17. A. Huag, *Composition and Properties of Alginates, Report No. 30*, Norw. Seaweed Res. Inst., Trondheim, 1964.

18. G. G. Polikarpov, *Radioecology of Aquatic Organisms*, North Holland, 1966.

19. H. Beckmann, *Pharmacology, Nature, Action, and Use of Drugs*, W. B. Saunders, 1961.

20. H. W. Nilson and J. A. Wagner, *Proc. Soc. Expt. Biol. Med.*, 1951, 76: 630.

21. S. C. Skoryna, Suppression of Intestinal Absorption of Radiostrontium by Substances Occurring in Phaeophyceae, *op. cit.*, pp. 396, 402-403.

22. R. Morgan, Progress Toward a Comprehensive Program in Radiation Safety, *Am. J. Roent. & Rad. Ther.*, 1958, 79: 349-351.

23. R. Morgan, Radiation Protection Standards, Joint Committee on Atomic Energy--Selected Materials on Radiation Protection Criteria and Standards: Their Basis and Use, May 1960, pp. 63-69.

24. R. Morgan, Radioactive Materials in Man and His Environment: The Character and Magnitude of the Problem, *Radioactivity in Man*, edited by George R. Meneely, M.D., C. C. Thomas, Publ., 1961.

25. R. Morgan, Radiation Protection and the Control of Ionizing Radiation, *The New Physician*, Dec. 1961, pp. 430-432.

26. R. Morgan, *The Control of Radiation Hazards in the United States*, NACOR Report #1, March 1959.

27. R. Morgan, *Radioactive Contamination of the Environment: Public Health Action*, NACOR Report #2, May 1962.

28. R. Morgan, Radiation Hazards of Primary Concern to Public Health—Present Status and Outlook, *Am. J. Public Health*, 1963, 53: 872-877.

29. H. Voltle, M. Alavaikko, and R. S. Piha, *Wein. Klin. Wochenschi*, Inst. Biochem., Univ. Oulu, Oulu, Denmark, 1979, vol. 91, no. 14, pp. 487-491.

30. E. Kvanta, *Acta Chemica Scandinavia*, 1968, vol. 22, no. 7, pp. 216-265.

31. P. Hernuss et al., *Strahlentherapie*, 1975, vol. 150, no. 5, pp. 500-506.

32. I. Osmanagic, M.D., Ph.D., Bee Pollen Protects Against Radiation Sickness Due to X-Ray Therapy, *Journal of the University Radiological Institute*, Sarajevo, Yugoslavia, 1973.

33. W. Robinson, Bee Pollen Arrests Cancerous Tumors in Mice, *Journal of the National Cancer Institute*, October 1948, pp. 119-123.

34. R. E. Keller and E. K. Prudnicenka, On the Composition of Propolis and Its Bactericidity, *Thesis of the Lectures of the Second Leningrad Scientific Conference on the Application of the Products of Apiculture in Medicine and Veterinary Medicine*, Leningrad, 1960, p. 53.

35. F. C. Porchum and A. J. Borovaja, Bactericidal Effects of Propolis and Its Use in Clinical Practice, *Military Medical Journal*, 1970, no. 9, p. 65.

36. P. V. Atkins et al., *Radiation Research*, 1967.

37. S. Graham and C. Mettlin, Fiber and Other Constituents of Vegetables in Cancer Epidemiology, *Nutrition and Cancer: Etiology and Treatment*, 1981, pp. 189-225.

38. R. Harvey et al., Effects of Increased Dietary Fiber on Intestinal Transit, *Lancet*, 1973, 1: 815.

39. B. Ershoff, Antitoxic Effects of Plant Fiber, *Amer. J. of Cl. Nut.*, 1974, 27: 1395.

40. D. Burkitt et al., Effect of Dietary Fiber on Stools and Transit Times and Its Role in the Causation of Disease, *Lancet*, 1971, 2: 1408-1412.

41. D. Burkitt et al., Dietary Fiber and Disease, *JAMA*, 1974, 229: 1068-1074.

42. D. Burkitt and H. Trowell, *Refined Carbohydrate Foods and Disease: Some Implications of Dietary Fiber*, Academy Press, 1975.

43. J. Hoveman, The Influence of pH on the Survival After X-Irradiation of Cultured Malignant Cells, *International Journal of Radiation Biology*, 1980, 37: 201-205.

44. E. L. David, *statement made at Eighth International Congress of Prophylactic Medicine*, Sept. 6, 1961.

45. J. R. Wolsieffer et al., *Journal of Dental Research*, 1973.

46. J. P. Ebel, G. Beck, G. Keith, H. Langendorff, and M. Langendorff, Study of the Therapeutic Effect on Irradiated Mice of Substances Contained in RNA Preparations, *Int. Jl. Radiat. Biol.*, 1969, no. 16, pp. 201-209.

47. *Dokl. Akad. Nauk., Bd.*, S. S. S. R., 1963, 126, p. 417.

48. J. Samachson et al., *Arch. Biochem. Biophys.*, 1960, 88: 335.

49. J. A. Miller, D. L. Miner, H. P. Rusch, and C. A. Baumann, Diet and Hepatic Tumor Formation, *Cancer Res.*, 1941, no. 1, p. 699.

50. K. Sugiura, On the Relation of Diets to the Development, Prevention and Treatment of Cancer, with Special Reference to Cancer of the Stomach and Liver, *J. Nutr.*, 1951, 44: 345.

51. G. W. Strandberg et al., Microbial Cells as Bioabsorbents for Heavy Metals: Accumulation of Uranium by Saccharomyces Cerevisial and Pseudomonas Aeruginosa, *Applied Environmental Microbiology*, 1981, 41 (1): 237-245.

52. A. Hutchens and N. Tretchikoff, *conversation with author (S.S.)*, Windsor, Ontario, 1966.

53. M. Lourau and O. Lartigue, *Experientia*, 1950, vol. 6, p. 25.

54. Duplan, Influence of Dietary Regimen on Radiosensitivity of the Guinea Pig, *Compt. Rend. Acad. Sc.*, 1953, vol. 236, p. 424.

55. S. Colloway, Reduction of X-Radiation Mortality by Cabbage and Broccoli, *Proc. Soc. Exptl. Biol. Med.*, 1959, vol. 100, p. 405.

56. S. Colloway et al., *Quartermaster Food and Container Institute for the Armed Forces Report*, N.R. 12-61, 1961.

57. J. Ibanez and A. Castellanos, Efecto de la Proteccion del Aceite de Oliva Virgin en Dosis Multiples Subletales de X-Irradiacion en la Rata, *Revista Clinica Espanola*, April 15, 1963, no. 1, pp. 14-20.

58. *Modern Nutrition* (Pasadena, Calif.), November 1960, p. 11.

59. S. D. Joshi et al., Effect of Ground Nut Oil on Radiation Injury in Mice, *Indian Journal of Experimental Biology*, May 1967, vol. 14, no. 3, pp. 263-267.

CHAPTER FIVE

1. W. O. Lindberg, *American Journal of Clinical Nutrition*, no. 6, 1958, p. 601.

2. *Nutrition Review*, 1955, no. 13, pp. 17-18.

3. R. Shekelle, M.D., J. Stamler, M.D. et al., *Lancet*, no. 8257, Nov. 28, 1981, pp. 1185-1189.

4. B. Szymezykowa, Influence of Local Application of Vitamin A Preparations in the Course of Post-Irradiation Skin Reactions in Man, *Pol. Przelgl. Radiol. Med. Nukl.*, no. 32, July/Aug. 1968, pp. 529-35.

5. D. W. D'Souza et al., *Environmental Physiology and Biochemistry*, 1974, pp. 400-485; Biochemistry and Food Technology Division of the Bhabha Atomic Research Center, Bombay, India.

6. E. Seifter et al., Morbidity and Mortality Reduction by Supplemental Vitamin A or Beta-Carotene in Mice Given Total-Body Gamma-Radiation, *Journal of the National Cancer Institute*, vol. 73, no. 5, 1984, pp. 1167-1177.

7. S. M. Levenson et al., Supplemental Vitamin A Prevents the Acute Radiation-Induced Defect in Wound Healing, *Annals of Surgery*, vol. 200, no. 4, 1984, pp. 494-512.

8. A. Morezek and W. Schmidt, Comparative Studies of the Influence of Various Active Substances of the Vitamin B Complex on the Radiation Syndrome in Rats Subjected to Whole-Body Irradiation, *Atomkernen*, 14, July/August 1969, pp. 237-241.

9. H. Mattie et al., *British Medical Journal*, July 1967.

10. I. Szoraolay, *Octa Paediatrica*, no. 4, 1963.

11. N. D. Egorova and S. R. Perepelkin, Protective Action of Pantothenic Acid in Rats with Radiation Sickness Given a Milk and Egg Diet, *Gigiena i Sanitoriya*, (Moscow: Meditsinskii Inst.), no. 10, 1979, pp. 25-28.

12. A. Morezek and W. Schmidt, Effect on the Radiation Syndrome of the Combined Administration of Vitamin B12 and Folic Acid in Whole-Body Radiation in Rats, *Folia Haematol*, (Leipzig), no. 90, 1968, pp. 401-410.

13. G. Barth and H. Graebner, The Treatment of Lethal Radiation Damage with Cobalamin,

Arzneimittel-Forsch, (Giessen, Germany: Universitat), no. 14, June 1964, pp. 665-668.

14. S. R. Perepelkin, N. D. Egorova et al., Prophylactic and Therapeutic Role of the B Vitamin Inositol in Radiation Disease, *Gigiena i Sanitoriya*, (Moscow: Meditsinskii Inst.), no. 10, 1979, pp. 96-98.

15. P. V. Atkin, *Radiation Research*, 1967.

16. K. A. Skulme, *Tr. Inst. Experim i Klinich Med.*, no. 28, 1962, pp. 171-244.

17. S. R. Perepelkin, Preventive and Therapeutic Role of Vitamins C, P, and B Complex in Radiation Diseases, *Gigiena i Sanitoriya*, (Moscow: Meditsinskii Inst.), no. 2, 1976, pp. 53-57.

18. G. Podusovskii et al., *L'Vovsk. Gos. Univ.*, no. 1, 1962, pp. 59-63.

19. K. A. Skulme, *op. cit.*

20. L. Ala-Ketola et al., Effect of Ascorbic Acid on the Survival of Rats After Whole-Body Irradiation, *Strahlentherapie*, (Dept. Radiotherapy, Univ. Oulu, 90220, Oulu 22, Finland), vol. 148, no. 6, 1974, pp. 643-644.

21. S. R. Perepelkin, N. D. Egorova et al., *op. cit.*

22. D. G. Devyatka and O. V. Yotsyna, Protective Effects of Ascorbic Acid During Exposure to Excessive Amounts of Ultraviolet Radiation, *Gigiena i Sanitoriya*, (Vinnitsa, Ukrania, U. S. S. R.: Meditsinskii Inst.), no. 10, 1977, pp. 99-101.

23. Y. Romantsev, Capillary Fragility and Vitamin P Protective Action Against Radiation, *Proc. Soc. Exptl. Biol. Med.*, no. 75, 1950, pp. 20-23.

24. M. K. O'Connor, J. F. Malone, M. Moriarty, and S. Mulgrew, A Radioprotective Effect of Vitamin C Observed in Chinese Hamster Ovary Cells, *British Journal of Radiology*, vol. 50, no. 596.

25. J. B. Field and P. E. Rekers, *Aecu-149*, January 19, 1949.

26. A. Morezek and W. Schmidt, *op. cit.*, pp. 237-241.

27. B. Sokoloff et al., *Journal of Clinical Investigation*, 1951, 30: 395.

28. H. Mattie et al., *op. cit.*

29. James A.Scott, M.D., and Gerald M. Kolodny, M.D., Interaction of Ionizing Radiation and Ascorbic Acid on 3T3 Mouse Fibroblasts, *International Journal for Vitamin and Nutrition Research*, vol. 51, no. 2, 1981, pp. 155-160.

30. A. DeCrosta, Natural Foods That Guard Against Radioactivity, *Organic Gardening*, July 1979, p. 120.

31. A. Tappel, Vitamin E Spares the Parts of the Cell and Tissues from Free Radical Damage, *Nutrition Today*, 1973, 8: 4.

32. M. A. Malic and R. Sternberg, R. M., Effect of Vitamin E on Post-Irradiation Death in Mice, *Experimentia* (Department of Biological Sciences, George Williams Campus, Concordia U., Montreal, Quebec), 1978.

33. H. Matsuura, Effect of Vitamin E on the Gamma Ray Irradiated Placenta-Histological Observations, *Vitamins*, no. 39, 1969, p. 262.

34. A. A. Majaj et al., Vitamin E Responsive Megaloblastic Anemia in Infants with Protein-Calorie Malnutrition, *American Journal of Clinical Nutrition*, no. 12, 1963, p. 378.

35. I. Kurokawa et al., Studies on the Effects of Vitamin E Upon the Preservation of Blood, *Vitamins*, no. 38, 1968, p. 10.

36. A. I. Hecht, M.S. and K. Mohrmann, M.S., Vitamin E and Low-Dose Irradiation, *The ACA Journal of Chiropractic*, August 1980, vol. 14, S-89-91.

37. W. O. Lindberg, *American Journal of Clinical Nutrition*, 1958, 6: 601.

38. M. T. Block, *Clinical Medicine*, 1950, 57: 112.

39. M. T. Block, *Insurance Medicine*, 1950, 5: 4.

40. F. Pascher et al., *Journal of Investigative Dermatology*, 1951, 17: 261.

41. E. V. Schute, *Annual of New York Academy of Science*, 1949, 52: 358.

42. B. Sokoloff et al., *op. cit.*.

43. J. B. Field et al., *American Journal of Medical Science*, 1949, 218: 1.

44. J. Domokos et al., *Inter. Rev. Vit. Res.*, 1950, 21: 444.

45. J. J. Wells et al., *Proc. Staff Meet. Mayo Clin.*, 1947, 22: 482.

Notes

46. W. S. Wallace, *South. Med. J.*, 1941, 34: 170.

47. W. B. Bean et al., *Am. J. Med. Sci.*, 1944, 108: 46.

48. M. Shinoda and Y. Takogi, Pharmacological Studies on Chemical Protectors Against Radiation, #4: Studies on Radioprotective Effects of Vitamin E and its Derivatives, *Yakugaku Lasshi* (National Inst. of Radiological Sciences, Chiba, Japan), no. 88, March 1968, pp. 278-82.

49. Shute and Taub, Vitamin E for Ailing and Healthy Hearts, *Drug Information Center Pharmacy Newsletter for Physicians*, 1971, no. 5, p. 11.

50. R. Palmer et al., Effect of Calcium Deposition on Strontium-90 and Calcium-45 in Rats, *Science*, 1958, 127: 1505.

51. H. Wasserman and C. Comer, Effect of Dietary Calcium and Phosphorus Levels on Body Burden of Ingested Radiostrontium, *Proceedings of the Society for Experimental Biology and Medicine*, 1960, 103: 124.

52. I. A. Sarapul'tsev and K. A. Koldoeva, *Inst. Biolozike Ministerstva*, 1974.

53. I. Ya. Pachenko et al., *Inst. Biofiziki Minzdrava*, 1974, Moscow, U.S.S.R.

54. W. Czosnowska et al., *Health Physics* (Inst. for Nuclear Res., Warsaw, Poland), 1972.

55. M. Alpert et al., *Chemical and Radionuclide Food Contamination*, MMS Information Corp., 1973.

56. J. Lenicham, *Strontium Metabolism*, Academic Press, 1967.

57. *International Journal of Applied Radiation and Isotopes*, 1967, 18: 407-415.

58. H. Spencer et al., Effect of Low and High Calcium Intake on Strontium-90 Metabolism in Adult Man, *International Journal of Applied Radiation and Isotopes*, 1967, 18: 605-614.

59. M. Alpert, *op. cit.*

60. S. Fox, *Journal of Food Science*, vol. 39, no. 2, 1974, pp. 321-324.

61. F. N. Marzulli et al., *Current Problems in Dermatology*, 1978, 7: 196-204.

62. *Int. Z. Klin. Pharmakol., Ther. Toxikol.*, no. 1, Oct. 1968, pp. 514-516

63. J. Remy et al., Changes in Intestinal Absorption after Acute Irradiation in the Pig, *Strahlentherapie*, vol. 148, no. 1, 1974, pp. 95-106.

64. D. P. Shapherd, *Dietary Protection Against Ionizing Radiation* (Thesis), 1970, Texas A & M University, College Station, Texas, University Microfilms Order No. 71-8912.

65. A. Breccia et al., Chemical Radioprotection by Organic Selenium Compounds in Vivo, *Radiat. Res.* (University of Bologna), June 1969, no. 38, pp. 483-492.

66. L. Wattenberg, *Journal of the National Cancer Institute*, 1972, 48: 1425-1431.

67. J. Harr, J. Exon, P. Whanger, and P. Weswig, *Clinical Toxicology*, 1972, 5 (2): 187-194.

68. R. Passwater, *American Laboratory*, 1973, 5 (6): 10-22.

69. G. Schrauzer and D. Ishmael, *Annals of Clinical Laboratory Science*, 1974, 4: 441-447.

70. M. Jacobs and D. Griffin, *Cancer Letters*, 1977, 2: 133-138.

71. C. Griffin and M. Jacobs, *Cancer Letters*, 1977, 3: 177-181.

72. G. Schrauzer, *Inorganic and Nutritional Aspects of Cancer*, Plenum Press, 1978, p. 330.

73. P. Whanger, I. Tinsley, J. Schmitz, and J. Exon, *Second International Symposium on Selenium in Biology and Medicine*, May 1980, Texas Tech University, Lubbock, Texas.

74. D. Medina, *J. American Med. Assoc.*, October 2, 1981, 246 (14): 1510.

75. R. Shamberger and D. Frost, *Canadian Medical Association Journal*, 1969, 100: 682.

76. R. Shamberger and C. Willis, *Journal of National Cancer Institute*, 1970, 44: 931.

77. R. Shamberger and C. Willis, *Critical Reviews in Clinical Laboratory Sciences*, June 1971, pp. 211-221.

78. G. Schrauzer and W. I. Rhead, *Experientic*, 1971, 27: 1069-1071.

79. J. Wedderburn, *New Zealand Veterinarian Journal*, 1972, 20: 56.

80. G. Schrauzer, W. Rhead, and G. Evans, *Bioinorganic Chemistry*, 1973, 2: 329-340.

81. G. Schrauzer, D. White, and C. Schneider, *Bioinorganic Chemistry*, 1977, 7: 36.

82. *Chemical and Engineering News*, January 17, 1977, p. 345.

83. G. Schrauzer, W. Rhead, and G. Evans, *op. cit.*, p. 334.

84. *Ibid.*, p. 336.

85. *Critical Reviews in Clinical Laboratory Science*, 2: 211-221.

86. J. Spallholz et al., *Proceedings of the Society of Experimental Biological Medicine*, 1973, 143: 685-698.

87. B. Sheffy and R. Schulz, *Cornell Veterinarian*, 1978, 68 (suppl. 7): 48-61.

88. R. S. Desowitz and J. W. Barnwell, *Infection and Immunity*, 1980, 27 (1): 87-89.

89. J. Martin and J. Spallholz, *Proceedings of the Symposium of Selenium-Tellurium in the Environment*, 1976, Pittsburgh, Penn., Industrial Health Foundation, pp. 204-225.

90. T. Berenshtein, Zdravookl. *Belorussia*, 1972, 18 (10): 34-36.

91. S. Fox, *Journal of Food Science*, 1974, 39 (2): 321-324.

92. S. Potter et al., *J. Nut.*, 1974, 104 (5): 638-647.

93. Anon., *Nature*, 1975, pp. 238-239.

94. Y. Sugiura et al., *J. Amer. Chem. Soc.*, 1976, 98 (8): 2339-2341.

95. G. F. Nordberg, *Effects and Dose Relationships of Toxic Metals*, pp. 88-91.

96. L. Szentkuti and W. Giese, Studies on the Binding Capacity of the Skeletal Muscle Constituents for Cesium-137, *Health Physics*, 1974, 26: 343-347.

97. G. Webb, J. Simmonds, and B. Watkins, Radiation Levels in Eastern Europe, *Nature*, 1986, 321 (6073): 821-822.

98. Committee on Food Protection, Food and Nutrition Board, National Academy of Sciences, *Radionuclides in Foods*, National Academy Press, 1973, pp. 22-56.

99. J. Cline, Effect of Nutrient Potassium on the Uptake of Cesium-137 and Potassium and on Discrimination Factor, *Nature*, 1962, 193: 1302-1303.

100. D. P. Shapherd, *op. cit.*

101. P. D. Gabovich and I. A Mikhalyuk, Metabolism of Iron, Copper, and Molybdenum and Ultraviolet Irradiation, *Voprosy Pitaniya*, 1976, no. 4, pp. 70-75.

102. Z. Prouza, J. Pospisil, and L. Dienstbier, Changes in Distribution of Iron in Rats after X-Irradiation of the Whole Body, *Sbornik Lakarsky*, 1975, 77 (2): 218-223.

103. K. P. Filin, Absorption in the Intestine of Labeled Lipids, Vitamin B-12 and Iron Citrate after Gamma-Irradiation, *Meditsinskaya Radiologiya*, 1974, 19 (10): 17-22.

104. J. Tache, A. R. Mehron, and Y. Tache, Intestinal Absorption of Iron in Irradiated Rabbits, *Revue Canadienne de Biologie*, 1973, 32 (3): 157-167.

CHAPTER SIX

1. I. I. Brekhman, L. I. Oskotsky, and A. I. Khakham, The Action of Some Preparations from the Oraliaceae Family in Experimental Radiation Sickness, *Izv. Akad. Nauk.*, U.S.S.R., Ser. Biol., 1970, 6: 33-36.

2. T. M. Khatnashvili, Trial of the Use of the Fluid Extract of Eleutherococcus in the Treatment of Patients with Lip and Mouth Cancer, *Materials for the Conference on Problems of Medicinal Therapy at the Oncology Clinic*, 1964, Leningrad, U.S.S.R., pp. 163-164.

3. G. Mainanski, The Healing Effect of Combined Eleutherococcus/antibiotics Treatment on Experimentally Induced Chronic Radiation Sickness, *The Symposium on Eleutherococcus and Ginseng*, 1962, edited by I. I. Brekhman, The Academy of Sciences, Vladivostok, U.S.S.R., pp. 26-28.

4. *Symposium on Eleutherococci and Ginseng*, edited by the Far Eastern Center of the Siberian Div. of the U.S.S.R. Academy of Sciences, Vladivostok, 1964; and, *Results of Eleutherococci Studies Carried Out in the Soviet Union*, edited by the Far Eastern Center of the Siberian Div. of the U.S.S.R. Academy of Sciences, Vladivostok, 1965.

5. A. R. Gvamichava et al., A Preliminary Result of Employment of Eleutherococcus in the Complex Therapy of Cancer of the Mammary Gland, *Eleutherococcus and Other Adaptogens Among the Far Eastern Plants*, edited by I. I. Brekhman, 1966, The Far Eastern Publishing House, Vladivostok, U.S.S.R., pp. 231-236.

6. I. A. Studentzova, The Effect of Eleutherococcus on the Toxicity of Certain Anticancer Preparations, *The Symposium on Eleutherococcus and Ginseng*, 1962, edited by I. I. Brekhman,

The Academy of Sciences, Vladivostok, U.S.S.R., pp. 33-34.

7. L. L. Maliugina et al., The Effect of Eleutherococcus on the Growth of Transplanted Tumor and on the Development of Its Metastases, *The Symposium on Eleutherococcus and Ginseng,* edited by I. I. Brekhman, 1962, The Academy of Sciences, Vladivostok, U.S.S.R., pp. 28-30.

8. E. V. Tzyrlina, On the Combined Effect of Eleutherococcus (Extract) and Thio-TEPA on the Metastasis of Sarcoma Tumors in Rats, *Eleutherococcus and Other Adaptogens Among the Far Eastern Plants,* edited by I. I. Brekhman, 1966, The Far Eastern Publishing House, Vladivostok, U.S.S.R., pp. 95-100.

9. L. L. Maliugina, Experimental Data on the Effect of Certain Adaptogens on the Metastasis of Tumors, *Eleutherococcus and Other Adaptogens Among the Far Eastern Plants,* edited by I. I. Brekhman, 1966, The Far Eastern Publishing House, Vladivostok, U.S.S.R., pp. 85-93.

10. N. M. Turkevich and I. D. Matreichuk, The Employment of Eleutherococcus in the Complex Treatment of Experimental Cancer of the Mammary Gland in Rats, *A Summarized Review of the Study of Eleutherococcus in the Soviet Union,* 1966, edited by Z. I. Gutnikova et al., The Academy of Sciences, Vladivostok, U.S.S.R., pp. 44-45.

11. I. I. Brekhman, *Eleutherococci—Experimental and Clinical Data,* 1970, U.S.S.R. Foreign Trade Publication, No. 28017/2, Moscow, p. 26.

12. F. K. Kzhioev and S. D. Prasol, The Effect of Eleutherococcus Liquid Extract on the Blood Serum Proteins Under the Condition of an Acute Blood Loss, *Eleutherococcus and Other Adaptogens Among the Far Eastern Plants,* 1966, edited by I. I. Brekhman, Far Eastern Publishing House, Vladivostok, U.S.S.R., pp. 69-72.

13. I. Y. Rusin, The Resistance of the Body to Different Types of Anesthetics When Dibazol, ACTH, Cortisone, and Eleutherococcus are Administered, *Lek Sredstva Dal'nego,* Vostoka 7: 27-31; Biological Abstracts 48: 107062.

14. T. M. Zyryanova, The Effect of Extracts of Leuzea, Ginseng Root, and Eleutherococcus on the Tonus of Vessels of the Retina, *Mater Teoret Klinich Med,* 5: 69-71; Biological Abstracts 48: 69689.

15. E. A. Pichurina, The Effect of Extracts of Ginseng Leuzea Carthomoides, and Eleutherococcus on the Course of Cobalt Erythremia, *Mater Teoret Klinich Med,* 5: 78-81; Biological Abstracts 49: 13012.

16. G. F. Golotkin and S. N. Bojko, Research on the Increased Resistance of Organisms Treated with Eleutherococcus Senticosus Preparations, *Materials to the Study of Ginseng and Other Far Eastern Plants,* 1963, edited by A. Oranskaia, The Academy of Sciences, Vladivostok, U.S.S.R., pp. 257-259.

17. O. I. Kirillov and I. V. Dardymov, The Effect of Eleutherococcus on the Catabolistic Changes Caused in Young Rats by Cortisone, Thyroidine, and 6-methylthiouracil, *Eleutherococcus and Other Adaptogens Among the Far Eastern Plants,* 1966, Far Eastern Publishing House, Vladivostok, U.S.S.R., pp. 55-62.

18. M. I. Zotova, A Comparative Characterization of the Stimulating and Adaptogenic Action of Extracts of Roseroot Sedum and Eleutherococcus, *Cent. Nerv. Syst. Stimul.,* 1966: 67-71; Biological Abstracts 48: 107086.

19. I. Gagarin, Prophylaxis of Eleutherococcus on Patients in Zanolajpyaj, *Adaptation and Adaptogens,* 1977, 2: 128.

20. A. P. Golikov and N. Ikonnikov, First Trial of the Prevention of Some Diseases with Eleutherococcus and with Other Medicinal Substances, *The Symposium on Eleutherococcus and Ginseng,* 1962, edited by I. I. Brekhman, The Academy of Sciences, Vladivostok, U.S.S.R., pp. 51-52.

21. G. Wikman, *The Use of Russian Root in Preventive Medicine in Industry,* Swedish Herbal Institute, Gothenburg, 1981, pp. 2-9.

22. O. I. Kirillov, The Effect of Eleutherococcus on the Involution of the Thymus with Cortisone and AKTG, *Materials from the 12th Science Session,* 1965, Ministry of Health RSFSR, Khabarovsk Regional Medical Institute, Khabarovsk, U.S.S.R., Nov. 1964, pp. 19-21.

23. O. I. Kirillov and I. V. Dardymov, *op. cit.*, pp. 55-62.

24. O. I. Kirillov et al., The Effect of Eleutherococcus on the Change in Weight of Adrenals and Thyroid Under the Condition of Prolonged Charge, *Eleutherococcus and Other Adaptogens Among the Far Eastern Plants*, 1966, edited by I. I. Brekhman, Far Eastern Publishing House, Vladivostok, U.S.S.R., pp. 13-16.

25. G. Wikman, *Research Conducted on the Effects of Eleutherococcus senticosus Maxim*, Swedish Herbal Institute, Gothenburg, 1980, p. 9.

26. G. V. Cherakashin, The Effect of an Extract of Eleutherococcus Senticosus and of a Preparation of Roseroot Sedum (Rodozin) on the Severity of Experimental Listeriosis, *Cent. Nerv. Syst. Stimul.*, 1966: 91-96; Biological Abstracts 48: 113118.

27. G. V. Cherakashin, The Effects of Eleutherococcus and Rhodosine Preparations on the Resistance of Animals to Experimental Listeriosis, *Izv. Sib. Otdel., Akad. Nauk., U.S.S.R., Ser. Biol. Med. Nauk.*, 1968, 1: 116-121; Biological Abstracts 50: 99491.

28. Y. V. Federov et al., Effect of Some Stimulants of Plant Origin on the Development of Antibodies and Immunomorphological Reactions During Acarid-Borne Encephalitis, *Cent. Nerv. Syst. Stimul.*, 1966: 99-105; Chemical Abstracts 69: 104731e.

29. M. I. Polozhentseva and T. L. Bykhovtzova, The Effect of Ginseng and Eleutherococcus Liquid Extract on the Formation of Antibodies (Agglutinins) in Rabbits, *Eleutherococcus and Other Adaptogens Among the Far Eastern Plants*, 1966, edited by I. I. Brekhman, Far Eastern Publishing House, Vladivostok, U.S.S.R., pp. 73-76.

30. M. I. Polozhentseva, The Influence of the Extracts of Eleutherococcus senticosus on Certain Nonspecific Immunological Indexes of Blood in the Rabbit, *Processes of Adaptation and Biologically Active Substances*, 1976, edited by I. I. Brekhman et al., Far Eastern Publishing House, Vladivostok, U.S.S.R., pp. 87-90.

31. M. I. Zotova, *op. cit.*, pp. 67-71.

32. A. S. Saratikov and R. A. Pichurina, Ability of Some Plant Stimulators to Stimulate Adaptation When There Are Pathological Reactions in the Peripheral Blood, *Izv. Sibir. Otdel., Akad. Nauk., U.S.S.R., Ser. Biol. Med. Nauk.*, 1965, 1: 113-119; Biological Abstracts 47: 62277.

33. T. I. Strokina, Modification of the Interaction of Transmission Systems in Nervous Disorders Following Treatment with Eleutherococcus, *Zhur Neuropathol. Psych.*, 1967, 67: 903-906.

34. V. V. Padkin and E. F. Baburin, The Excretion of Vitamins from Male Subjects Under the Conditions of Joint and Separate Treatment with Eleutherococcus and Polyvitamin Complex, *Eleutherococcus and Other Adaptogens Among the Far Eastern Plants*, 1966, edited by I. I. Brekhman, Far Eastern Publishing House, Vladivostok, U.S.S.R., pp. 185-190.

35. K. A. Mescherskaia and V. M. Nosyrev, The Effect of the Extract from Eleutherococcus on the Excretion of Ascorbic Acid, *A Summarized Review of the Study of Eleutherococcus in the Soviet Union*, 1966, edited by Z. I. Gutnikova, The Academy of Sciences, Vladivostok, U.S.S.R., pp. 51-53.

36. N. Tretchikoff and Alma R. Hutchens, *conversation with author (S.S.)*, Windsor, Ontario, 1969.

37. M. Yonezawa, A. Takeda, and N. Katoh, *Restoration of Radiation Injury by Ginseng Extract*, Department of Medical Biology and Hygiene, Radiation Center of Osaka Prefecture, Shinke-cho, Sakai, Osaka 593, Japan.

38. A. Takeda, M. Yonezawa, and N. Katoh, *J. Radiat. Res.*, 1981, 22: 323.

39. A. Takeda, N. Katoh, and M. Yonezawa, *J. Radiat. Res.*, 1982, 23: 150.

40. M. Yonezawa, N. Katoh, and A. Takeda, *J.Radiat. Res.*, 1985, 26: 436.

41. L. G. Lajtha, *Current Topics in Radiation Research*, 1965, edited by M. Ebert and A. Howard, North-Holland Publishing Co., Amsterdam, Vol. 1, pp. 141-163.

42. M. Yonezawa, N. Katoh, and A. Takeda, *J. Radiat. Res.*, 1985 26: 436.

43. K. Hirashima, *The Shai-Shin Igaku*, 1973, 128: 1720.

44. H. Oura, S. Nakashima, K. Tsukudo and Y. Ohta, *Chem. Pharm. Bulletin*, 1972, 29: 930.

45. H. Oura, S. Hiai, Y. Odaka, and T. Yokazawa, *J. Biochem.*, 1975, 77: 1057.

46. M. Yonezawa, *Radiation Research*, 1976, 17: 111.

47. M. Yamamoto, U. Hayashi, H. Ohshima, E. Makino, T. Itaya, Y. Suzuki, and A. Kumagai, *Symposia for Wakan-Yaku*, 1972, 6: 49.

48. G. A. Vasil'ev, A. N. Ukshe, and V. I. Sokolov, Radioprotective Action of Acclimatization to Hypoxia in Conjunction with Cysteamine and a Ginseng Root Extract, *Radiobiology*, July/August 1969, 9: 570-573.

49. E. E. Collins, M.D. and C. Collins, Fresh Aloe Vera Used for X-Ray Dermatitis, *American Journal of Roentgenology*, vol. 33, no. 1, March 1935, pp. 396-397.

50. E. E. Collins, M.D. and C. Collins, Aloe Vera and Alvagel as a Therapeutic Agent in the Treatment of Radiation, *The Radiological Review*, 1935.

51. E. L. S. Reynolds, D. Sc. and G. Westacott, Discovery That Aloe Arborescens Would Work on X-Ray Burns as Well as Aloe Vera, *The Aloes of Tropical Africa and Madagascar*, September 1966, no. 384, p. 34.

52. N. P. Mordvinova and B. K. Rostotskii, A Comparative Assessment of the Action of Emulsion from the Juice of Aloe arborescens and Aloe striatula for the Prevention of Radium Injuries, *Med. Radiol.*, (State Scientific Research Inst. of Roentgen-Radiology, Ministry of Public Health, U.S.S.R. and All-Union Scientific Research Inst. of Medicinal and Aromatic Plants, U.S.S.R.), vol. 6, no. 11, Nov. 1961, pp. 16-20.

53. N. Mordvinova and B. Rostotskii, Extract of Aloe, Supplement to Clinical Data, *Medexport*, (Moscow, U.S.S.R.), 1962.

54. J. B. Brown, M.D., F.A.C.S. and J. Barrett, Use of Aloe Vera on Radiation Burns, *CA-A Cancer Journal for Clinicians*, no. 14, 1963, pp. 14-15.

55. C. C. Lushbaugh, M.D. and D. B. Hale, B.S., Animal Research on Acute Radiation Damage, *Cancer*, vol. 6, no. 4, July 1953, pp. 690-698.

56. G. Gjerstad and T. D. Riner, Current Status of Aloe as Cure-All, *American Journal of Pharmacy*, no. 140, 1968, p. 62.

57. J. Flagg, Aloe Vera Gel in Dermatological Preparations, *American Perfumer*, no. 74, 1959, p. 27.

58. M. Lafavore, Aloe Verified, *Organic Gardening*, August 1981, p. 46.

59. M. C. Robson, J. P. Heggers and W. J. Hagstrom, Myth, Magic, Witchcraft, or Fact? Aloe Vera, *The Journal of Burn Care and Rehabilitation*, May/June 1982, pp. 157-163.

60. J. E. Crewe, Aloes in the Treatment of Burns and Scalds, *Minnesota Medicine*, August 1939, pp. 538-539.

61. N. P. Knowlton, M.D. et al., Beta Ray Burns of Human Skin, *JAMA*, vol. 141, no. 4, September 24, 1949.

62. A. B. Loveman, M.D., Leaf of Aloe Vera in Treatment of Roentgen Ray Ulcers, *Archives of Dermatology and Syphilology*, no. 36, 1937, pp. 842-843.

63. F. B. Mandeville, Aloe Vera in Treatment of Radiation Ulcers of Mucous Membranes, *Radiation Review*, no. 32, 1939, pp. 538-539.

64. R. Rovatti, Aloe Vera Ointment Tested on Third Degree Burns, *Industrial Medicine and Surgery*, no. 28, August 1959, pp. 364-368.

65. T. D. Rowe, Effects of Fresh Aloe Vera Gel in Treatment of Third Degree Roentgen Reactions on White Rats, *Journal of Am. Pharm. Assoc.*, no. 29, 1940, pp. 348-350.

66. T. D. Rowe, Further Observation on the Use of Aloe Vera Leaf in Treatment of Third Degree X-Ray Reactions, *J. Am. Pharm. Assoc.*, no. 30, p. 266.

67. C. S. Wright, M.D., Aloe Vera in Treatment of Roentgen Ulcers and Telangiectasis, *JAMA*, vol. 106, no. 16, April 18, 1936, pp. 1363-1364.

68. C. W. Waller and O. A. Gisvold, A Phytochemical Investigation of Larrea Divaricata, *American Pharm. Assoc.*, no. 34, 1945, pp. 78-81.

69. J. L. Hartwell, Plant Remedies for Cancer, *Cancer Chemotherapy Reports*, no. 7, May 1960, pp. 19-24.

70. C. R. Smart, M.D., H. Y. Hogle, M.D., et al., An Interesting Observation on NDGA and a Patient with Malignant Melanoma, *Cancer Chemotherapy Reports*, no. 53, April 1969, p. 148.

71. R. S. Pardini et al., Inhibition of Mitochondrial Electron Transport by Nordihydro-guaiaretic Acid—NDGA, *Biochemical Pharmacology*, no. 19, 1970, p. 2699.

72. Bio-Strath is produced in Zurich, Switzerland and distributed exclusively by Naturally Vitamin Supplements, Inc., 14851 North Scottsdale Road, Scottsdale, Arizona 85254.

73. H. Fritz-Niggli, Untersuchungen uber die Beeinflussung des Strahlensyndroms der Maus durch Verfutterung von Bio-Strath Elixier, *Hippokrates*, heft 20, 1967, p. 812-814.

74. H. Sporri and M. Dobeli, Untersuchungen uber den Einfluss von gekochtem and ungekochtem Bio-Strath auf weisse Rattan, *Zwischenbericht fur das eerste Halbjahr*, July 26, 1968.

75. H. Sporri, Untersuchungen uber den Einfluss von Bio-Strath auf das Korperwachstum, das Blut und dei Lebensdauer weisser Ratten, *Zwischenbericht*, 5, February 18, 1963.

76. J. D. Ireson, G. B. Leslie, D. Bunn, and J. Roberts, The Effect of Three Health Food Supplements on Rat Body Weight and Health, *Research on Bio-Strath*, 1970, p. 11.

77. J. M. Bagshaw and G. B. Leslie, Comparison of Various Dietary Supplements and Their Effect Upon the Growth Rate of Young Rats, *Laboratory Animals*, no. 8, 1974, pp. 189-197.

78. H. Fritz-Niggli, *op. cit.*

79. C. Michel and H. Fritz-Niggli, Die Beeinflussung der Fertilitat der weissen Maus durch kleine Strahlenmengen und ein Hefepraparat (Bio-Strath), *Druckfertiges Manuskript*, vol. 8, no. 3, 1972.

80. C. Michel and H. Fritz-Niggli, Effects of a Yeast Preparation (Bio-Strath) and Low Dosage Irradiation on Fertility in White Mice, *International Radiological Review*, vol. 42, no. 3, 1973, pp. 3-13.

81. F. H. Schwarzenbach, Die Wirkung von Bio-Strath auf die Fertilitat bestrahlter Mause, *Auswertung der Versuche*, 1970/71, von Frau Prof. Dr. H. Fritz-Niggli, (January 14, 1972).

82. H. Fritz-Niggli and C. Michel, Effects of a Yeast Preparation (Bio-Strath) on Radiation-Induced Developmental Anomalies, *Swiss Med.* 5, no. 11, 1983, pp. 42-44.

83. K. W. Brunner and F. H. Schwarzenbach, Die Wirkung Einesstandardisierten Hefeex-raktes (Bio-Strath-Elixier) auf den Allgemeinzustand therapeutisch bestrahlter Tumorpatien-ten, *Druckfertiges Manuskript*, vol. 10, June 10, 1972.

84. J. D. Ireson, G. E. Conway, and F. H. Schwarzenbach, The Effect of a Complex Yeast Preparation, as a Food Supplement, on the Growth of Ehrlich's Ascites Tumor in Mice, *European Journal of Cancer*, vol. 8, no. 2, April 1972.

85. *Atomikernenegie*, no. 3, 1976.

86. A. R. Boden, G. B. Leslie, and G. K. Salmon, The Effect of an Herbal Yeast Food Supplement (Bio-Strath) on the Response of Mice to Bacterially Induced Leucophenia, *Swiss Med.*, vol. 6, no. 5, 1984, pp. 82-83.

87. J. J. Farrow and G. B. Leslie, The in Vivo Protective Effect of a Complex Yeast Preparation (Bio-Strath) Against Bacterial Infections in Mice, *Medita*, vol. 8, no. 6/7, 1978.

88. M. A. Bokuchova and N. I. Skobeleva, Chemistry and Biochemistry of Tea and Tea Manufacture, *Advan. Food Res.*, 1969, 17: 215-292.

89. R. O. Asplund, M.D. et al., Isolation of Antitumor Polysaccharide Fractions from Yucca Glouca, *Growth*, vol. 4, no. 2, 1978, p. 223.

CHAPTER SEVEN

1. R. D. Barhard, M.D. and J. F. Barhard, M.D., *Lancet*, September 8, 1965.

2. *Journal of Digestive Diseases*, April 1952.

3. *Australian and New Zealand Journal of Medicine*, June 1977.

4. *Current Therapeutic Research*, August 1973.

5. *Current Therapeutic Research*, August 1978.

6. *Nutrition and Metabolism*, 1974, vol. 17, no. 6.

7. C. Marinescu, M. Popla, and O. Covulea, Radioprotection Experiments with Nucleic Acids, *Rev. Sanit. Mil.*, Jan.-Feb., 1969, 72: 61-64.

Notes

8. H. Langendorgg, Der bisherige Beitrag der Radiobiologie zur Therapie von Strahlenschaden (The Contribution to Date of Radiobiology to the Therapy of Radiation Lesions), *Roentgenpraxis* 20, 1967, no. 1, pp. 3-8.

9. R. E. Libinzon et al., Effectiveness of the High-Molecular DNA in the Treatment of Acute Radiation Sickness, *Radiobiologiza*, 1963, 3: 111-116.

10. *M. Suvrem. Med.* 21, 1970, no. 6, pp. 12-18.

11. S. Akaboshi, M. Shikita, E. Matsui, and H. Hoshina, Radiation Protection By Oral Administration of L-Cysteine In Mice, *Chem. Pharm. Bull.*, 20 (4), 1972, pp. 721-724.

12. I. Gozdash, T. Szesszardy, I. Szorady, and M. Erostyzk, Radiation Protection by Combinations of Pantothenic Acid and Cysteamine in Animal Experiments, *Kiserl. Orvostud.*, 26 (1), 1974, pp. 66-69.

13. Z. Ikamal, K. Wihorto, and H. Muryono, Cysteine as a Radiation Protecting Agent in White Mice with Respect to Cobalt-60 Gamma Radiation, *Medika*, 6 (11), 1980, pp. 678-680.

14. P. Lohman, O. Vos, C. Van Sluis, and J. Cohen, Chemical Protection Against Breaks in DNA of Human and Bacterial Cells by X-Irradiation, *Biochem. Biophys. Acta*, 224 (2), 1970, pp. 339-352.

15. M. Lafleur, J. Woldhuis and H. Loman, Effects of Sulfhydryl Compounds on the Radiation Damage in Biologically Active DNA, *Int. J. Radiat. Biol. Relat. Stud. Phys., Chem. Med.*, 37 (5), 1980, pp. 493-498.

16. H. Moenig and E. Abd-Ghani, Biological Radiation Protection: Effect of Sulfur-Containing Organic Compounds on X-Ray-Induced Radicals in Freeze-Dried Rat Liver, *Strahlentherapies*, 135 (6), 1968, pp. 731-738.

17. O. Wheeler, M. Santos, R. Amparo Ribot, and M. Ramos, *Radiat,*, 36 (3), 1968, pp. 601-609.

18. Xue-Peng Li et al., ESR Studies of Radiation Protection Effect by Cysteine and Cysteomine, *Radiat. Phys. Chem.*, 16 (4), 1980, pp. 319-320.

19. C. Nagata and T. Yamaguchi, Electronic Structure of Sulfur Compounds and Their Protecting Action Against Ionizing Radiation, *Radiation Research*, 1978, 73: 430-439.

20. A. Petkau and W. S. Chelock, Radioprotective Effects of Cysteine, *International Journal of Radiobiology*, 25, 1974, p. 321.

21. Cysteomine as a Protective Agent, *Radiation Research*, 82, 1979, p. 74.

22. E. Copeland, Mechanisms of Radioprotection: A Review, *Photochemistry and Photobiology*, 1978, 128: 839-844.

23. Xue-Peng Li et al., ESR Studies of Mechanisms of Radiation Protection Effect By Cysteine and Cystine, *Radiat. Phys. Chem.*, 17 (5), 1981, pp. 273-277.

24. G. Rathsen and H. Lieser, Significance of Gluthione in Radiation Effect and in Chemical Radiation Protection, *Strahlentherapie*, 143 (6), 1972, pp. 670-676.

25. Ford Heritage, *Composition and Facts About Foods*, Health Research (70 Lafayette Street, Mokelumne Hill, California), 1968, p. 41.

26. *Food Irradiation Information* 4: 65, 1975; *Food Science and Technology Abstracts* 8, 1976, 5R251.

27. B. Underdal, J. Nordal, G. Lunde, and B. Essum, *Lebensmittel Wissenschaft & Technologie*, 6 (3), 1973, pp. 90-93.

28. A. A. Rubanovskaya, M.D., *Journal of the American Medical Association*, Nov. 18, 1962.

29. *Nutrition Research*, Sept. 1955.

30. *Organic Consumer Report*, Aug. 8, 1972.

31. Stantchev et al., Administration of Granular Pectin to Workers Exposed to Lead, *Leit Ges Hygiene Gregebiet* 25, 1979, pp. 585-587.

32. *Unconventional Sources of Dietary Fiber*, Ivan Furda, editor, ACS Symposium Series 214, American Chemical Society, Washington, D.C., 1983.

33. S. Reiser, Metabolic Effects of Dietary Pectins Related to Human Health, *Food Technology*, Feb. 1987, p. 91.

34. H. E. Hamilton, G. S. Melville and S. A. Moss, Radioprotection of Rodents with Papain, *Report for Sept. 1967-Sept. 1968, Aerospace Medicine*, March 1969, Brooks AFB, Texas.

35. Vavrova et al., The Effect of Thymusin Application Upon Radiation Sickness in Mice, *Folia Biol.*, 22 (5), May 1977, pp. 320-329.

36. G. Valesini et al., Clinical Improvement and Partial Correction of the T-Cell Defects of Acquired Immunodeficiency Syndrome (AIDS) and Lymphadenopathy Syndrome (LAS) by a Calf Thymus Lysate, *European J. Clin. Oncol.*, 22: 531-2.

37. P. Cozzola, P. Mozzanti, and G. Bossi, In Vivo Modulating Effect of a Calf Thymus Acid Lysate on Human T Lymphocyte Subsets and CD4+/CD8+ Ratio in the Course of Different Diseases, *Curr. Ther. Res.*, 1987, 42: 1011-17.

38. H. Zenker and W. Rossbandre, *Fruehjahrsschule Kernchem.*, Zentralinst, Kernforsch., Rossendorf Dresden, E. Germany, 1974, pp. 102-4.

39. *Clinical Toxicology 3 (1): 1-4, March 1970.*

40. *Acta Pharmacologica et Toxicologica*, 1948, 4: 275.

41. *Bulletin de la Societe de Chime Biologique*, October-December, 1945, 27: 513-518.

42. *Journal of Animal Science*, February, 1972, 34: 322-325.

43. *JAMA*, 210 (10), December 8, 1969, 1846.

44. P. M. Kidd, Ph.D., *Ge-132: Research Breakthrough from the Orient*, 1986, manuscript available from the Germanium Institute of North America, P.O. Box 8207, Berkeley, CA 94707.

45. *Niwa Manuscript*, unpublished, from Asai Germanium Research Institute Co., Ltd., Izumihon-cho 1-6-4, Komae-Shi, Tokyo, Japan.

46. H. Mochizuki and T. Kada, Antimutagenic Effect of Ge-132 on X-Ray Induced Mutations in *Escherichia coli, International Journal of Radiation Biology*, 1982, 42 (6): 652-659.

47. Kidd, *op. cit.*, p. 4.

48. K. Loren, *The Report on Germanium*, Life Extension Educational Service (1759 Cosmic Way, Glendale, CA 91201), pp. 76-77.

49. M. Machisu et al., Analgesic Effect of Novel Organogermanium Compound, Ge-132, *The Journal of Pharmacobio-Dynamics*, 1983, 6: 814-820.

50. Y. Mizushima et al., Restoration of Impaired Immunoresponse by Germanium in Mice, *International Archives of Allergy and Applied Immunology*, 1980, 63: 338-339.

51. F. Suzuki and R. B. Pollard, Prevention of Suppressed Interferon Gamma Production in Thermally Injured Mice by Administration of a Novel Organogermanium Compound, Ge-132, *The Journal of Interferon Research*, 1984, 4 (2): 223-233.

52. T. Suzuki et al., Suppression and Acceleration of Experimental Amyloidosis in Mouse Model, *Acta Pathol. Japan*, 30 (4): 557-564.

53. Kidd, *op. cit.*, p. 4.

54. M. T. Saito et al., Germanium Research of Surgical Patients, 1976 International Medical Convention of Surgeons, available from Dr. Parris Kidd, Germanium Institute of North America, P.O. Box 8207, Berkeley, CA 94707.

55. Niwa Manuscript, *op. cit.*, p. 61.

56. H. Mochizuki and T. Kada, *op. cit.*, pp. 653-659.

57. M. T. Saito et al., *op. cit.*

58. R. Takashima and Y. Mitsui, *Germanium as Stabilizer of Cysteine Eye Drop*, abstract available from the Germanium Institute of North America.

59. L. Lee-Benner, *Physician's Guide to Aging, the Immune System, and Free Radical Damage*, World Health Foundation, 1986.

60. F. Suzuki and R. B. Pollard, *op. cit.*, pp. 223-233.

61. H. Aso et al., Induction of Interferon and Activation of NK Cells and Macrophages in Mice by Oral Administration of Ge-132, an Organic Germanium Compound, *Microbiological Immunology*, 19 (1): 65-74.

62. F. Suzuki et al., Importance of T-cells and Macrophages in the Antitumor Activity of Carboxyethylgermanium Sesquioxide (Ge-132), *Anticancer Research*, 185, 5: 479-484.

CHAPTER EIGHT

1. David Blankenhorn et al., Beneficial Effects of Combined Colestipol-Niacin Therapy on Coronary Atherosclerosis and Coronary Venous Bypass Grafts, *Journal of the American Medical Association*, June 19, 1987, 257 (23): 3233-40.

2. K. Pavlus, Decontamination of Vegetables and Fruit, *Ind. Obst.-Gemueseverwert* (Bundesforschungsanstalt Lebensmittelfreschhaltung, Karlsruhe, W. Germany), Feb. 15, 1968, 53: 85-88.

CHAPTER NINE

1. Peter Pohl, M. D., Zur Therapie der Strahlenbedingten Leukopenie mit Esberitox, *Medizinische Klinik*, August 29, 1969, vol. 64, issue 35, pp. 1546-7.

2. A. J. Stoll and A. Brack, Antibacterial Substances II, Isolation and Constitution of Echinacoside, a Glycoside from the Roots of *Echinacea angustifolia*, *Helv. Chim. Acta.*, 1950, 33: 1877-93.

3. E. Koch and H. Uebel, Experimental Studies Concerning the Local Action of *Echinacea purpurea* on Tissues, *Arzneimittel Forschung*, 1953, 3: 16-19.

4. E. Koch and H. Uebel, Experimental Studies on the Local Influence of Cortisone and Echinacin upon Tissue Resistance Against Streptococcus Infection, *Arzneimittel Forschung*, 1954, 4: 551-60.

5. O. Kuhn, Echinacea and Phagocytosis, *Arzneimittel Forschung*, 1953, 3: 194-200.

6. E. Koch and H. Haase, A Modification of the Spreading Test in Animal Assays, *Arzneimittel Forschung*, 1952, 2: 464-7.

7. I. Bonadeo, G. Bottazzi, and M. Lavazza, Echinacin B, an Active Polysaccharide from Echinacea, *Riv. Ital. Essenze, Profumi, Piante Offic.*, 1971, 53 (5): 281-95.

8. K. H. Busing, Inhibition of Hyaluronidase by Echinacin, *Arzneimittel Forschung*, 1952, 2: 467-9.

9. K. H. Busing, The Effect of Extracts from *Echinacea purpurea* on the Properdin Levels in Rabbits, *Z. Immunitatsforsch*, 1958, 115: 169-76.

10. B. Chone, Gezielte Steuerung der Leukozytentinetik durch Echinacin, *Arzneimittel Forschung*, 1965, 11: 611.

11. S. A. Quadripur, *Ther. Ggw..*, 1976, 115: 1072.

12. D. J. Voaden and M. Jacobson, Tumor Inhibitors 3: Identification and Synthesis of an Oncolytic Hydrocarbon from American Coneflower Roots, *J. Med. Chem.*, 1972, 15 (6): 619-23.

13. A. Wacker and A. Hilbig, Virus Inhibition by *Echinacea purpurea*, *Planta Medica.*, 1978, 33: 89-102.

14. F. J. Reith, Pharmaceuticals Containing Lactic Acid Derivatives and Echinacea, *Ger. Ofen.*, 1978, p. 10.

15. H. Wagner and A. Proksch, Isolation of Polysaccharides with Immunostimulating Activity from *Echinacea purpurea*, *Int. Conf. Chem. Biotechnil. Biol., Act. Nat. Prod. (Proc.)*, B. Atanasova, ed., 1981, 3 (1): 200-2.

16. H. Wagner and A. Proksch, An Immunostimulating Active Principle from *Echinacea purpurea*,A. *Angew. Phytother.*, 1981, 2 (5): 166-8, 171.

17. J. L. Hartwell, Plant Remedies for Cancer, *Cancer Chemotherapy Reports*, No. 7, May 1960, pp. 19-24.

18. J. Ostrenga and D. Perry, Golden Seal, *The Pharm Chem Newsletter*, vol. 4, no. 1, Jan. 1975.

19. J. Hammond, Golden Seal: A Blessing in Disguise, *U.S. Journal of Drug and Alcohol Dependence*, vol. 2, no. 2, March 1978.

20. J. Hoveman, The Influence of pH on the Survival After X-Irradiation of Cultured Malignant Cells, *International Journal of Radiation Biology*, no. 37, 1980, pp. 201-205.

21. C. Bullock, Two Chinese Herbs Show Blooming Anticancer Potential, *Medical Tribune*,

March 28, 1984, p. 5.

22. D. W. D'Souza et al., Effects of Nutritional Status on Gastric Secretion and Composition in X-Irradiated Rats, *Environmental Physiology and Biochemistry*, vol. 4, no. 6, pp. 270-79, Biochemistry and Food Technology Division, Bhobba Atomic Research Center, Bombay, India.

23. D. Toreva, G. Slovcev et al., On the Protective Effect of the Michelle of High Fungi Upon Acute Radiation Sickness, *Folio Med.*, 1968, no. 10, pp. 110-14.

24. J. Tache, A. R. Mehron, and Y. Tache, Intestinal Absorption of Iron in Irradiated Rabbits, *Revue Canadienne de Biologie*, 1973, 32 (3): 157-167.

Optimal Nutrient Combining

In natural whole foods, vitamins, minerals, proteins, fats, carbohydrates, and other nutrients always occur in complementary combinations—they are never found alone isolated from other nutrients. Similarly, when nutrients are taken in supplemental form, they function best when taken together in particular combinations. That is, nutrients work in a complementary or *synergistic* manner. The presence of one nutrient improves the function of other nutrients. Nutrients work cooperatively so that the total effect is greater than the sum of the effects if each nutrient were taken alone.

Some nutrients are so closely interrelated that if they were taken alone, not only would they be ineffective, but the results may be more harmful than beneficial. For example, all B vitamins should be taken together. They are so interrelated that large doses of any single B vitamin may be therapeutically valueless or may cause a deficiency of others. As you will see in the Optimal Nutrient Combining and Common Deficiency Factors table, all the nutrients function best when combined with other synergistic nutrients.

This table also lists some common factors that can cause a deficiency of each nutrient discussed in Part II of this book. Optimal dosages and additional nutrient combining recommendations are presented in Chapters 5 and 8.

Optimal Nutrient Combining and Common Deficiency Factors

	Complementary Synergistic Nutrients		Common Depleting or Antagonistic Factors	
Vitamin A	Calcium	Vitamin B complex	Air pollution	Infections
	Choline		Alcohol	Lactation
	Iodine	Vitamin B$_{12}$	Arsenicals	Liver
	Phosphorus	Vitamin C	Aspirin	disorders
	Unsaturated	Vitamin D	Coffee	Mineral oil
	fatty acids	Vitamin E	Cold weather	Nephritis
		Zinc	Corticosteroid	Nitrates
			drugs (such as	Obstructed
			cortisone and	bile duct
			prednisone)	Phenobarbital
			Diabetes	Pneumonia
			Dicumarol	Pollution
			Disease	Pregnancy
			Drugs	Stress
			Excess iron	Thyroid
			Fat deficient	disorders
			diet	Tobacco
			Gastrointestinal	Trauma
			disorders	
Vitamin B Complex	Calcium	Vitamin C	Alcohol	Infection
	Magnesium	Vitamin E	Antibiotics	Insecticides
	Phosphorus	Zinc	Aspirin	Processed
			Caffeine	foods
			Corticosteroid	Sleeping
			drugs	pills
			Diuretics	Stress
			Estrogen pills	Sugar
			Excessive	Sulfonamides
			carbohydrates	(antibiotics)
			Heavy	
			perspiration	

	Complementary Synergistic Nutrients		Common Depleting or Antagonistic Factors	
Vitamin B₁ (Thiamine)	Folic acid Manganese Niacin Sulfur	Vitamin B complex Vitamin B₂ Vitamin C Vitamin E	Alcohol Antiobiotics Boiling with acids Caffeine Exposure to heat, air, or water during cooking Fever	Raw clams and oysters Raw fish Stress Sugar Surgery Tobacco
Vitamin B₂ (Riboflavin)	Niacin Phosphorus Vitamin B complex	Vitamin B₆ Vitamin C	Alcohol Alkalies Antibiotics Caffeine Copper toxicity	Light (especially ultraviolet) Oral contraceptives Sugar Stress Tobacco
Vitamin B₃ (Niacin)	Phosphorus Vitamin B complex Vitamin B₁	Vitamin B₂ Vitamin C	Alcohol Antibiotics Caffeine Excess water	Excessive starches in diet Infection Stress Sugar Trauma
Vitamin B₅ (Pantothenic acid)	Biotin Calcium Folic Acid Sulfur	Vitamin B Complex Vitamin B₆ Vitamin B₁₂ Vitamin C	Alcohol Acids (such as vinegar) Alkalies (such as baking soda) Antibiotics Aspirin	Caffeine Excess heat (as in cooking and milling) Insecticides Methylbromide (a fumigant) Stress

	Complementary Synergistic Nutrients		Common Depleting or Antagonistic Factors	
Vitamin B6 (Pyridoxine)	Linoleic acid (an unsaturated fatty acid) Magnesium Potassium Sodium Vitamin B Complex	Vitamin B1 Vitamin B2 Vitamin B5 Vitamin C Unsaturated fatty acids	Aging Alcohol Birth Control Pills Caffeine Cortisone Estrogen Fasting	Lactation Light Oral contraceptives Pregnancy Radiation Reducing diets Tobacco X-rays
Vitamin B12 (Cyanoco-balamin)	Biotin Calcium Choline Cobalt Folic Acid Inositol Iron	Optimal thyroid function Potassium Proper hydrochloric acid Sodium Vitamin B complex Vitamin B6 Vitamin C	Aging Alcohol Autoimmune reactions Caffeine	Deficient "intrinsic factor" in g.i. tract Dilantin Laxatives Oral Contraceptives Tobacco
Vitamin B15 (Pangamic acid)	Vitamin A Vitamin C	Vitamin E Vitamin B Complex	Diaphoretics Diuretics	Laxatives
Biotin	Folic Acid Pantothenic Acid Sulfur	Vitamin B Complex Vitamin B12 Vitamin C	Alcohol Antibiotics Avidin (a protein in raw egg white) Caffeine	Lactation Oxidation Pregnancy Sulfa drugs
Choline	Folic acid Inositol Linoleic acid Manganese	Vitamin A Vitamin B complex Vitamin B12	Alcohol Caffeine	Insecticides Sugar

	Complementary Synergistic Nutrients		Common Depleting or Antagonistic Factors	
Folic Acid	Biotin	Vitamin B12	Aging	Leukemia
	Vitamin B complex	Vitamin C	Alcohol	Mental retardation
	Vitamin B5		Anticonvulsants	Oral contraceptives
			Caffeine	
			Diarrhea	Phenobarbital
			Disease	Pregnancy
			Exposure to heat	Streptomycin
			Exposure to light	Stress
				Sulfa drugs
			Hodgkin's disease	Vomiting
Inositol	Choline	Vitamin B2	Antibiotics	Diuretics
	Folic acid	Vitamin B5	Caffeine	Excess water
	Linoleic	Vitamin B6	Diabetes	Sulfonamides (sulfa drugs)
	PABA	Vitamin B12		
	Phosphorus	Vitamin C		
	Vitamin B complex	Vitamin E		
	Vitamin B1			
PABA	Folic Acid	Vitamin C	Alcohol	Sulfanomides
	Vitamin B complex		Caffeine	

	Complementary Synergistic Nutrients		Common Depleting or Antagonistic Factors	
Vitamin C	Bioflavonoids	Manganese	Aging	Fatigue
	Calcium	Vitamin A	Air pollution	Fever
	Copper	Vitamin B12	Alcohol	High copper
	Magnesium		Antibiotics	High iron
			Antihistamines	High protein
			Anxiety	diet
			Aspirin	Hypoglycemia
			Baking soda	Infection
			Barbiturates	Injury
			Burns	Menstruation
			Canning	Mercury
			Cooking in	Oral
			copper	contraceptives
			Cortisone	Oxidation
			DDT	Pain killers
			Estrogen	Pasteurization
			Excess water	Petroleum
			intake or	Pregnancy
			elimination	Schizophrenia
			Exposure to	Stress
			light	Surgery
			Exposure to	Tobacco
			air	
Vitamin D	Calcium	Unsaturated	Air pollution	Dilantin
	Choline	fatty acids	Alcohol	Mineral Oil
	Phosphorus	Vitamin A	Clothing	Oral contraceptives
		Vitamin C	Clouds	Window glass
			Corticosteroid	
			drugs	
Vitamin E	Inositol	Vitamin A	Air pollution	Hypolipidemic
	Magnesium	Vitamin B	Antibiotics	drugs
	Manganese	complex	Chlorine	Inorganic iron
	Selenium	Vitamin B1	Estrogen	Mineral oil
	Unsaturated	Vitamin C	Excessive	Oral
	fatty acids		unsaturated	contraceptives
			fats or	Oxidation
			oils	Rancid fats
			Food milling	and oils
			and processing	

	Complementary Synergistic Nutrients		Common Depleting or Antagonistic Factors	
Vitamin F	Biotin Phosphorus Selenium Vitamin A	Vitamin B5 Vitamin B6 Vitamin C Vitamin D Vitamin E Zinc	Excessive carbohydrates Exposure to air	Oxidation Radiation

Bioflavo-noids	Calcium
	Magnesium
		Vitamin C	Air pollution
			Aspirin
			Canning
			Cortisone
			DDT
			Diaphoretics
			Diuretics
			Excess salt
				Excess water
				  intake or
				  elimination
				Fever
				Heat
				Oxidation
				Pasteurization
				Stress
				Tobacco

Calcium	Appropriate
	  production of
	  hydrochloric
	  acid
	Iron
	Magnesium
	Manganese
	Phosphorus
		Vitamin A
		Vitamin C
		Vitamin D
		Vitamin E
		Unsaturated
		  Fatty Acids
			Anxiety
			Aspirin
			Corticosteroid
			  drugs
			Deficient exercise
			Deficient
			  hydrochloric
			  acid
			Deficient
			  vitamin D
				Depression
				Diarrhea
				Excessive fats
				Oxalic acid
				  in food
				Phytic acid
				  in food
				Stress
				Thyroid disorders

Cobalt	Copper Iron	Vitamin B12 Zinc	None currently known	
Copper	Cobalt Iron	Vitamin C Zinc	Excess Zinc	

Iodine	None
	  currently
	  known
			Perspiration	

Fighting Radiation

	Complementary Synergistic Nutrients		Common Depleting or Antagonistic Factors	
Iron	Calcium	Phosphorus	Alkalies	Excess
	Cobalt	Protein	Antacids	manganese
	Copper	Vitamin B6	Aspirin	Excess
	Folic Acid	Vitamin B12	Bleeding	phosphorus
	Hydrochloric	Vitamin C	Caffeine	Excess zinc
	acid		Diarrhea	Menstruation
	(appropriate		Deficient	Oxalic acid
	amounts)		hydrochloric	Phytic acid
	magnesium		acid	in food
			EDTA (a food	Pregnancy
			preservative)	Synthetic
			Excess cellulose	vitamin E
Magnesium	Calcium		Alcohol	Fluorine
	Phosphorus		Coffee	High cholesterol
	Protein		Corticosteroid	High protein diet
	Vitamin B6		drugs	Oxalic acid
	Vitamin C		Diuretics	in food
	Vitamin D		Drugs	Phytic acid
			Excess	in food
			commercial	
			cow milk	
Manganese	Calcium	Vitamin B	Antibiotics	Excess
	Phosphorus	complex	Excess calcium	phosphorus
		Vitamin E		
Phosphorus	Calcium	Vitamin A	Alcohol	Excess fats
	Iron	Vitamin D	Aluminum	Excess
	Magnesium	Unsaturated	Antacids	magnesium
	Manganese	fatty acids	Aspirin	Excess iron
	Protein	Zinc	Corticosteroid	Sugar
			drugs	Thyroid
			Diuretics	disorders

	Complementary Synergistic Nutrients		Common Depleting or Antagonistic Factors	

Potassium	Magnesium
	Sodium
		Vitamin B6	Alcohol
			Aspirin
			Caffeine
			Corticosteroid
			  drugs
			Diarrhea
			Diuretics
			Excess salt
			High
			  cholesterol
				Laxatives
				Low blood
				  sugar
				Stress
				Sodium
				Sugar
				Sweating
				Vomiting

Selenium	Iron	Vitamin E	Mercury	Other toxic metals
Sodium	Potassium Vitamin B6	Vitamin D	Diarrhea Excessive perspiration	Vomiting

Sulfur	Biotin
	Pantothenic Acid
		Vitamin B
		  complex
		Vitamin B1
			None currently
			  known	

Zinc	Calcium
	Copper
	Phosphorus
		Vitamin A
		Vitamin B6
		Vitamin E
			Alcohol
			Cadmium
			Corticosteroid
			  drugs
			Diuretics
			Excess calcium
			Excess copper
			Hodgkin's
			  disease
				Lack of phosphorus
				Leukemia
				Oral
				  contraceptives
				Phytic acid
				  in food
				Synthetic
				  chelating
				  compounds
				  (such as
				  used to
				  remove excess
				  copper)
				Unbalanced diet

The Amazing Spiderwort

There are promising indications that the plant spiderwort, *Tradescantia ssp*, is one of the best biological or living indicators of radiation and chemical pollution. Studies have shown that in just twelve to thirteen days after being contaminated with even low "safe" doses of radiation or hazardous chemicals, its normally blue stamen hairs begin mutating pink. The greater the contamination by toxins, the more the flower mutates. The great advantage of the spiderwort is that it absorbs toxins internally and can even store them, much like a mammal. Mechanical indicators measure only temporary external levels of contamination. Hence, spiderwort may give a more meaningful measure of the cumulative effect of contamination on all living biological systems.

Since 1974 spiderwort has been successfully and repeatedly tested in Japan as a reliable indicator of radiation. The research studies performed by radiation geneticists at the Kyoto and Saitama Universities in Japan and the Biology Department of Brookhaven National Laboratory in Upton, New York, have shown that this plant has the unique characteristic of being able to detect low levels of radiation and dangerous chemical mutagens in the environment.[1, 2]

A graphic illustration of the potential importance of spiderwort is a series of investigations carried out in Japan in 1974 - 1977. Research scientists placed a species of spiderwort, *Tradescantia ohiensis*, near a nuclear power plant. They observed how many stamen hairs of the spiderwort plant mutated pink and then calibrated an index in order to determine both the amount of radiation absorbed and the extent of mutation.

Before concluding that the increase in mutations in the spiderwort was due to radiation from the nuclear power plant, the researchers used controlled experiments to examine other environmental factors that might have caused the changes such as pesticides, car exhaust, and atmospheric fallout. But the only connection they could find was with wind direction from the nuclear power plant.

The researchers pointed out that the type of devices (dosimeters) used to monitor routine emissions measured only gamma radiation, not alpha or beta. Also, the dosimeters were measuring the external gamma ray dose for living organisms. The spiderworts, on the other hand, were showing the absorbed dose. The researchers observed that the amount of radiation absorbed by plant or animal tissue is "very much greater" than the amount measured mechanically. They noted, "Therefore, the. . . radiation level monitored (by the dosimeters) represents only a part, probably a minor part, of the actual absorbed dose, (external and internal) in living organisms. In fact, the increase of pink mutations detected in the spiderwort stamen hairs corresponded with intensities 56 times larger than reported by monitoring devices."[3]

These spiderwort experiments illustrate the important biological aspects of radiation exposure: attachment, absorption, and then cumulative concentration of absorbed doses into the tissues. These experiments demonstrate that low levels of radiation can accumulate and concentrate in living tissue, causing extensive genetic damage, including genetic mutations.

At several nuclear power plants in Europe, Japan, and the U.S., groups are planting certain clones of *Tradescantia* to monitor the increasing amounts of radiation that routinely flow downwind in their own local area and to serve as an active biological indicator of the cumulative effects of dangerous chemical mutagens.

Research has currently pinpointed three clones or species of *Tradescantia* that prove to be accurate indicators of absorbed radiation and mutagenic environmental pollutants. They are *Tradescantia ohiensis*, *T. virginiana*, and *T. paludosa*. These spiderworts are native to North America and can be grown in many parts of this continent and Europe.

Friends, a nuclear resource group on Long Island, is planting spiderwort around the Shoreham One nuclear plant. This group distributes information on spiderwort, including a comprehensive bibliography of research performed on *Tradescantia* as a biological indicator of radiation.[4]

Notes

1. S. Ichikawa, *The Spiderwort Strategy*, Saitama University Laboratory of Genetics (255 Shimo-Okubo, Orawa, Saitama 338, Japan).

2. A. G. Underbrink et al., "Tradescantia Stamen Hairs: A Radiobiological Test System Applicable to Chemical Mutagenesis," *Chemical Mutagens: Principles and Methods for their Detection*, Volume II, Plenum Press, 1973, pp. 171-207.

3. S. Ichikawa, *Nuclear Power Plant Suspected to Increase Mutations*, revised report by

Fighting Radiation

Motoyuki Nagata, Shizuo Oki, and Sadao Ichikawa (Laboratory of Genetics, Faculty of Agriculture, Kyoto University, Kyoto 606 Japan).
  4. *Spiderwort Bibliography*, Friends, P. O. Box 663, East Quogue, Long Island, NY 11942.

Radiation Detection & Measurement: Products & Services

Personal radiation detectors and measuring devices are available to consumers who want to monitor fallout levels, or emissions from microwave ovens, TV screens, video display terminals, and x-ray apparatus. There are also mail-order testing services which supply monitoring devices that measure radon in the home, x-ray exposure, and other types of radiation. After being left at potential sites of exposure, these devices are sent back to the mail-order service for laboratory analysis. When the test results come back, one then has the knowledge to choose the proper protective foods, herbs, and supplements, and it is possible to assess what must be done to avoid future exposure.

Below are three listings—of testing services and information sources, of radiation detectors and precision measuring devices for personal use, and of protective shields for screens which emit radiation. (The prices of all products and services are subject to change.)

I. Radiation Testing Services and Information

1. **CompuRad** Available from Personal Monitoring Technologies, Inc. (PMT)
Metro Center
88 Elm St.
Rochester, NY 14604
(800) 4-DETECT
New York State residents, call (716) 232-1600
Price: $39 per year

The CompuRad monitoring system was developed by Derace Schaffer, M.D., a radiologist and clinical associate professor at the University of

Rochester School of Medicine. According to Schaffer's article, "Medical and Dental X-Rays: How to Keep Track and Cut Back," which appeared in *Healthfacts* (the newsletter of the Center for Medical Consumers), "If we keep meticulous records of prescription drugs and we don't prescribe drugs that are known to cause cancer, how can we not keep track of radiation exposure we prescribe for patients at medical offices and dental offices around the country and hospital facilities? Studies conducted around the country have shown a more than 200-fold variation in radiation exposure for the very same types of examination."

CompuRad subscribers receive a year's supply of tiny paper dosimeters, which are put on the skin of the target area during x-ray examinations. Dosimeters measure the amount of exposure to radiation. After an x-ray exam, subscribers mail the dosimeter to PMT for a laboratory analysis of exposure levels. CompuRad's dosimeters can be carried easily in a wallet. They also measure natural background radiation, such as that received from a jet flight or from the presence of radon in the home. When readings are too high, PMT sends a questionnaire that helps evaluate the exact cause.

2. On-Guard Radiation Detection Test
Radiation Safety Corporation
140 University Avenue
Palo Alto, CA 94301
(415) 321-8986 or
(800) 443-0100 ext. 264
Price: $35

The On-Guard testing device monitors x-ray emissions from the screens of operating video display terminals and television sets. The device is placed on a screen for fifteen hours total operating time and is then mailed back to Radiation Safety Corporation for analysis. The company then sends a report which clearly explains the consumer's test results. If emissions exceed EPA standards, the consumer is notified at once.

3. Radon Testing and Information
Radon Technical Information Service
Research Triangle Park
P.O. Box 12194
Research Triangle Park, NC 27709
Price: Free

A number of testing laboratories and businesses offer radon analysis to concerned homeowners. In 1986, the EPA published a list of labs that perform radon tests. All the labs listed are certified by the EPA for quality assurance. There are 75 organizations on the current list, including state laboratories and the EPA's own facilities.

4. Radon Project (home radon measurement)
P.O. Box 90069
Pittsburgh, PA 15224
Price: $12 per test

Dr. Bernard Cohen and colleagues at the Department of Physics, University of Pittsburgh, have developed an accurate, inexpensive way to get an estimate of household radon levels. For a $12 check (made out to the University) the consumer receives a small container of activated charcoal. A strip of tape is removed to admit air, and the container is placed in the house for a week. It is then resealed with tape and returned to the lab with a fairly long questionnaire (which must be filled out). Test results are sent back with a clearly written interpretation of their meaning. The Radon Project is studying all test results in an effort to learn more about radon—the exact locations of soil deposits that emit it, its effects on human health, and how to better block its entry upwards into homes in radon risk areas.

5. EPA Publications on Radon
U.S. EPA
Center for Environmental Research Information
26 West St. Clair Street
Cincinnati, OH 45268
Price: free

1. *A Citizen's Guide to Radon—What It Is and What to Do About It*
(Environmental Protection Agency publication OPA-86-004, August 1986)

This booklet covers the origins of radon from natural uranium deposits; the risks it poses to health (mainly lung cancer); common entry points into the home; how to use radon detectors; how to interpret test results to evaluate radon risk; and appropriate actions to take at different levels of exposure. A helpful list of ways to reduce risk from radon is given.

2. Those homeowners with the tools and initiative to do radon-reduction work on their own homes may want more detailed information. See *Radon Reduction Techniques for Detached Houses* (EPA/625/5-86/019). You can also obtain copies of 1) and 2) by writing or calling the EPA office in your region.

6. EPA Regional Offices
EPA Region 1: Room 2203, JFK Fed. Bldg., Boston, MA 02203; (617) 223-4845
EPA Region 2: 26 Federal Plaza, New York, NY 10278; (212) 264-2515
EPA Region 3: 841 Chestnut St., Philadelphia, PA 19107; (215) 597-8320
EPA Region 4: 345 Courtland Street NE, Atlanta, GA 30365; (404)

881-3776
EPA Region 5: 230 South Dearborn St., Chicago, IL 60604; (312) 353-2205
EPA Region 6: 1201 Elm Street, Dallas, TX 75270; (214) 655-2200
EPA Region 7: 726 Minnesota Ave., Kansas City, KS 66101; (913) 236-2803
EPA Region 8: Suite 1300, One Denver Place, 999 18th Street, Denver, CO 80202; (303) 283-1710
EPA Region 9: 215 Fremont Street, San Francisco, CA 94105; (415) 974-8076
EPA Region 10: 1200 Sixth Avenue, Seattle, WA 98101; (206) 442-7660'
State—EPA Region

Alabama-4 Alaska-10 Arizona-9 Arkansas-6 California-9 Colorado-8 Connecticut-1 Delaware-3 District of Columbia-3 Florida-4 Georgia-4 Hawaii-9 Idaho-10 Illinois-5 Indiana-5 Iowa-7 Kansas-7 Kentucky-4 Louisiana-6 Maine-1 Maryland-3 Massachusetts-1 Michigan-5 Minnesota-5 Mississippi-4 Missouri-7 Montana-8 Nebraska-7 Nevada-9 New Hampshire-1 New Jersey-2 New Mexico-6 New York-2 North Carolina-4 North Dakota-8 Ohio-5 Oklahoma-6 Oregon-10 Pennsylvania-3 Rhode Island-1 South Carolina-4 South Dakota-8 Tennessee-4 Texas-6 Utah-8 Vermont-1 Virginia-3 Washington-10 West Virginia-3 Wisconsin-5 Wyoming-8

The EPA offers a number of services that citizens can use to watchdog and reduce environmental pollution. It may take persistence to make initial contact with an employee who can help you with your particular problem or complaint, but the effort can be well worthwhile.

II. *Personal Radiation Detectors and Measuring Devices*
1. Detectors
Personal Radiation Detector (for x-rays)
Available from Micon
Route 7, Box 4500C
Joplin, MO 64801
(417) 623-7083
Price: $14.95

Detectors register the presence of radiation but do not measure the precise rates or amounts of exposure to it. This device shines a soft green warning light when .4 rem per hour or higher levels of x-radiation are present in one's environment. Used for measuring emissions from televisions, VDT's, computer screens, and x-ray apparatus.

Microwave Leak Detector
Available from Radio Shack stores
Catalog # 22-2001
Price: $14.95

This small detector checks for leakage around the door seals of microwave ovens. It is slowly moved along outside the door seal when the oven is operating.

2. Measuring Devices

A. *Geiger Counters*

Available from Dosimeter Corporation
11286 Grooms Road
Cincinnati, OH 45242
(513) 489-8100 or
(800) 322-8258
Prices: $370-$600 for Geiger counters to measure gamma and x-ray exposure rates
$150 for attachable probes to measure alpha and beta radiation exposure

The more alpha, beta, x-ray, or gamma radiation a Geiger counter registers, the faster it clicks and/or displays digital readouts, measuring the exact rate of radiation exposure per minute. The basic Geiger counters measure x-rays and gamma radiation. Probes to measure alpha and beta radiation exposure rates can be attached to Geiger counters to extend their range. Some models only give digital readouts, other models only click, and yet others have both visual and auditory features.

B. *Personal Dosimeters Available from:*

Victoreen, Inc.
10101 Woodland Avenue
Cleveland, OH 44104
(216) 795-8200
Prices: $82.50 for dosimeter (Model #541 R)
$91.00 for dosimeter charging unit (Model #2000 A)

Dosimeter Corporation

11286 Grooms Road
Cincinnati, OH 45242
(513) 489-8100 or (800) 322-8258
Prices: $82.50 for dosimeter (Model #862)
$110 for battery operated charging unit with plastic case (Model #909)
$400 for plug-in charging unit with metal case (Model #910)

Personal dosimeters measure the amount of exposure to radiation, while Geiger counters measure the rate. Small dosimeter badges are routinely worn in workplaces where radiation tends to exceed background levels. They are read indirectly—that is, periodically taken off and analyzed in a lab. These badges are relatively inexpensive. More costly (around $80 and up) direct reading dosimeters can be purchased from the two companies listed above. These dosimeters measure exposure to x-rays and gamma rays. Some study and practice are necessary to take readings and evaluate them accurately with a direct reading dosimeter. After measuring for the amount of exposure, the dosimeter must be attached to a "charging unit," which removes an electrical charge that is stored in an ion chamber in the dosimeter. When incoming radiation enters this chamber and interacts with the electrical charge there, the dosimeter needle moves upscale to measure radiation. After removing the "old" charge from the ion chamber, the charging unit replaces it with a new one so the dosimeter can take a new measurement.

III. Protective Shields for Video Display Terminals, Home Computer Screens, and Television Sets

Design West
2532 Dupont Drive
Irvine, CA 92715
(714) 859-3533
Prices: $140 for 6" x 8" shield (Model #0900)
$150 for 8" x 10 1/2" shield (Model #1200)
$200 for 10" x 13" shield (Model #1500)
$630 for 17" x 21" shield (Model #2500)

Shields can be special ordered in any size. Call to inquire about special order prices.

Langley-St. Clair Instrumentation Systems, Inc.
132 West 24th Street
New York, NY 10011
(212) 989-6876
and 2635 Sandy Plains Road
Atlanta, GA 30066
(404) 977-4508 or (800) 221-7070
Prices: $129.95 for shields which block high frequency radiation
$159.95 for shields which block low frequency radiation
$169.95 for shields which block both high and low frequencies
Sizes are 8 1/2' x 11" (Model #85)
9 1/2" x 11 1/2" (Model #95)

10″ x 13″ (Model #10)
All three sizes are the same price for each type of shield.

Transparent leaded acrylic shields can be purchased in different sizes to block emissions of ultraviolet, electromagnetic, and x-ray radiation from VDT's, computer screens, and television sets. These shields can be attached to any operating terminal or screen, and are easily detachable for use on other radiation-producing appliances.

Unorthodox Approaches to Radiation Protection Deserving Further Research

BY GEOFFREY OELSNER

The following survey presents some of the research findings on unorthodox, speculative approaches to protection against radiation and environmental pollution which may be worthy of further scientific study. Research with promising implications for health protection has been done by experts in areas of study as varied as bioelectricity, naturopathy, homeopathy, bacteriology, and psychoneuroimmunology (the study of how emotional and mental attitudes affect the immune system). While no claims are being made or implied that these unorthodox approaches will provide consistent or reliable protection against toxins, further research and testing may prove beneficial in some areas.

One line of recent medical research has focused on how organisms are affected by electromagnetic (em) fields. The authors of a study on "magnetic fields and the number of blood platelets" found that mice suffered from less of a radiation syndrome when they were exposed to a magnetic field before being irradiated.[1] The researchers found an increased number of platelets in the mice's blood after the magnetic exposure and speculated that the increase may have been responsible for the reduced death rate from intestinal hemorrhages in the irradiated mice. However, bioelectric researcher Robert Becker, M.D., author of *The Body Electric* (William Morrow, 1985), and the Russian scientist A. S. Presmann, have both found that relatively weak em fields can disturb human regulatory functions. Therefore, the use of electromagnetic fields for therapy or self-treatment should be approached with caution until further research has been conducted.

As nutrition author Jeffrey Bland, Ph.D., has said, "Energy in medicine is here to stay. We recognize its diagnostic and therapeutic value, and we are concerned about the potential impacts of low level radiation of a nonionizing type on subtle physiologic functions including circadian rhythms, hormonal secretions, immune function, cell regeneration and nervous system function."[2]

Nature cures, like spiritual healing practices, are part of an age-old body of traditional healing knowledge which may offer some protection against the modern problems of radiation and chemical toxins. Interesting experiments have been conducted on the radioprotective value of negative air ions, clinical hydrotherapy, natural hot springs, clay treatments, and quartz crystals. Just as our human energies may interact to catalyze physical healing, so also natural substances may help hasten recovery from toxin related damage.

Negative ions are produced in the air by natural atmospheric changes and can also be generated by mechanical means. Clinicians at hospitals in Israel, Hungary, Switzerland, and other countries have employed negative ion generators to successfully ease the breathing of patients with a range of respiratory problems. High concentrations of negative ions have been shown in laboratory experiments to help neutralize damage to the cilia of the lungs caused by many kinds of atmospheric contaminants, including cigarette smoke. Negative ions fortify health by improving blood circulation.

The use of high concentrations in the air of negative ions merits further attention as an aid to the treatment and prevention of overexposure to radiation. The results of a Russian study, "On the Preventive Action of Aero-Ionization in Acute Radiation Sickness," suggest that the oxygen-enhancing properties of negative air ions could help the body to repair and resist cellular injury from radiation.[3] The authors conclude that "negative aero-ionization may prevent radiation injury in lethal gamma-irradiated animals."

The use of hydrotherapy (treatments using water) in combination with EM fields was shown to improve peripheral blood circulation in the treatment of Russian patients who had been chronically exposed to ionizing radiation.[4]

Hot mineral springs have long been known to have drawing and soothing effects. Health-preserving effects of hot spring hydrotherapy were examined in twenty Japanese farmers from villages near Hiroshima and Nagasaki.[5] The men, aged sixty to eighty-two years, came periodically to a mountain spring for a "cure." They were examined there by researchers from Kyushu University for measurable changes in physical strength before, during, and after the hot spring therapy. Improvements in physical strength were observed in about half of the patients. No other treatments were given concurrently.

Homeopathy, a modality of healing developed by Dr. Samuel

Hahnemann in the late eighteenth century, is currently being practiced and researched most enthusiastically in India, Great Britain, France, Greece, Germany, Brazil, Mexico, and Russia. It works on the principle of "like cures like." In its *Materia Medica* are substances which produce disease symptoms in healthy persons, but which can act as remedies for the same symptoms in the event of illness. When taken in minute dosages specified by a qualified practitioner, homeopathic remedies are said to counter disease by helping to activate the body's defense mechanisms.

Hahnemann believed that there are three basic "miasms," or underlying pervasive causes of all chronic diseases. In the 1880s, certain homeopaths debated that tuberculosis was a fourth inherited miasm. Now, some practitioners have added radiation and petrochemical miasms to this list, and homeopaths are currently researching a number of approaches to protection from radiation and chemical toxins.

Rokan-K is a radioprotectant developed by Schwabbe, a West German manufacturer of homeopathic remedies. It is a combination of *Nux Vomica* (traditionally given by homeopaths for stomach disorders, nervous troubles, vomiting, and as an antidote to toxic chemicals, alcohol, and drugs) with an extract of oats and grains in a vitamin-rich medium. A series of experiments with eighty German patients indicated the beneficial effects of this preparation in treating radiation sickness.[6] There were "no detrimental side effects." Testing did not reveal any alteration in the blood's protein fraction, as expected after irradiation.

Correspondence with several journals and clearinghouses of homeopathic research revealed no further information on established radioprotective remedies. However, Richard Moskowitz, M.D., a physician practicing homeopathic and allopathic medicine in the Boston area, suggested that certain homeopathic preparations derived from radioactive elements or radiant energy processes be investigated for potential use after extreme radiation exposures. Moskowitz thinks that the remedies X-Ray[7], Uranium Uranium Nitricum[8], and Radium might be relevant to the radiation problem, "insofar as they can reproduce and therefore cure some of the symptoms of exposure." Moskowitz advised that researchers study the "symptom-pictures" of these three remedies, in addition to those of the well-known "polychrest" (from a Greek word meaning "many uses") remedies. He advised against taking these or any other homeopathic preparations without consulting a licensed homeopathic physician, and noted that although the Uranium and Radium preparations usually are administered in such dilute form that no amount of the original radioactive substance is left, these remedies should nevertheless be approached with extra caution.

Other homeopathic-type preparations which may be worthy of further research into their ability to protect against radiation and toxins are the biochemical tissue salts. In particular, Australian nutritionist and naturopath Mira Louise's claims for tissue salts should be scientifically tested and evaluated.

In 1957, Louise began using the salts to cure her patients' radiation symptoms after they had been exposed to radioactive fallout from nuclear tests in the Pacific. Among other symptoms, she noted fatigue, weakness, breathlessness, light-headedness and vertigo, dimming vision, headaches, falling hair, skin rashes, parched skin, bone disorders, mental confusion, and impaired memory. She analyzed patients' blood to check for deficiencies, then prescribed the necessary tissue salts. According to Esther Chapman in *How to Use the Twelve Tissue Salts* (Pyramid Books, 1971), many patients recovered from their symptoms in a matter of hours or days; others with more severe symptoms felt some relief in a short time but took six weeks to three months to feel well again. The tissue salts along with dietary changes produced recovery in most of Louise's patients after their exposure to fallout containing strontium-90 and other radioactive particles. Further research is needed to determine how much the dietary changes alone contributed to recovery, independent of any benefits from the tissue salts.

Certain species of bacteria may provide protection from ionizing radiation. These species, Radiodurans, Radiokevrans, *Pseudomonas aeruginosa*, and others, can live in various radioactive environments, including amid high concentrations of plutonium and even within reactor cores. This is due to natural chelating agents which allow them to metabolize certain radioactive substances.

Bacteria are tiny biochemical laborers. A group of bacteria big enough to be seen can contain millions of individual microbes. They reproduce by growing until they are large enought to split in two. Bacteria break down dead plant and animal matter by means of enzymatic proteins which metabolize nutrient molecules. Bacteria often live symbiotically with other creatures, as harmful or helpful parasites. Some kinds live on our skin; intestinal varieties are necessary for food digestion. Some bacteria can metabolize more than a hundred kinds of chemicals.

Edible yeast bacteria (*Saccharomyces cerevisine*) and *Pseudomonas aeruginosa* have been compared for their ability to accumulate and absorb uranium.[9] Eugene Premuzic, Ph.D., and others have been researching bacterial species that grow in radioactive environments so as to isolate and apply their chelating powers to human and environmental radiation protection. Premuzic, working at the federal Brookhaven National Laboratory in Massachusetts, told us in 1984 that his findings since about 1981 on natural chelatants in bacteria have been "tremendously promising." He was critical of the attempts of chemists to derive synthetic protectants while overlooking natural ones.

Researchers have tested many natural chelating agents in plutonium therapy. These include ascorbic acid, citric acid, lactic acid, the amino acids cysteine and methionine, and nicotinic acid.[10] Premuzic predicted that natural chelating agents would attract wider interest as research with bacteria continues. His own tests with non-pathogenic varieties of *Pseudomonas aeruginosa* bacteria since 1984 seem to confirm their value and long-term safety as remedies after exposure to certain radioactive elements.

Many species of *Pseudomonas* are pathogenic. They are a problem in hospital environments, where they develop a high resistance to antibiotics. Non-pathogenic varieties are abundant in certain soils, but this would not be a significant dietary factor for those eating fruits and vegetables grown in these soils.

Premuzic is isolating the natural chelating products that *P. aeruginosa* strains produce in the presence of radiation and some toxic metals. He postulates that eventually an extract of these natural chelating products could be taken orally by humans after exposure to plutonium and other radioactive contaminants. At this stage, however, his research focuses on the biochemical effects of these chelating agents on mice which have been exposed to various kinds of radiation. Studies to date indicate that the bacteria's effects are nontoxic. The bacteria may also prove efficient for treatment of heavy metal contamination.

Premuzic and associates note, "*Pseudomonas aeruginosa* species are resistant to some heavy metals, and can live in thorium, uranium, and plutonium contaminated environments. 10, 100, and 1,000 ppm (parts per million) of uranium and thorium salts added to *Pseudomonas* cultures slowed the growth of the culture medium. Actual reductions in growth occurred only at concentrations of 1,000 ppm or higher. Uranium inhibited growth more than thorium. Subsequent analyses of the cultures revealed that the bacteria produced several new chelating agents for thorium and uranium.[11]

These new chelating agents somewhat resemble chelatants found in iron which enhance its solubility and bioavailability in the environment. Premuzic et al. hypothesize that these agents, and the byproducts of other highly adaptive bacteria, may eventually be used to enhance the dissolution and elimination of radioactive thorium, uranium, plutonium, and other heavy metals in the treatment of people or at waste disposal sites.

The work of radiologist O. Carl Simonton, M.D., Ernest Lawrence Rossi, Ph.D., Gerald Jampolsky, M.D., and others in the infant field of psychoneuroimmunology suggests that immunological resistance can be strengthened by visualization practices, hypnotherapy, and attitudinal changes. Cancer patients receiving radiation, chemotherapy, or nutritionally oriented treatments have experienced accelerated improvements and cure after practicing Simonton's technique.

The patient begins with a progressive relaxation exercise and goes on to visualize in a personally meaningful, symbolic way healthy cells ousting and replacing the cancerous ones. Simonton has observed that visualization accelerates cure and can reduce side effects from concurrent treatments with radiation or chemotherapy, as practitioners of the healing modality known as "therapeutic touch" have also noted.

Therapeutic touch is an interactive system of healing similar to the traditional healing practice of laying on of hands. Developed by Dolores Kreiger, Ph.D., R.N., of the New York University School of Nursing, and her colleagues, therapeutic touch has been documented in a number of experiments to raise hemoglobin and hematocrit levels in the blood, help premature babies gain weight more quickly, reduce pain and stress, and accelerate healing of a wide variety of diseases.[12]

Therapeutic touch is on the curriculum of over thirty schools of nursing in the U.S. and is practiced in twenty-six other countries. According to Kreiger's close associate Dora Kunz, in a 1984 study, therapeutic touch treatments reportedly reduced nausea and other side effects in about thirty cancer patients receiving radiotherapy or chemotherapy. When patients were taught a procedure involving the visualization of a deep blue color, the therapeutic touch treatments were even more successful.

Similar positive results have been obtained with cancer patients by the practice of c'hi kung (literally "breath work"), a traditional Chinese system of self-care and healing which combines visualization with movement, breathing, and vocalization. Harvard Medical School professor David Eisenberg, M.D., documented in *Encounters with Qi* (W.W. Norton, 1985) the astounding cases of anesthesia and healing he saw demonstrated by chi kung masters (some of whom were also physicians) on his visit to China. The entire world of traditional healing knowledge beckons to researchers in the field of psychoneuroimmunology today.

The cross-pollination of knowledge from these and other areas of learning may eventually result in the blossoming of new ways to maintain and regain our health in this nuclear age. The approaches discussed in this survey need to be rigorously tested. No claims are being made that these unorthodox approaches will now provide reliable or consistent protection to a significant portion of the general population. Only with further testing will we know whether any of these approaches, alone or in combination, might develop into a useful therapeutic agent against damaging radiation or chemical contaminants. Our only lasting protection, of course, can come from following suggestions similar to those provided in the main part of this book, and from a collective change of heart, a determination to minimize the sources of radiation and the silent spring of environmental contamination.

Notes

1. M. F. Barnothy and J. M. Barnothy, "Magnetic Fields and the Number of Blood Platelets," *Nature*, no. 255, pp. 1146-1147.

2. J. Bland, "Energy in Medicine," *Complementary Medicine*, vol. 2, no. 4.

3. L. V. Serova and M. I. Fedotova, "On the Preventive Action of Aero-Ionization in Acute Radiation Sickness," *Biull. Eskp. Biol. Med.*, no. 57, pp. 60-63.

4. V. Bragina and G. Kipsanova, "Chamber Bath Therapy with Napthalene Emulsions in Disorders of the Peripheral Blood Circulation in Patients Chronically Exposed to Ionizing Radiation," *Gig. Tr. Prof. Zabol*, no. 12, pp. 43-45.

5. H. Tsuji, O. Aso et al., *Hot Spring Therapy of Atomic Bomb Exposed Patients*, Institute of Balneotherapeutics, Kyushu University, Japan.

6. J. Lackner, *Strahlentherapie*, no. 89, pp. 283-287.

7. H. C. Allen, M.D., *The Materia Medica of the Nosodes with the Proving of the X-Ray*, Sett Dey and Co. (Calcutta, India), 1973, pp. 526-555.

8. J. H. Clarke, M.D., *A Dictionary of Practical Materia Medica, Vol. 3*, Health Science Press, 1977, pp. 1477-1478.

9. G. W. Strandberg, S. E. Shumate and J. R. Parrott, "Microbial Cells as Biosorbents for Heavy Metals: Accumulation of Uranium by *Saccharomyces cerevisiae* and *Pseudomonas aeruginosa*," *Appl. Environ. Microbiol.*, vol. 41, no. 1, pp. 237-245.

10. K. N. Raymond and W. L. Smith, "Actinide-Specific Sequestering Agents and Decontamination Applications," *Structure and Bonding, Vol. 43*, Springer-Verlag, (Berlin), 1981, pp. 159-186.

11. E. T. Premuzic, A. J. Francis, M. Lin and J. Schubert, "Induced Formation of Chelating Agents by *Pseudomonas aeruginosa* Grown in Presence of Thorium and Uranium," *Archives of Environmental Contamination and Toxicology, Vol. 14*, Springer-Verlag, (New York), 1985, p. 759.

12. D. Krieger, *The Relationship of Touch, with Intent to Help or Heal, to Subjects' In-vivo Hemoglobin Values: A Study in Personalized Interaction*, American Nurses Association Ninth Nursing Research Conference, San Antonio, Texas, March 21, 1973.

Suggested Readings

A Nuclear Waste Primer by the League of Women Voters Education Fund, 1730 M St. N.W., Washington, DC 20036, 1980. #391. $1.95. Gives basic information on types of radioactive waste and its storage, and describes ways to help reform our government's waste management policies.

Fear at Work: Job Blackmail, Labor, and the Environment by Richard Kazis and Richard L. Grossman, Pilgrim Press, 1982. Ever since the major environmental legislative advances of over a decade ago, industry has blamed "EPA regulations" for shutting down plants and costing workers jobs. This notion has taken such a hold that unions often side with industry against environmentalists. This rift threatens to widen ever further if unemployment increases. Kazis and Grossman refute the industry arguments, and they back their statements with substantive and detailed research. They make a well-documented case for the common interests of labor and environmental activists.

Food Irradiation: Who Wants It? by Tony Webb, Tim Lang, and Kathleen Tucker, Thorsons Publishers, 1987, $5.95. "This clearly written book explains the facts of food irradiation, its proposed uses, and its potential hazards to our health and environment," Michael Jacobson, Ph.D., notes in the introduction. This is not only the first book-length treatment of the topic, but an authoritative report that will serve as a handbook for years to come.

Justice Downwind: America's Atomic Testing Program in the 1950's by Howard Ball, Oxford University Press, 1986, $21.95. Tells the astonishing story of how the U.S. government exploded atomic weapons on its own soil and what happened in the wake of those tests. This is a well-researched accounting of a sad episode in American history.

Killing Our Own: The Disaster of America's Experiment with Atomic Radiation by Harvey Wasserman et al., Delacorte Press, 1982. $16.95; $12.95 paper. Tells the stories of nuclear victims, from the survivors of Hiroshima and Nagasaki to participants in early A-bomb tests, from employees at nuclear reactors to residents of the Three Mile Island area. It contains a cogent summary of the effects of radiation on health.

No Nukes: Everyone's Guide to Nuclear Power by Anna Gyorgy and Friends, South End Press, 1979. $15; $10 paper. Gyorgy explains the nuclear fuel cycle and the dangers it poses to human and environmental health, and discusses alternatives to nuclear power. Clearly written and well illustrated, *No Nukes* is the primer of the anti-nuclear movement.

Nuclear Madness by Helen Caldicott, M.D., Bantam, 1981. $3.50. A passionate call to mobilize against nuclear power and arms, from a pediatrician who has played an international role in the anti-nuclear cause.

Nuclear Power: The Bargain We Can't Afford by Richard Morgan, Environmental Action Foundation (724 Dupont Circle Building, N.W., Washington, DC 20036), 1977. $4.95. A well-documented analysis of the faulty economics of nuclear power, this concise book reveals how the hidden costs of nuclear power generation make for higher utility rates.

Peace Resource Book: A Comprehensive Guide to Issues, Groups, and Literature by Elizabeth Bernstein et al., Ballinger Publishing Company, 1986. $14.95. A readable survey of key peace issues, with resources for citizen involvement and self-education.

Radiation and Human Health by John W. Gofman, M.D., Ph.D., Sierra Club Books, 1981. $29.95. Gofman is widely acknowledged as one of the world's foremost authorities on radiation and human health. Drawing on his forty years of experience and from reliable studies, he presents overwhelming evidence that there is no safe level of exposure to radiation, and that even low levels of ionizing radiation increase the likelihood of cancer, leukemia, genetic damage, and other diseases.

Radon: The Invisible Threat by Michael Lafavore, Rodale Press, 1987, $12.95. This book provides a clear and readable introduction to radon—what it is, where it is, and how to keep your house safe from it. The author offers timely and sensible answers to tough questions about this major threat to our health.

Stop Nuclear War: A Handbook by David Barash, Ph.D., and Judith Lipton, M.D., Grove Press, 1982. $7.95. This empowering book contains many suggestions for effective citizen action. It includes a good section on the escalating arms race and its economic consequences.

The Fate of the Earth by Jonathan Schell, Knopf, 1982. $11.95. This eloquent book on nuclear weapons and their threat to our planet describes the global devastation that would result from a major nuclear attack. Schell exhorts us to "break through the layers of our denials, put aside our faint-hearted excuses, and rise up to cleanse the earth of nuclear weapons."

Well Body, Well Earth: The Sierra Club Environmental Health Source-book by Mike Samuels, M.D., and Hal Zina Bennett, Sierra Club Books, 1983. $12.95. An information sourcebook for understanding why some of the changes imposed on the planet by modern technologies alter the natural environment so dramatically that the health of the earth as well as of the millions of species it supports is deeply threatened. This book describes the dangers of radiation, water and air pollution, and many chemicals and poisons. The book does fall short, however, of being the comprehensive personal self-help manual it claims to be. It gives a prescription though for the environmental health of our society.

Resource Groups

The optimum diet and health program presented in Part III can strengthen us and shield us from radiation and chemical toxins, but it is equally necessary to minimize the sources of these hazards if we want lasting security. Personal and planetary protection go hand in hand. Individual health and fulfillment can be achieved only when basic human rights are ensured for everyone. As anthropologist Margaret Meade once said, "Never doubt that a small group of thoughtful, committed citizens can change the world; indeed it's the only thing that ever has."

If you want to lend a hand, there are over 9,000 groups in this country working for peace, nuclear disarmament, environmental protection, and the use of safe, renewable energy sources. These groups are dependent upon citizen involvement and action for their success, and many function in a decentralized, non-bureaucratic manner that invites the full participation of all.

The first groups listed below are national in scope, though they may also have state and local chapters. Information on contacting regional and local grassroots organizations is given in a second section, followed by a listing of educational sources for teachers and peace activities for young people. There's also a listing of some good resources for further information on herbs.

I. National Groups and Organizations
ACCESS
1755 Massachusetts Ave. N.W.
Suite 501
Washington, DC 20036

(202) 328-2323

ACCESS provides a clearinghouse of information on issues pertaining to peace and international security, including arms control, regional conflicts, nuclear power, and medical and psychological issues of the nuclear age. ACCESS offers an inquiry service for specific questions; nonpartisan briefing papers on important security debates like nuclear testing and the Star Wars Defense Initiative; and a speaker referral service. Occasional calls are free of charge as a public service. (For other clearinghouses, see listings on the Nuclear Information and Resource Service, Nuke Watch, Peace Net computer service, and the Topsfield Foundation.)

American Friends Service Committee
1501 Cherry Street
Philadelphia, PA 19102
(215) 241-7000

The A.F.S.C. has been involved in peace and disarmament work since 1917. Among its many outreach activities, the A.F.S.C. sponsors a Peace Program. A Program Resources Book offers for sale slide shows, pamphlets, and a series of maps on the military-industrial complex.

Center for Defense Information
1500 Massachusetts Ave. N.W.
Washington, DC 20005
(202) 862-0700

The C.D.I. provides up-to-date reports on military issues like nuclear weapons and the arms race. A newsletter, *The Defense Monitor*, is published ten times each year.

Center for Science in the Public Interest
1501 16th St. N.W.
Washington, DC 20036
(202) 332-9110

This organization lobbies to reform government policies on health and food quality and offers the public information on improving health through changes in diet.

Citizen's Clearinghouse for Hazardous Wastes
P.O. Box 926
Arlington, VA 22216
(703) 276-7070

Founded by veterans of the Love Canal toxic waste site, C.C.H.W. teaches individuals and grassroots organizations how to mobilize against local environmental hazards.

Clergy and Laity Concerned
198 Broadway, Rm. 302
New York, NY 10038
(212) 964-6730

C.A.L.C. is a religious organization that stresses peace and jobs as alternatives to military spending. It actively supports bilateral disarmament and a nuclear freeze.

Committee for Nuclear Responsibility
P.O. Box 11207
San Francisco, CA 94101
(415) 776-8299

Dr. John Gofman, who is both a physician and a doctor of nuclear/physical chemistry, is director of this group, which is concerned with addressing the dangers of x-ray treatments, other routine medical procedures involving radiation, and all other sources of radiation.

Common Cause
2030 M St. N.W.
Washington, DC 20036
(202) 833-1200

This is a national, nonprofit, nonpartisan citizens lobbying group of more than 270,000 members working to make federal and state governments more responsive to citizens. Nuclear arms control and military spending issues are top priorities.

Environmental Action
1525 New Hampshire Ave. N.W.
Washington, DC 20036
(202) 745-4870

E.A. chapter members work to eliminate chemical and atomic hazards from our water and air and to promote safe and more affordable technologies for generating power. E.A. lobbyists at the Washington office are working to influence legislators to back environmentally sane policies.

Fellowship of Reconciliation
P.O. Box 271
Nyack, NY 10960
(914) 358-4601

Members practice citizens' diplomacy and seek to affect government policy in their national and international work for peace and for nuclear disarmament. F.R. publishes a newsletter, *Fellowship*, eight times yearly.

Freeze
220 I St. N.E.
Suite 130
Washington, DC 20002
(202) 544-0880

Focuses on nuclear disarmament. Provides support for the development of local peace organizations and sponsors public educational and media programs.

Friends of the Earth
530 Seventh St. S.E.
Washington, DC 20003
(202) 543-4312

A citizens-based group that promotes the preservation, restoration, and rational use of the earth. Their continuing concerns include acid rain, the ozone layer, renewable energy, and other environmental issues.

Greenpeace, U.S.A.
1611 Connecticut Ave. N.W.
Washington, DC 20009
(202) 462-1177

On land and at sea, Greenpeace takes direct action to block the dumping of toxic wastes and protect all forms of life in the environment. It aims for an end to nuclear testing and for bilateral arms reduction.

Ground Zero
P.O. Box 19329
Portland, OR 92719
(503) 245-3519

This group conducts education and citizens action programs in an effort to ban nuclear war and weaponry. It publishes a monthly newsletter, *Report from Ground Zero.*

Health and Energy Institute
236 Massachusetts Ave. N.E.
Suite 506
Washington, DC 20002
(202) 543-1070

This group offers a speakers bureau and printed information on the damaging effects of ionizing radiation from sources like nuclear power plants and medical treatments. It is also a reliable source for information on food irradiation.

National Audubon Society
950 Third Ave.
New York, NY 10022
(212) 832-3200

A nonprofit group with 560,000 members, it works to preserve the quality of life through the protection of wildlife, land, water, and other natural resources. Also promotes rational strategies for energy development and use.

National Coalition to Stop Food Irradiation
Box 59-0488
San Francisco, CA 94159
(415) 566-2734

N.C.S.F.I is in the forefront of the efforts to expose food irradiation as the dangerous, unnecessary technology it is. The Coalition is active on the federal, state, and local levels, and distributes valuable information on all aspects of the food irradiation issue.

National Mobilization for Survival
853 Broadway
New York, NY 10003
(212) 533-0008

A major coalition of local antinuclear, safe energy, peace, and religious groups, Mobilization for Survival strives to put an end to the arms race, phase out nuclear power, and shift national priorities from military to human needs.

National Wildlife Federation
1412 16th St. N.W.
Washington, DC 20036
(202) 797-6800

This organization of almost five million members promotes environmental and animal protection through education and political action. Its national network of affiliates focuses on local environmental issues.

Nuclear Information and Resource Service
1616 P St. N.W.
Suite 160
Washington, DC 20036
(202) 328-0002

NIRS is a national clearinghouse and action group concerned with all aspects of nuclear power. It provides an information inquiry service by telephone, mail, and through NIRSNET, a versatile "computerized bulletin board." NIRS monitors Congress, the NRC, state regulatory bodies, the courts, and the nuclear industry and sends out alerts to its members and the media on upcoming issues and votes. It gives legal and technical assistance to activist lawyers and grassroots groups, and publishes a wide range of educational materials for teachers. NIRS' book *Teaching Nuclear Issues* gives a full listing of information on background reading, curriculum guides, film catalogues, hands-on projects, games, and children's peace organizations. NIRS also publishes a quarterly newsletter called *Groundswell*.

Nuke Watch
315 W. Gorham St.
Madison, WI 53703
(608) 256-4146
   Nuke Watch functions as a clearinghouse on nuclear power and arms issues and advises other antinuclear groups.

Peace Net
3228 Sacramento
San Francisco, CA 94115
(415) 923-0900
   Peace Net computer service offers a clearinghouse of computerized data pooled by over 1,200 peace, environmental, and social justice organizations.

Physicians for Social Responsibility
1601 Connecticut Ave. N.W.
Suite 800
Washington, DC 20009
(202) 939-5750
   Since 1979, the P.S.R. has educated medical professionals and the public about the grave physical, psychological, social, and economic consequences of the nuclear arms buildup and of the nuclear industry. The quarterly *Physicians for Social Responsibility Report* gives current legislative information and bulletins on P.S.R. activities. Membership is open to everyone.

Public Citizen—Critical Mass Energy Project
215 Pennsylvania Ave. S.E.
Washington, DC 20003
(202) 546-4996
   The Critical Mass Energy Project supplies grassroots groups and the public with factsheets on nuclear power, and lobbies for safe alternatives to nuclear power plants. Critical Mass helps local grassroots organizations make an impact on nuclear issues.

Public Citizen—Health Research Group
2000 P St. N.W.
Washington, DC 20036
(202) 293-9142

An advocacy group for safe food and drugs, and for occupational health and safety, the Health Research Group is an outreach arm of Public Citizen, which Ralph Nader founded in 1971. It opposes the irradiation of food and many other health-threatening practices through petitions, lobbying, and litigation.

SANE: A Citizens Committee for Sane Nuclear Power
711 G St. S.E.
Washington, DC 20003
(202) 546-7100

Appealing to human and economic common sense, SANE conducts lobby, media, and citizen action campaigns for peace, arms reduction, and a re-ordering of economic priorities. It publishes the bimonthly magazine *Sane World*.

Sierra Club
730 Polk St.
San Francisco, CA 94109
(415) 776-2211

The largest grass-roots organization in the U.S. dedicated to conservation and environmental protection by influencing public policy decisions. A bimonthly magazine is available.

Union of Concerned Scientists
26 Church St.
Cambridge, MA 02238
(617) 547-5552
and
1616 P St. N.W.
Suite 310
Washington, DC 20036
(202) 332-0900

A consortium of scientists and laypeople addressing the health and societal issues raised by nuclear policies and technologies, the U.C.S. supports nuclear power safety and arms control.

War Resisters League
339 Lafayette St.
New York, NY 10012
(212) 228-0450

The War Resisters League is a pacifist organization founded in 1923. It provides antinuclear groups with training and assistance in the uses of peaceful civil disobedience for protest at nuclear power and waste disposal sites.

Women's International League for Peace and Freedom
1213 Race St.
Philadelphia, PA 19107
(215) 563-7110

The largest women's peace group, WILPF was founded in 1915 by Nobel Peace Prize winners Jane Addams and Emily Greenbalch. WILPF stands for social equality, disarmament, and a nuclear-free world. Peace programs include their Stop the Arms Race project, a nuclear weapons freeze campaign, a women's speaking tour on Central America, and a comprehensive test ban campaign. WILPF has chapters in 45 countries, an international office in Geneva, and offices at the U.N. in New York.

II. Contacting Regional and Local Grassroots Organizations

The Topsfield Foundation—Grassroots Peace Directory
P.O. Box 203
Pomfret, CT 06258
(203) 928-2616

The Topsfield Foundation maintains a computer-based *Grassroots Peace Directory* of organizations and networks (religious and secular) working in this country within the fields of international security, peace, and disarmament. The directory contains over 9,000 listings. It is printed in ten regional editions, which are updated biannually. Topsfield encourages telephone calls from anyone wishing to order volumes of its directory or to contact peace, social justice, or environmental groups working near them. The staff offers a research service for specialized information. Topsfield also provides grants and support to organizations promoting peace, disarmament, and social justice. The Foundation launched the ACCESS information service in 1984 to act as a clearinghouse on key national security issues. Options, a University outreach program on nuclear policy, was started as a pilot program on nine campuses in 1985. It mobilizes faculty members to initiate public debate and discussion programs on national security issues within their host communities.

III. *Educational Resources for Teachers and Peace Activities for Young People*

Children's Campaign for Nuclear Disarmament

Contact: Hannah Rabin
Box 550, R.D. #1
Plainfield, VT 05667
(802) 454-7119

A children's network started by two young Vermont sisters. Their campaign office now serves as a support for 50 or so chapters around the country involved with a range of activities for children. The group's major project has been a children's campaign to write letters of opposition to nuclear arms to President Reagan. Thousands of children attended two presentations of these letters to the White House. Brochures describing the campaign are 10 cents each.

Children's Creative Response to Conflict

Box 271
Nyack, NY 10960
(914) 358-4601

Established in 1972 to provide teachers with workshops and individual training in the communications skills and conflict resolution, C.C.R.C. also publishes a newsletter, *Sharing Space*, designed to keep teachers up-to-date and to share new techniques and experiences.

Children's Peace Network

1346 Connecticut Ave. N.W.
Suite 1126
Washington, DC 20036
(202) 835-0777

A clearinghouse for information and resources for children, parents, and educators. CPN's major outreach project is through their resource guide *The Peace Book* and a musical production based on it. CPN answers requests for information by telephone or mail.

Educators for Social Responsibility

639 Massachusetts Ave.
Cambridge, MA 02139
(617) 492-1764

Established to educate teachers, parents, and school administrators about the issues of nuclear war and the arms race. ESR conducts major conferences for teachers and offers the *Day of Dialogue Planning Manual*, a book of innovative teaching ideas and resources.

The Jane Addams Peace Association and
the Women's International League for Peace and Freedom
1213 Race St.
Philadelphia, PA 19107
(215) 563-7110

WILPF offers many resource materials for teachers. (Send a stamped, self-addressed envelope for a list of publications.) The annual Jane Addams Children's Book Award is named after one of the founders of WILPF, the first woman to win the Nobel Peace Prize.

Nuclear Education Project
26 Granite St., #3
Somerville, MA 02143

A group of five women from the Boston area produced the handbook *Parenting in a Nuclear Age: A Support Book.* The book is aimed at parents who want a primer on the nuclear threat with positive ideas for family education and action.

Nuclear Information and Resource Service
1616 P St. N.W.
Suite 160
Washington, DC 20036
(202) 328-0002

NIRS offers two comprehensive resource guides for teachers. For the elementary school teacher there is *Growing Up in a Nuclear Age: A Resource Guide for Elementary School Teachers*, 32 pp., $5 each plus 85 cents postage. For the secondary school teacher they offer *Nuclear Dangers: A Resource Guide for Secondary School Teachers*, 32 pp., same price. These two guidebooks provide annotated listings of educational materials on nuclear issues, including background reading for teachers, classroom materials (curriculum guides, kits, simulation games, etc.), books for students to read on their own, relevant organizations and government agencies, and audio-visual resources. The two guides give detailed descriptions and full ordering information on all items listed. NIRS also offers curriculum materials for secondary teachers.

The Riverside Church Disarmament Program
490 Riverside Drive
New York, NY 10027
(212) 749-7000

The church supplies an excellent resource list entitled "Peace Teaching and Children" with classroom activities, cooperative games, and more. The focus is on teaching peaceful conflict resolution.

Sierra Club
730 Polk St.
San Francisco, CA 94109
(415) 776-2211
They offer an "Environmental Education Packet" ($4) with resources for teachers, reading lists for students, articles, and policy statements.

Student/Teacher Organization To Prevent Nuclear War
P.O. Box 232
Northfield, MA 01360
(413) 498-5311 ext. 264 or 418
This is a national organization of high school students and teachers who are educating themselves and their local communities about the dangers of the nuclear arms race and the concrete actions young people can take toward averting the threat of nuclear war. Membership is $7 for students and $15 for adults and includes a unique newsletter of articles and resource information by both teachers and students. The group's many autonomous chapters around the country are aided by the central office in Massachusetts.

United Campuses to Prevent Nuclear War
1346 Connecticut Ave. N.W.
Washington, DC 20036
(202) 223-6206
A nationwide organization of college faculty and students which seeks to introduce new courses on the arms race and the threat of nuclear war. Co-sponsor of the annual convocation on nuclear war.
Acknowledgement and thanks go to ACCESS, NIRS, the Topsfield Foundation, and all the other groups which helped compile this resource listing.

IV. *Herbal Information*
The American Herb Association
P.O. Box 353
Rescue, CA 95672
(916) 626-5046
The A.H.A. is composed of lay people, health professionals, and businesses involved in medical herbology. It publishes an informative quarterly newsletter describing important current research into herbs. It also sponsors symposia of international scope, and can tap into a network of knowledgeable consultants about herbs.

Herb Research Foundation
P.O. Box 2602
Longmont, CO 80501

A nonprofit research and educational organization, the H.R.F. is primarily made up of professional herbalists. The Foundation seeks to increase the quality of information available on herbs as medicines, foods, and cosmetics. The publication *HerbalGram* (P.O. Box 12006, Austin, TX 78711; (512) 331-4244) is sent to all members, and it provides up-to-date information on herbs in the media, herb-related workshops and conferences, herbal research and data bases, and so forth.

Optimal Health for the Nuclear Age Newsletter and Network (OHNA)

Optimal Health for the Nuclear Age is a newsletter edited and published four times per year by Steve Schechter, N.D. Contact OHNA, P.O. Box 294, Encinitas, CA 92024. Rates are $11.00 per year, $13.50 overseas.

Each issue of Optimal Health for the Nuclear Age focuses on scientifically documented, effective, and safe natural therapies for attaining optimal health. Learn self-help techniques for detoxifying from radiation, chemical toxins, and drugs. The emphasis is on self-treatment for specific health problems caused by these toxins relating to the organs, glands, blood, and lymph, and the immune, reproductive, nervous, and skeletal systems. Self-help therapies are provided for adults and children that can easily be used at home, work, school, and during recreational activities. Similar in format to *Fighting Radiation & Chemical Pollutants with Foods, Herbs, & Vitamins*, the OHNA newsletter is a presentation of foods, herbs, supplements, and other natural therapies documented both to counteract toxins and to boost the immune system. New research findings are synthesized for the reader into an optimal diet and health program for the nuclear age.

The newsletter includes inspirational discussion of how we can evolve personal, social, and political transformations that would affect the causes of the problems. And there are recipes, new book reviews, resource groups, and discussion of unorthodox approaches that deserve further research. The newsletter also contains specific information for individuals, small businesses, and corporations on how to make the workplace healthier, thus increasing quality of life and productivity, and decreasing absenteeism.

By subscribing to the OHNA newsletter, you will gain access to the Optimal Health for the Nuclear Age Network. OHNAN will be available to do computer searches and international networking to provide self-help information for members who have a health disorder relating to a specific radioisotope, pollutant, or drug. Your membership in, and any further contribution to, the Network will help provide for further dissemination of information on how we can obtain optimal health in the nuclear age.

About the Author

Steven R. Schechter, N.D., T.T.I., is a naturopathic health counselor, a clinical nutritionist, a licensed therapy technology instructor, and a licensed massage therapy instructor. He began studying naturopathy, natural self-healing, and massage therapies in 1966 while enrolled in a pre-medicine program at the University of Michigan. As an undergraduate, he was chosen to conduct research at the first medical laser laboratory in the world, and he graduated cum laude with majors in clinical psychology and religion. He also graduated with highest honors from two naturopathic schools, attended a one-year school on religious mysticism, and has apprenticed with several internationally renowned naturopaths and healers. He has taught clinical nutrition at major universities, directed holistic health programs in three states, and had feature articles published in *Let's Live, Health Foods Business, Natural Health, East West, Alive, Delicious!, Natural Foods Merchandiser, E Magazine, Vegetarian Times, Spectrum,* and other national health magazines.

Schechter regularly presents seminars and workshops on various aspects of holistic health at symposia and learning centers. Each of the last seven years, he was a featured speaker at the three largest health industry trade conventions and seven largest consumer health expos in the United States.

He is on the Medical Advisory Boards and regularly writes for both *Let's Live* and *Health Foods Business.* He and this book are listed in *Who Is Who In Service To The Earth.*

He founded and directs the Vital-Life Training Institute of Southern California, a detoxification retreat center and state-approved school of holistic health, clinical nutrition, medical herbology, and massage therapies near his home in Encinitas, California. He advises corporations and health care providers on vitality, immunity, detoxification, and optimal health. He is currently working on his next book.

Schechter is available for personal health consultations either on the telephone or at his office. He has developed a procedure for *personal, individualized tele-*

phone health consultations. Call his office in Encinitas, CA to schedule a consultation. He is also available to teach workshops in your area.

Contact Vital-Life/Vitality, Ink for further information and to be on his mailing list.

VITAL-LIFE TRAINING INSTITUTE/VITALITY, INK
P.O. Box 294
Encinitas, CA 92024
(619) 943-VITL (8485)

Index